Women's Mental Health

A Clinical Guide *for* Primary Care Providers

Joan C. Urbancic, PhD, PMHNP-BC
Professor Emeritus
University of Detroit Mercy
Detroit, Michigan

Carla J. Groh, PhD, PMHNP-BC
Professor
University of Detroit Mercy
Detroit, Michigan

Wolters Kluwer | Lippincott Williams & Wilkins
Health
Philadelphia • Baltimore • New York • London
Buenos Aires • Hong Kong • Sydney • Tokyo

Acquisitions Editor: Jean Rodenberger
Managing Editor: Helen Kogut
Senior Production Editor: Marian A. Bellus
Director of Nursing Production: Helen Ewan
Senior Managing Editor / Production: Erika Kors
Senior Designer: Joan Wendt
Art Director, Illustration: Brett MacNaughton
Manufacturing Coordinator: Karin Duffield
Production Services / Compositor: Aptara, Inc.

9 8 7 6 5 4 3 2 1

Printed in China

Library of Congress Cataloging-in-Publication Data

Women's mental health : a clinical guide for primary care providers / [edited by] Joan C. Urbancic, Carla J. Groh.
p. ; cm.
Includes bibliographical references and index.
ISBN 978-0-7817-6828-3
1. Women—Mental health. 2. Primary care (Medicine) I. Urbancic, Joan C. II. Groh, Carla J. [DNLM: 1. Mental Disorders. 2. Primary Health Care. 3. Women's Health. WM 140 W8723 2009]
RC451.4.W6W6595 2009
616.890082—dc22

2008031750

Care has been taken to confirm the accuracy of the information presented and to describe generally accepted practices. However, the authors, editors, and publisher are not responsible for errors or omissions or for any consequences from application of the information in this book and make no warranty, expressed or implied, with respect to the currency, completeness, or accuracy of the contents of the publication. Application of this information in a particular situation remains the professional responsibility of the practitioner; the clinical treatments described and recommended may not be considered absolute and universal recommendations.

The authors, editors, and publisher have exerted every effort to ensure that drug selection and dosage set forth in this text are in accordance with the current recommendations and practice at the time of publication. However, in view of ongoing research, changes in government regulations, and the constant flow of information relating to drug therapy and drug reactions, the reader is urged to check the package insert for each drug for any change in indications and dosage and for added warnings and precautions. This is particularly important when the recommended agent is a new or infrequently employed drug.

Some drugs and medical devices presented in this publication have Food and Drug Administration (FDA) clearance for limited use in restricted research settings. It is the responsibility of the health care provider to ascertain the FDA status of each drug or device planned for use in his or her clinical practice.

LWW.com

Dedication

To our female patients for their courage and willingness to embark with us on a collaborative journey in mental health healing

Acknowledgments

We are indebted to many people who have been directly or indirectly instrumental in the development and publication of this book. But, foremost, we must acknowledge the women who were our patients for mental health services at both the McAuley Health Center, a nurse-managed center funded by the HRSA, Division of Nursing, and Mercy Primary Care Center, a physician primary care facility supported by the Trinity Health System. Both of us were inspired and gratified to be able to practice as psychiatric/mental health nurse practitioners in a primary care setting with patients referred to us from the health care providers in these two centers. But it was the women themselves who were so instrumental in our recognition of the degree to which mental health disorders can and must be diagnosed and treated in the primary care setting.

The majority of our patient population consisted of the working poor, mostly women, whose incomes were too high for Medicaid but too poor to afford health insurance. Some of the women had a schizophrenic disorder for many years with persistent psychotic symptoms that were undiagnosed and untreated until they sought treatment at our primary care centers. Many women had severe depression with suicidal ideation. A significant number of these depressed women also experienced psychotic symptoms due to the severity of their depression. Others had bipolar and anxiety disorders that were undiagnosed and untreated. Most had problems of daily living that required a sympathetic and knowledgeable professional to assist them to cope with these problems, many of which were insurmountable. By collaborating with the women in providing psychotherapy, therapeutic listening, medication as needed, and community resources, we believe that we made a significant difference in their lives. It has been a privilege and honor to work so closely with these women on their journey to mental health wellness.

While our work with the women was both a challenge and a joy, it was the staff at McAuley Health Center and Mercy Primary Care Center that provided the environmental context that our patients so sorely needed. The warm, nurturing, and welcoming atmosphere created by the staff at both centers instilled a sense of trust that allowed the women to seek therapy and share their life stories.

The nurse practitioners and physicians in both settings contributed to the inspiration for this book by their willingness to refer their patients who were in need of psychiatric services and then to collaborate on the treatment of these patients. Dr. Margaret Meyers, the Medical Director, and Aiisya Williamson, the Executive Director of Mercy Primary Care Center, have consistently facilitated our practice at their center, as has Tracy Chan, Nurse Practitioner and Clinical Coordinator of McAuley Health Center and Dr. Pamela Williams, Family Practice physician.

Acknowledgment of our contributors is essential. They have been diligent and patient in reviewing and returning repeated drafts of their work. Their expertise is clearly demonstrated in each of their chapters. Also, our many reviewers are to be commended for their astute and conscientious reviews of our chapters. Their comments have strengthened the book significantly, and we are sincerely appreciative of their efforts. One reviewer in particular, Dr. Manual Dumlao, our consulting psychiatrist, reviewed many chapters of the book and gave us invaluable feedback during the development of the book.

We have also been very fortunate to have exceptional editors, Helen Kogut and Audrey Alt, who have provided us with excellent editing, guidance, and feedback during the book development process.

Finally, our husbands, Bill and Manny, are to be commended for their ongoing support, feedback, good humor, and patience during the challenging book development period.

Contributors

Carolyn Baird, RN-BC, DNP(s), MBA, CARN-AP, CCDP-D
Nursing Instructor
Waynesburg University
McMurray, Pennsylvania

Toni Baird, BS, CCDP
Therapist
Wesley Spectrum Services
Coraopolis, Pennsylvania

Janet Baiardi, PhD, FNP-BC
Associate Professor
Coordinator, FNP Program
University of Detroit Mercy
Detroit, Michigan

Marquerite Baty, PhD (c), MSN, MPH, RN
PhD candidate
Johns Hopkins University School of Nursing
Baltimore, Maryland

Jacquelyn C. Campbell, PhD, RN, FAAN
Anna D. Wolf Chair and Professor
Johns Hopkins University School of Nursing
Baltimore, Maryland

Sharon Morgillo Freeman, PhD, RN, APRN-CS, CARN-AP
Executive Director, Center for Brief Therapy, PC;
Associate Faculty, Indiana-Purdue University;
Visiting Professor
Babes-Bolyai University School of Psychology
Cluj, Napoca, Romania

Carla J. Groh, PhD, PMHNP-BC
Associate Professor
University of Detroit Mercy
Detroit, Michigan

Rosa Gonzalez Guarda, PhD, MSN, MPH, RN
University of Miami, School of Nursing and Health Studies
Coral Gables, Florida

M. Linda Hoes, PhD, PMHNP-BC
CEO
Mental Health Associates;
Assistant Professor
Wayne State University
Detroit, Michigan

Catherine Judd, MS, PA-C
Psychoneuroendocrine Research Program
Department of Psychiatry
UT Southwestern Medical Center at Dallas
Parkland Health & Hospital System
Jail Mental Health Program
Dallas, Texas

Shane M. LaGore, MSN, APRN-BC, CGNP
John A. Hartford Foundation and American Academy of Nursing Building Academic Geriatric Nursing Capacity Scholar
Geriatric Nurse Practitioner
Foote Health System at the Senior Resource Center
Jackson, Michigan

Bernadette Longo, PhD, RN
Assistant professor
Orvis School of Nursing
University of Nevada–Reno
Reno, Nevada

Jody Lori, MS, CNM
Lecturer IV
School of Nursing
Nurse-Midwifery Education Program
University of Michigan
Ann Arbor, Michigan

Patricia J. Lutz, MEd, CAC, CCDP, SAP
Director of Abstinent Living
The Turning Point Halfway House for Women in Recovery
Washington, Pennsylvania

Carol Mallory, MSN, RN, MA, APN
Certified Healing Touch Practitioner
Certified Holistic Nurse
Minden, Nevada

Margaret Meyers, MD
Medical Director
Mercy Primary Care Center
Detroit, Michigan

Sharon Moser, MS, PA-C, LLP
Associate Professor
College of Health Professions
University of Detroit Mercy
Detroit, Michigan

Katherine Nash, MSN, RN, SANE-A, D-ABMDI
PhD student
Johns Hopkins University School of Nursing
Baltimore, Maryland

Michelle O'Grady, MS, CNM
Lecturer IV
School of Nursing;
Director
Health Sciences Scholars Program
College of Literature, Science, and the Arts
University of Michigan
Ann Arbor, Michigan

Juliann V. Pancari, RNBC, BSN, MEd, CAC Diplomate, CCS, CCDP Diplomate
Continuous Quality Improvement Manager
Odyssey HealthCare of Pennsylvania
Pittsburgh, Pennsylvania

David Rosen, MD, MPH
Clinical Professor, Pediatrics, and Communicable Disease
CS Mott Children's Hospital
University of Michigan Health System
Ann Arbor, Michigan

Alice Running, PhD, APRN
Associate Professor, Nurse Practitioner
Post Masters Certificate in Integrated Therapies
Orvis School of Nursing
University of Nevada
Reno, Nevada

Prevesh K. Rustagi, MD
Clinical Associate Professor
Department of Psychiatry
Indiana University School of Medicine;

President
Fort Wayne Psychiatry, PC
Fort Wayne, Indiana

Judy T. Sargent, RN, MS
Doctoral Candidate
University of Michigan
Ann Arbor, Michigan

Mary Serowoky, MSN, FNP-BC
Nurse Practitioner
Oakwood Inkster Teen Health Center
Inkster, Michigan

Karen Stein, PhD, RN, FAAN
Associate Professor
University of Michigan
Ann Arbor, Michigan

Joan C. Urbancic, PhD, PMHNP-BC
Professor Emeritus
University of Detroit Mercy
Detroit, Michigan

Ann L. Whall, PhD, RN, FAAN, FGSA
Professor
The University of Michigan School of Nursing
Ann Arbor, Michigan;
Associate Director
The Michigan Geriatrics Center;
Allesee Endowed Chair in Gerontologic Nursing, and Visiting Professor
Oakland University School of Nursing
Rochester Hills, Michigan

Jessica Roberts Williams, PhD, MPH, RN
PhD Candidate
Johns Hopkins University School of Nursing
Baltimore, Maryland

Peter C. Wolf, MDiv, LMSW, ACSW
Psychotherapy Private Practice
Heron Ridge Associates, PLC
Bloomfield Hills, Michigan

Suzanne York, PA-C, MPH
Associate Professor
Program Director & Chairperson
Physician Assistant Program
University of Detroit Mercy
Detroit, Michigan

Reviewers

Jill Allard Ross, RN, PhD, MLS
Assistant Professor of Nursing
University of Alabama at Birmingham
Birmingham, Alabama

Patricia T. Alpert, PhD, MSN
Assistant Professor; MSN Coordinator; St. Jude Program Director
University of Nevada, Las Vegas
Las Vegas, Nevada

Sharon Elaine Ballard, MSN, APRN, BC, FNP
Associate Clinical Professor
Texas Woman's University
Dallas, Texas

Rebecca Baron, RN
Staff Nurse
St. Elizabeth Hospital
Appleton, Wisconsin

Kathryn A. Blair, RN
Professor
University of Colorado-Colorado Springs
Beth El School of Nursing
University of Colorado, Colorado Springs
Colorado Springs, Colorado

Geraldine Collins-Bride, RN, MS, ANP
Clinical Professor and Vice Chair
Department of Community Health Systems
University of California, San Francisco
San Francisco, California

Fran Dreier, RN, FNP, MHS
Assistant Clinical Professor
University of California, San Francisco, School of Nursing
San Francisco, California

Robert W. Jarski, PhD
Professor
Oakland University School of Health Sciences
Rochester, Michigan

Gloria Joachim, RN, MSN, NP(F)
Associate Professor
University of British Columbia School of Nursing
Richmond, British Columbia, Canada

Sandra Keavey, MPAS, PA-C
Physician's Assistant Private Practice
Great Lakes Heart Center of Alpena
Alpena, Michigan

William J. Lorman, PhD, MSN, PsyNP, CARN-AP
Chief Clinical Officer
Livengrin Foundation, Inc
Bensalem, Pennsylvania; Assistant Professor
Drexel University Graduate Nursing Department
Philadelphia, Pennsylvania

Sandra Maas, RN, MSN
Residential Nursing Faculty
Estrella Mountain Community College Nursing Program
Avondale, Arizona

Don Porter, PharmD
Assistant Dean for Professional Affairs
Harding University College of Pharmacy
Searcy, Arkansas

Shirley Repta, PhD, APRN, BC, MBA
EX Director, Behavioral Health Inova Health System
Inova Health System
Alexandria, Virginia

Barbara Rideout, MSN, APRN, BC
Nurse Practitioner
Student Health Center
Drexel University College of Medicine
Philadelphia, Pennsylvania

Belinda Seimer, RN, MSN, CFNP
Clinical Instructor
Ohio State University
Columbus, Ohio

Wendy Sellers Cambell, MSW, MA, PhD
Clinical Faculty
University of South Carolina
Columbia, South Carolina

Cornelia Walsh, RN, BC, BSN, MSHS
Nurse Manager
Newton Emergency Dept;
Nurse Manager
IV Infusion Teams
Boston Medical Center
Boston, Massachusetts

Nicole Whitson, RN, MSN
Complex Nursing Instructor
Jones County Junior College
Ellisville, Mississippi

Paige Wimberly, RN
Assistant Professor of Nursing
Arkansas State University
Jonesboro, Arkansas

Michael E. Zychowicz, DNP, RNFA, NP-C
Assistant Professor of Nursing
Mount Saint Mary College
Newburgh, New York

Preface

This book is written for all primary care providers who would like to be more proficient and knowledgeable in treating their female patients who present with mental health problems. This includes nurse practitioners, physician assistants, nurse midwives, and physicians. Today the majority of mental health disorders are being diagnosed and treated by these providers. For example, 90 percent of depressed patients are diagnosed and treated by a non-psychiatrist. At the same time, the majority of patients with mental disorders remain untreated or undertreated. Because women comprise the bulk of primary care patients and are overrepresented in many major mental health disorders such as mood, anxiety, and eating disorders, it stands to reason that primary care providers will encounter a significant number of women with mental health problems in their practice. Therefore, it is essential that providers are skilled and knowledgeable about the diagnosis, treatment, resources, and referral process for these women.

Data consistently indicate that women suffer from a lifetime prevalence of mood disorders at twice the rate of men. However, the majority of six million women with major depression or dysthymia remain undiagnosed and often present differently than men on signs and symptoms of mental health disorders. Furthermore, women have higher rates of comorbid disorders than men as well as different patterns of comorbidity.

Despite these serious concerns, the existing literature that focuses on male/female differences in mental health is limited. When we began researching the literature prior to the initiation of this book in 2006, a number of books existed on mental health problems in primary care, but there was only one book on *women's mental health in primary care settings*. To our knowledge there are no current books on the market that focus on women's mental health in *primary care settings*. Furthermore, while books do exist on women's mental health, these books are written from the perspective of a psychiatric practice rather than a primary care practice. Patients often present quite differently in these two settings with more severe symptoms presenting to the psychiatric as opposed to the primary care setting.

The number of PAs, NPs, and CNMs in primary care has been increasing each year. The majority of these midlevel providers practice in primary care settings and can be expected to be the providers of mental health care services to their female patients. We believe that this book will serve as a gender-specific clinical guide for midlevel providers as well as primary care physicians and will assist these professionals in making more accurate diagnosis and effective treatment plans. Educators of these professionals will also find this book to be useful and appropriate for their students because core competencies for accreditation in psychiatric/mental health services are required in all of these professions. Furthermore, our book has a multidisciplinary approach with contributors from a variety of professions, including nurses, physician's assistants, nurse midwives, psychiatrists, primary care physicians, social workers, and psychologists.

We have included 16 chapters in this book and, while the topics are not inclusive of all women's mental health disorders, they represent the most common mental health problems seen among women patients in primary care settings. Each chapter uses the same format, thereby facilitating readers in quickly finding the information they are seeking. Each chapter also contains well-organized tables and boxes for quick assimilation of important points. Resources, including commonly used instruments appropriate for primary care settings, and their websites are at the end of each chapter. Chapters are also distinguished by being research-based and originating from a variety of professional disciplines. Finally, all of our contributors are experts in their fields, and we are proud to have them as contributors to our book.

Drs. Joan Urbancic and Carla Groh

Contents

Carla J. Grob

chapter 1

Foundations of Women's Mental Health

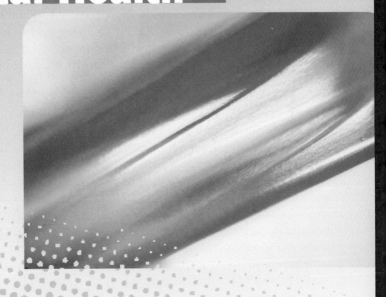

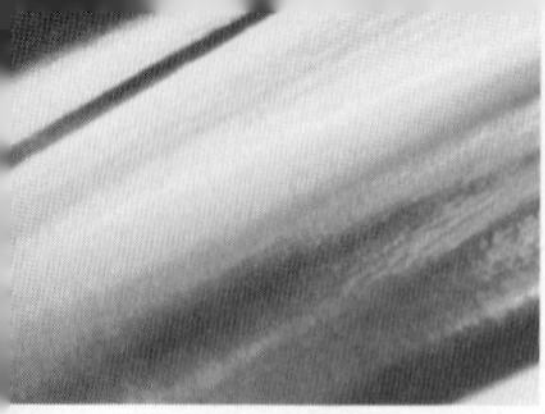

Women's mental health needs can create a conundrum for primary care practitioners (PCPs) as they strive to balance the increasing demands of providing health care in the 21st century with the desire to respond to the real-life needs of women in their clinical practices. Findings from the National Ambulatory Medical Care Survey (Woodwell and Cherry, 2004) estimated that Americans made 890 million office visits in 2002, a 17-percent increase from 1992 through 2002. The majority of those visits (62.7 percent) were to primary care specialists, with midlevel practitioners (physician assistants, nurse practitioners, and/or nurse midwives) being seen at 3.1 percent of those visits. Women continue to have a higher percentage of office visits than men, and findings have shown that as women age, the number of office visits rise. One finding of particular interest was the significant increase (48 percent from 1995 through 2002) in the drug mention rates for antidepressants during office visits. Moreover, antidepressants ranked in the top three therapeutic drug classes mentioned during visits (along with nonsteroidal anti-inflammatory drugs and antihistamines) (Woodwell and Cherry).

Previous studies have shown that women take more psychotropic medications than men. About two thirds of antidepressants and tranquilizers dispensed in the United States are prescribed to women, and more women than men take multiple medications (Roe, McNamara, and Motheral, 2002). Yet despite the increased awareness of mood disorders and increased use of antidepressants, mental health disorders remain underdiagnosed and undertreated in primary care. The National Comorbidity Survey Replication Study (Wang, Lane, Olfson, et al., 2005) reported two significant findings with clinical implications for primary care practitioners. First, of those respondents who reported anxiety, mood, impulse control, and/or substance abuse disorders as defined by the *Diagnostic and Statistical Manual of Mental Disorders, Fourth Edition* (*DSM-IV*), in the 12 months before the interview, 22.8 percent were treated by a general medical provider (others received services by mental health specialty providers, employees of human services departments, and alternative medicine practitioners). Second, respondents treated by the general medical provider received fewer visits (1.7 vs. 7.4) and treatment that less frequently met minimal standards of care than those treated by the mental health specialty providers (12.7 vs. 48.3 percent). Wang et al. (2005) concluded that "most people with mental disorders in the United States remain either untreated or poorly treated" (p. 629).

Based on the above information, it is increasingly obvious that PCPs are major providers of mental health services in the United States. As greater emphasis is placed on clinical outcomes, it becomes even more imperative for

PCPs to focus on strategies for addressing mental illnesses in women that integrate the female mind and body in the daily practice of health care. Satcher (U.S. Department of Health and Human Services [DHHS], 1999) proclaimed that mental health is fundamental to health, yet the burden of mental illness on health and productivity has not been fully recognized (Wisner, 2004).

The remainder of this chapter will focus on mental health factors that PCPs need to be aware of and sensitive to when providing health care to women patients. The relative contributions of these factors will vary across individuals as well as across phases of the life cycle.

WOMEN AND THE MENTAL HEALTH SYSTEM

Historically, the mere possession of a female body was thought to increase one's vulnerability to mental illness. Mental illness was believed to be related to disruptions of the reproductive system—such as neurasthenia and hysteria (Chrisler and Caplan, 2002)—and a likely consequence if women transgressed the "laws of nature" and stepped outside their proper social roles (Tomes, 1990). This belief is evident in one of the earliest accounts of women's experience in mental institutions, *Women of the Asylum: Voices from Behind the Walls, 1840–1945* by Geller and Harris (1994). Twenty-six women told their stories of being incarcerated against their wills for holding views or behaving in ways that deviated from the norms of their day. Treatment for mental illness during this period was an amalgam of different approaches. Women received gender neutral treatments (e.g., bloodletting, purging, mechanical restraints, wet packs, vitamin and mineral tonics, and opiates) as well as gender-specific treatments (e.g., the "rest" cure, removal of the ovaries, electrical charges applied to the uterus, hot water injections into the vagina, and clitoral cauterization (Geller and Harris).

The first decades of the 20th century ushered in a new generation of women—and the mental health reform movement. Women were more independent, more rebellious, and better educated; they advocated for suffrage and for the rights and concerns of those less fortunate. This was also the first generation of women who were openly sexual. The reform movement gained force with the publication of *A Mind That Found Itself* (Beers, 1908), an autobiography chronicling Beers' struggle with mental illness and the shameful state of mental health in the United States. The theories and underlying causes of mental illness became the focus of renewed interest and research during this time. There was a shift from mental illness being viewed as impaired action of the mind, instincts, and sentiment to the belief that for every mental state, there was a correlated physical concomitant believed to have caused the psychiatric dysfunction (Barnes, 1912).

Although the reform movement advocated for more humane treatments, the 1930s to 1950s saw some of the most radical physical interventions. During this period, prefrontal lobotomies, prolonged narcosis, insulin shock, electroconvulsive therapy (ECT), and enforced sterilization were common somatic therapies (Geller and Harris, 1994). Women outnumbered men as recipients of insulin shock, ECT, and lobotomies (Showalter, 1985) even though women did not outnumber men in mental institutions (Tomes, 1990).

The dominant theories that shaped the understanding and treatment of women during the early and mid-decades were based on the male-privileged theories of Freud, Erikson, Bettelheim, and Kohlberg (as well as others). The common theme was expert male authority and a subordinate female patient (Bentley, 2005). The early decades also saw the development of psychoanalysis (e.g., "talking cure") for the treatment of mental disorders, which according to Freud were rooted in life experiences and the internal dynamics of lust and desire.

The feminist movement in the late 1960s and early 1970s challenged the theories of male dominance/female submission, sparking a new era of theorizing about women's experience with respect to mental health. Chesler's (1972) classic work *Women and Madness* exposed our culture's practice of defining women's experience as pathologic and its use of the mental health system to maintain the status quo in terms of gender roles and in the allocation of power and status (Bentley, 2005). Early feminists such as de Beauvoir (1952), Friedan (1963), Millett (1969), and Brownmiller (1975) paved the way for the reconceptualization of women's psychological development posited by Chodorow (1978, 1989), Gilligan (1982), and Miller (1986). This new psychology argued that women's development is different from that of men, recognizing that women build on and develop in a context of attachment and affiliation with others (Miller), whereas men tend to value separation and individuation. Furthermore, women's connectedness (as opposed to men's value of independence) and sense of shared empathy lead to strength and health (Miller and Stiver, 1997). At the same time, there was increased acknowledgment that women's mental health is impacted by a myriad of social, political, and economic factors.

Despite these advances, there are still fragments of sexism and bias in the 21st century. Women's biology is once again being questioned as a cause of mental illness. Considerable controversy exists over the status of premenstrual dysphoric disorder (PMDD) and premenstrual syndrome (PMS) as valid diagnostic categories for inclusion in the *DSM*. Those who object to the diagnosis argue that menstruation is a normal bodily function, and any psychological changes associated with this function should be seen as normal as well. Further, they argue that classifying PMS or PMDD as a mental disorder stigmatizes women and raises questions about the social construction of mental illness (Caplan, 1995; Caplan, McCurdy-Myers, and Gans, 1992; Chrisler and Caplan, 2002; Figert, 1996). Although PMS was dropped from the 1994 edition of *DSM-IV* because of insufficient scientific evidence, PDD was included in an appendix labeled "Needing Further Study." What will happen with the next revision of the *DSM* remains to be seen.

HEALTH DISPARITIES AMONG WOMEN

Women and girls made up 50.9 percent of the total United States population in 2000 (Smith and Spraggins, 2001). It is projected that the female population will continue to increase, with just under half of females projected to be members of racial or ethnic minority groups by the year 2050 (Campbell, 1996). This projection is important for PCPs since it is well documented that racial and ethnic minorities often experience poorer access to health care and lower quality of preventive, primary, and specialty care than do whites (National Healthcare Disparities Report, 2005).

Women of Racial and Ethnic Minority Groups

Some of the documented health disparities suggest that black women have higher death rates due to heart disease, diabetes, cancer, and stroke as well as the shortest life expectancy compared with other groups of women. Hispanic women have the highest incidence of cervical cancer, while American Indian/Alaskan Native women fare the worst of all groups studied for smoking, binge drinking, cirrhosis mortality rate, and violence against them. Poor or near poor women are more likely to report fair or poor overall health; limitations in activity; and having anxiety or depression, arthritis, asthma, diabetes, hypertension, obesity, and osteoporosis. Additionally, poor or near poor women are more likely to report lack of health insurance, dissatisfaction with their health plan when insured, and not having a consistent source of care (Making the Grade, 2004; National Healthcare Disparities Report, 2005). Women of color are more likely than white women to experience poverty and to be uninsured (Table 1.1).

There are striking disparities in mental health among women as well. Racial and ethnic minorities have less access to mental health services; are less likely to receive needed services; and, when they do receive care, it is more likely to be poor in quality (DHHS, 2001). Further, minorities are overrepresented among the

Table 1.1 • Socioeconomic Characteristics for U.S. Women by Race and Ethnicity*

	White	Black	American Indian/ Alaskan Native	Asian American/ Pacific Islander	Hispanic
Uninsured (%)	12.0	21.0	27.2	20.3	36.9
Poor (%)**	8.8	22.8	21.4	10.0	21.2
High School Completion (%)	89.4	80.2	79.6	86.7	58.8

*"African American" is used to describe all black women living in the United States, regardless of country of origin or immigrant status; Hispanic/Latina women are primarily from Mexico but may come from other regions, including Central and South America, Puerto Rico, and Cuba, and nearly two thirds are born outside of the United States; Asian American women may be from China, the Philippines, Asia, Korea, Vietnam, or Japan, whereas Pacific Islander women come from more than 22 islands (Polynesian, Micronesian, Melanesian) and Hawaii; and American Indian/Alaskan Native women come from more than 561 recognized tribes and 300 spoken languages.
**Women 18 years of age and older whose family income level falls below the federal poverty threshold (2001–2002).
From *Making the grade on women's health: A national and state-by-state report* (2004).

nation's vulnerable, high-need groups (e.g., adults who are homeless, incarcerated, or in foster care). These subpopulations are usually at higher risk for mental illness and have a higher need for mental health services, yet they are at the greatest risk for not receiving those services. Taken together, the evidence suggests that racial and ethnic minorities bear a greater burden from unmet mental health needs and thus suffer a greater loss to their overall health and productivity (DHHS).

Although more is known about the disparities than the reasons behind them, several barriers have been suggested that deter women in general from reaching treatment: cost, fragmentation of services, lack of availability of services, and societal stigma toward mental illness (DHHS, 1999). Additional barriers specific to minority women include mistrust and fear of treatment, racism and discrimination, and differences in language and communication (DHHS, 2001).

Women with Disabilities

It is estimated that 28.2 million women (19.5 percent of all females) have some level of disability, with 18.4 million being severely disabled. Black women have the highest rates for severe disability (14.6 percent), followed by white women (13.2 percent) and Hispanic women (10.1 percent). Furthermore, as women age, their rates of disability increase significantly: 55.9 percent of all females 65 years of age and older report some level of disability (Steinmetz, 2006). Women with disabilities face multiple barriers to health care: physical inaccessibility to medical offices and equipment, lack of transportation, limited health information, and discrimination by health care providers (Making the Grade, 2004). Also, women with disabilities are at greater risk for living in poverty and receiving government-funded health insurance, which often restricts the services most needed by these women. Further, disabled women and girls are more likely to experience emotional, physical, and sexual abuse; depression; and discrimination in employment and housing than nondisabled women (Making the Grade).

Women Living in Rural Areas

Women living in rural areas comprise about 20 percent of the U.S. female population (U.S. Census Bureau, 2000), with approximately 10 percent being women of color (Hargraves, 2002). Rural women are faced with economic, cultural, and behavioral challenges. They experience high rates of poverty, unemployment, and geographic isolation as well as limited educational and vocational opportunities. Rural women report being more likely to smoke (especially during pregnancy), drink alcohol, and be obese compared with urban women. Moreover, along with being under- or uninsured, rural women frequently lack access to both health care options and various supportive, ancillary services (Coward, Davis, Gold, et al., 2006). Women of color experience all of the mentioned issues in addition to cultural differences that further fragment health care services, such as health beliefs, racism, language barriers, migratory patterns, and abject poverty (Hargraves).

Immigrant and Refugee Women

Women are migrating to the United States at an unprecedented rate and currently represent 11.1 percent of the total female population in the United States (U.S. Census Bureau, 2002). About half of the immigrants in the United States were born in Latin America and about one quarter in Asian countries, with the remaining born in other parts of the world (Making the Grade, 2004). Women may emigrate for a number of reasons. Some come voluntarily, while others undergo forced migration (e.g., refugees, asylum seekers, and stateless persons).

Numerous barriers discourage immigrant women from accessing health care services, including cost, provider relationships, lack of female physicians, women's lower status and men's gatekeeping, time constraints, transportation, language, and lack of health insurance (Aroian, 2001). Immigrant women with the greatest barriers are those who are unemployed, less acculturated, more recent to the country, less educated, poorer, of lower social status, and uncomfortable with their language skills (Aroian). Immigrant women are also reported to have higher rates of psychological distress than their male counterparts as well as their host population (Webster, McDonald, Lewin, et al., 1995). Correlates of psychological distress for immigrant women include low income; unemployment or not working in one's field; less education; low acculturation, or retention of traditional values; language difficulty; old age; poor health; and lack of social supports (Aroian).

Women refugees are at an even higher risk for poor health outcomes than immigrant women, especially serious mental health disorders (Chung and Bemak, 2002). Many refugee women experience posttraumatic stress disorder following one or several of the following events: rape and sexual violence, threats of mass genocide, torture or witnessing torture, death of family members, persecution, starvation, dangerous escapes from their home countries, or extreme hardship in refugee camps (Chung and Bemak).

Lesbians

Lesbians are a heterogeneous group of women of various ages, ethnicities, and socioeconomic levels who may have little more in common than their sexual orientation (Klinger, 2002). However, as a subgroup, lesbians are less likely to seek, or more likely to delay seeking, health care than other women. Lesbians' access to health care may be affected by such factors as the lack of culturally competent providers and the presence of homophobia among providers, more limited access to health insurance because lesbians cannot share in spousal benefits, and financial barriers that may impede access to health insurance coverage (Solarz, 1999). Stress may be a major health issue for lesbian women who face multiple forms of discrimination; this may be especially true for those who are also members of ethnic or racial minority groups. The combination of homophobia, racism, and sex-based discrimination puts the health of these women in "triple jeopardy" (Solarz).

CULTURE AND MENTAL ILLNESS

Culture plays a pivotal role in mental illness. It influences whether people seek help in the first place, the type of help they seek, what coping styles and social supports they have, and how much stigma they attach to mental illness (DHHS, 2001). Culture is broadly defined as a common heritage or set of beliefs, norms, and values shared by one group (DHHS, 1999). There are a variety of ways to define a cultural group—by ethnicity, religion, geographic region, age group, sexual orientation, or profession. As such, many people consider themselves as having multiple cultural identities (DHHS, 2001). Although the culture of the patient is important, the culture of the PCP and service system are equally important since they affect diagnosis, treatment, and the organization and reimbursement of services (DHHS, 2001). The divergent cultures between patient and PCP (and health care system) can create barriers to effective health care and leave patients feeling misunderstood and marginalized.

In recent years, there has been a proliferation of articles and conference presentations on the clinical aspects of culture as it relates to health care, particularly in the areas of assessment and treatment. Several racial, ethnic, and underrepresented groups have been the focus of this effort: Asians, blacks, Hispanics, Native Americans, Arab Americans, women, gays, lesbians, transgendered, and bisexuals. This effort has resulted in a better understanding of the multifaceted ways in which culture influences mental illness and the presentation of symptoms. The identification of culture-bound syndromes (i.e., local specific patterns of symptoms) has been invaluable for health care providers in understanding mental health problems and disorders within and among cultures (Boxes 1.1 and 1.2).

Box 1.1 • Asian Culture-Bound Syndromes

Neurasthenia (Shenjang Shuaruo)

- Lack of nerve strength, neurologic weakness, exhaustion of nervous system.
- Chinese syndrome characterized by mental and physical fatigue, poor concentration, poor memory, dizziness.
- Physical symptoms such as changes in appetite and sleep, headaches, sexual dysfunction.

Shin-Byung

- Korean syndrome characterized by anxiety and physical complaints such as weakness, dizziness, poor appetite, insomnia. Dissociation may present.
- Attributed to possession by ancestral spirits.

Hwa-Byung

- Most common in middle-aged Korean women ("anger sickness").
- Sense of epigastric/upper abdominal mass/heaviness, shortness of breath, indigestion, fatigue, flushing, palpitations, vomiting, cold hands or feet, panic.
- Thought to be due to suppression of anger, disappointment, grudges, and unfulfilled expectations.

From Lim, R. F., & Lu, F. (2005).

Box 1.2 • Hispanic Culture-Bound Syndromes

Ataque de Nervious (Attack of Nerves)

- Similar to panic attacks but often accompanied by more violent behavior and may occur without fear or apprehension; often precipitated by an upsetting event.
- Uncontrollable shouting, trembling, palpitations, heat in chest rising to head, fainting, seizurelike episodes.
- Two thirds may have depressive or anxiety disorder.
- Generally treated symptomatically; no solid data on optimal treatment.

Nervios (Nerves)

- More generalized state compared with *ataque de nervious.*
- Analogous with generalized anxiety disorder.
- Emotional upset, somatic distress, social isolation, restlessness, feeling out of control, mood/affective instability.
- External stressors are a major factor.

Susto (Fright)

- A sudden fright or trauma, causing the soul or spirit to leave the body and making one vulnerable to various ills.
- Anxiety, irritability, anorexia, insomnia, trembling, sweating, tachycardia, diarrhea, depression, vomiting.
- Spiritists may be very helpful.

Atypical Psychotic Symptoms

- Psychotic symptoms described by Hispanic patients often present differently from those seen in other populations.
- May include atypical auditory and visual hallucinations in the context of an otherwise unremarkable mental status exam.
- Symptoms include a knocking at door, doorbell ringing, shadows, spots, children's voices calling name.
- Seldom part of chief complaint.

From Lim, R. F., & Lu, F. (2005).

Although this knowledge is fundamental in delivering culturally competent care, several issues related to culture are important to bear in mind. First, there is tremendous diversity within each cultural group. For example, the Asian American category is extremely diverse, with about 43 different ethnic subgroups and over 100 languages and dialects spoken (DHHS, 2001). That is, what might be true for Cambodians may not be true for Chinese. Second, generalizations about culture are meant to provide a starting point for health care providers and are not meant to invoke cultural stereotypes or reduce pathology to a cultural phenomenon (Lim and Lu, 2005). Thus, it is critical to not make assumptions based on culture alone but to verify the meaning of symptoms for each person. Third, the stigma of mental illness and the "conspiracy of silence" within the family transcend most cultural and ethnic groups. To address the issue of stigma, it is critical for PCPs (as well as other health care providers) to reflect on their own view of mental illness and what it means to them. It is with this insight that PCPs can then begin to help patients and their families deal more openly and effectively with mental illness. Fourth, many cultures use traditional healing practices that often supersede the treatment prescribed by PCPs (Box 1.3).

Since patients rarely share this information unless asked, it is the responsibility of the PCP to learn about indigenous treatments and to ask appropriate questions. Last, there is no doubt that PCPs need to become more culturally competent and be able to work effectively and sensitively within various cultural contexts. There are several published sets of guidelines that can guide PCPs to ask questions about the presentation of symptoms that recognize the centrality of culture in understanding those symptoms. Box 1.4 lists nine questions that may be helpful to PCPs in clinical practice.

Spirituality and Religion

Spirituality and religion play a prominent role in the lives of most Americans, including members of many racial and ethnic minorities (DHHS, 2001). Although there is no precise definition of spirituality, it is commonly thought to include transcendence, meaning and purpose in life, connection with others and the universe, and inner resources. Spirituality may (or may not) be experienced and expressed through religion, which is characterized by beliefs, rituals, social organization, and cumulative traditions (Fukuyama and Sevig, 1999). Further, individual conceptualizations of spirituality are greatly influenced by culture, gender, and socioeconomic class (Wade-Gayles, 1995).

The intersection of spirituality and women's health is an important area of query for PCPs. It is becoming increasingly evident that spirituality is a critical

Box 1.3 • Traditional Health and Healing Practices

Native Americans
- Teas, roots, and other herbal remedies
- Sweat lodge ceremonies
- Seek advice from herbalists, spiritual healers, medicine men

African Americans
- Voodoo
- Herbs
- Prayer

Hispanic/Latino
- Advice from spiritual healers (*espiritistas* and/or *curanderos*)

Asian Americans
- Coining
- Pinching
- Cupping
- Moxibustion
- Acupuncture
- Medicated paper
- Healing ceremonies
- Advice of healer and/or shaman

life factor and frame of reference for many women who seek primary care services. Evidence suggests that spirituality has a significant influence on health behaviors (Banks-Wallace and Parks, 2004) and is a constitutive element of optimal health in women (Maloy, 2000). However, spiritual and religious beliefs about mental illness may be different from beliefs about physical illness and can influence a woman's decision to seek or avoid professional help. For example, a study examining the Pentecostal perspective on depression's causes and treatments found that Pentecostals endorsed a variety of causal factors for depressions (contrary to Pentecostal theologic literature), yet faith was endorsed as the most effective treatment option (Trice and Bjorck, 2006). Similar findings have been

Box 1.4 • Questions to Ask Related to Mental Health Symptoms

1. What do you call your problem?
2. What has caused it?
3. Why do you think it started when it did?
4. What does it do to you?
5. How severe is it?
6. What do you fear most about it?
7. What are the chief problems it has caused you?
8. What kind of treatment do you think you should receive?
9. What are you currently doing to deal with the problem?

From Kleinman, A. (1981).

reported among black women, who reported a greater likelihood of seeking mental health services from religious sources (Brown, 2004) and informal community support than from professional providers (Primm, Cabot, Pettis, et al., 2002).

Another challenge for many PCPs is how religion and spiritual beliefs have been viewed in the United States. Historically, Western religions have been valued more and are better understood than Eastern religions. Judaism, Christianity, Islam, and the Baha'i faith are monotheistic faiths (i.e., belief in one God) practiced by about half of the world's population. Believers of Eastern religions, on the other hand, seek to find enlightenment by looking within themselves. Hinduism and Buddhism are common faiths in India, Southeast Asia, and Japan; Taoism and Confucianism are religious philosophies practiced in China; and Shinto is the traditional religion of many Japanese people. Indigenous religions are practiced throughout the world, particularly in sub-Saharan Africa, and are similar to the traditional beliefs of the Native Americans in North and South America. Primary care practitioners who do not strive to broaden their understanding of *all* world religions and spiritual beliefs will be at a severe disadvantage in their attempts to maximize therapeutic effectiveness and health outcomes for our increasingly diverse patient population. It is not compulsory that practitioners endorse patient belief systems or other aspects of their spirituality, but practitioners do need to acknowledge said systems as a critical point in a patient's frame of reference (Hall and Livingston, 2006).

WOMEN AND PSYCHOPHARMACOLOGY

Women are the primary consumers of psychotropic medications in the United States (Robinson, 2002), yet it is unclear to what extent PCPs consider sex differences in psychopharmacology when prescribing. These differences are important since about two thirds of antidepressants and tranquilizers dispensed are prescribed to women, and more women than men take multiple medications (Roe et al., 2002). Further, women tend to have more side effects and adverse effects with psychotropic medication than do men (Hamilton and Yonkers, 1996).

Increasing data show that sex differences exist in the absorption, distribution, metabolism, and excretion of many medications (Table 1.2). Although the effect of the menstrual cycle on psychotropic medication levels is unclear, data suggest that medication levels may vary across the cycle (Burt and Hendrick, 1997). The use

Table 1.2 • Sex Differences in Psychotropic Pharmacokinetics

Drug Mechanism	Effect on Women	Effect on Psychotropics
Absorption	Slower gastric emptying	↑ Residual volume Slower absorption Delayed peak levels ↓ Peak serum concentrations
Bioavailability	Lower gastric acid secretion	↑ Absorption of bases such as TCA, benzodiazepines, and phenothiazines ↓ Gastric absorption of acids such as phenytoin and barbiturates
Distribution	Lower body weight Lower total blood volume Higher percent body fat Higher brain blood flow	↑ Blood levels ↑ Blood levels ↓ Blood levels initially, ↑ later due to storage in fat ↑ Blood flow
Metabolism	Slower clearance for drugs	↓ Blood levels ↑ Side effects and adverse effects at optimal doses ↑ Rates of tardive dyskinesia

From Hamilton, J. A., & Yonkers, K. A. (1996); Robinson, G. E. (2002).

of oral contraceptives (OCs) may additionally influence levels of psychotropic medication. OCs differentially affect the blood levels of various benzodiazepines, decreasing levels of temazepam (Restoril) but increasing levels of others, such as chlordiazepoxide (Librium), diazepam (Valium), and nitrazepam (Alodorm, Mogadon, Nitredon, Nilandron). OCs also decrease serum tricyclic levels and may potentate the prolactin response of antipsychotics. Further, drugs such as carbamazepine (Tegretol) and phenobarbital (Luminal) may reduce the efficacy of OCs (Hamilton and Yonkers, 1996; Robinson, 2002). The effect of OCs on levels of psychotropic medication is important information for PCPs since they are used by approximately 11 million women between 15 and 44 years of age in the United States ("Aim Toward Success," 2006).

Age also affects the pharmacodynamics and pharmacokinetics of medications. As women age, they may require lower doses of psychotropic medication due to diminishing levels of estrogen and other age-related biologic changes, including decreased levels of serum albumin, decreased lean body mass, lower hepatic blood flow, and decreased renal excretion and elimination (Hamilton and Yonkers, 1996). All of these processes may result in an increase in serum levels and half-lives for many psychotropic medications in older women.

Another factor that influences response to medication is ethnicity. Ethnopharmacology is a relatively new area of research that focuses on how people in diverse ethnic groups metabolize certain drugs (Munoz and Hilgenberg, 2005). Much of the research has focused on the cytochrome P-450 (CPY) enzymes that are responsible for phase 1 metabolism of most antipsychotic and antidepressant medications. Research findings suggest that genetic variations in one or more of the CYP enzymes may cause differing drug responses (Lin, Smith, and Lin, 2003) and that certain ethnic groups have more of these variations than do others (Munoz and Hilgenberg) (Box 1.5).

One of the most widely studied enzymes is CYP2D6. Genetic changes in this enzyme have been shown to affect the rate of drug metabolism, which in turn affects drug plasma levels at a given dosage. For example, people who have more than two functional copies of the CYP2D6 gene have faster than normal enzyme activity and are known as "ultrarapid metabolizers," whereas those with two nonfunctional copies of the gene have slower than normal enzyme activity and are known as "poor metabolizers." Ultrarapid metabolizers will metabolize a drug quickly, resulting in lower serum concentrations, whereas poor metabolizers metabolize the drug more slowly and have higher serum levels at the same dose. In general, Asians tend to be poor metabolizers and often need substantially lower doses of psychotropic medications (Lim and Lu,

Box 1.5 • Ethnopharmacologic Findings Related to Psychotropic Medication

Traditional Antipsychotic Medication*

- Hispanics require lower doses compared with whites (Ruiz et al., 1996).
- Blacks are at greater risk for tardive dyskinesia than whites (Glazer et al., 1994; Trans et al., 1999).
- Asians require lower doses to achieve response than whites (Lin & Poland, 1989).
- Asians experience more extrapyramidal symptoms than whites at the same dose (Lin et al., 1989).

Atypical" Antipsychotic Medication**

- Preferable in ethnic minorities because fewer adverse effects occur (Frackiewicz et al., 1999).

Tricyclic Antidepressants***

- Blacks are likely to have faster therapeutic response, higher serum concentrations, and more adverse effects than whites (Lawson, 1996; Strickland et al., 1991).
- Blacks are at greater risk of delirium than whites (Strickland et al., 1991).
- Hispanics report adverse effects at lower doses than whites (Mendoza et al., 1991).
- Hispanic women achieved comparable clinical outcomes at half the dose prescribed to white women (Mendoza et al., 1991)

Lithium and Lithium Derivatives

- Blacks require lower doses than whites (Strickland et al., 1995).
- Blacks reported more adverse effects (lethargy, dizziness) than whites at similar doses (Strickland et al., 1995).

*Typical antipsychotics include chlorpromazine (Thorazine), perphenazine (Trilafon), prochlorperazine (Compazine), thioridazine (Mellaril), trifluoperazine (Stelazine), and haloperidol (Haldol).

**Atypical antipsychotics include clozapine (Clozaril), olanzapine (Zyprexa), risperidone (Risperdal), quetiapine (Seroquel), ziprasidone (Geodon), and aripiprazole (Abilify).

***Tricyclic antidepressants include amitriptyline (Elavil, Endep, Tryptanol), clomipramine (Anafranil), desipramine (Norpramin, Pertofrane), doxepin (Sinequan), imipramine (Tofranil), nortriptyline (Pamelor), protriptyline (Vivactil), and trimipramine (Surmontil).

Table 1.3 • Factors Affecting the Drug-Metabolizing Enzymes

Factor	Effect
Smoking	Significantly reduces blood levels of psychotropics
Grapefruit juice	Increases blood level of nefazodone (Serzone) and alprazolam (Xanax)
St. John's wort	↑ Metabolism, resulting in ↓ blood levels when combined with alprazolam (Xanax) and midazolam (Versed) ↑ Possibility of serotonin syndrome when combined with MAOIs, TCAs, SSRIs, mirtazapine (Remeron), and venlafaxine (Effexor)

2005). Additional factors that may affect the drug-metabolizing enzymes are included in Table 1.3.

CONCLUSION

Women with mental illness in primary care settings present with a vast array of treatment challenges for the busy primary care practitioner. Some of these challenges are related to the complexity associated with mental illness, and other challenges are related to how health care is delivered in the United States. Women do not always realize that they are experiencing a mental illness, and if they do, they may minimize the symptoms. PCPs do not routinely assess for mental illness or emotional distress, so these disorders often go undetected and untreated.

This chapter has identified several factors that can alert the PCP to situations where a woman might be more vulnerable to the development of a mental illness or mental health problems. Race, ethnicity, socioeconomic class, and where one lives, as well as spiritual and religious beliefs, can either buffer the effects of stress or confound the effects of stress.

Although mental disorders are found worldwide, diagnosis continues to be extremely challenging because the manifestations of mental disorders vary with age, gender, race, ethnicity, and culture (DHHS, 2001). Even when a mental disorder is diagnosed, treatment can be complicated by a multitude of factors (e.g., hormones, aging, prescription medications, stigma, fear of discrimination, religious beliefs).

As Charles Dickens (1859) states in the beginning of his novel *A Tale of Two Cities*, "It was the best of times, it was the worst of times" (p. 1). Women who experience mental illness or mental health problems in the 21st century have a tremendous number of treatment options and mental health resources available to them, yet the majority of these mental illnesses are either undiagnosed or, if diagnosed, undertreated. The goal of this book is to provide primary care practitioners important assessment, diagnostic, and treatment options as they provide primary care services to women who might also experience mental illness or mental health problems. Primary care practitioners are in a position to positively impact the lives of women and their families.

References

Aim toward success in OC compliance, better communication improves use: More than 33% have sex when OC reliability may be compromised. (2006). *Contraceptive Technology Update, 27*(2), 13–15.

Aroian, K. J. (2001). Immigrant women and their health. *Annual Review of Nursing Research, 19*, 179–225.

Banks-Wallace, J., & Parks, L. (2004). It's all sacred: African American women's perspectives on spirituality. *Issues in Mental Health Nursing, 25*, 25–45.

Barnes, F. M. (1912). Chemistry of nervous and mental diseases. *American Journal of Insanity, 68*, 431–472.

Beers, C. W. (1908). *A mind that found itself: A memoir of madness and recovery.* Pittsburgh: University of Pittsburgh Press.

Bentley, K. J. (2005). Women, mental health, and the psychiatric enterprise: A review. *Health and Social Work, 30*(1), 56–63.

Brown, J. A. (2004). African American church goers' attitudes toward treatment seeking from mental health and religious sources: The role of spirituality, cultural mistrust, and stigma toward mental illness. Ann Arbor, MI: ProQuest Information and Learning Company (UMI No. 3129678).

Brownmiller, S. (1975). *Against her will: Men, women and rape.* New York: Ballantine Books.

Burt, V. K., & Hendrick, V. C. (1997). *A concise guide to women's mental health.* Washington, DC: American Psychiatric Press, Inc.

Campbell, P. R. (1996). *Population projections for states by age, sex, race, and Hispanic origin: 1995 to 2025.* U.S. Bureau of the Census, Population Division, PPL-47.

Caplan, P. J. (1995). *They say you're crazy: How the world's most powerful psychiatrists decide who's normal.* Cambridge, MA: Perseus Books.

Caplan, P. J., McCurdy-Myers, J., & Gans, M. (1992). Should "premenstrual syndrome" be called a psychiatric abnormality? *Feminism & Psychology, 2*, 27–44.

Chesler, P. (1972). *Women and madness.* New York: Avon Books.

Chodorow, N. (1978). *The reproduction of motherhood: Psychoanalysis and the sociology of gender.* Los Angeles: University of California Press.

Chodorow, N. (1989). *Feminism and psychoanalytic theory.* New Haven: Yale University Press.

Chrisler, J. C., & Caplan, P. (2002). The strange case of Dr. Jekyll and Ms. Hyde: How PMS became a cultural phenomenon and a psychiatric disorder. *Annual Review of Sex Research, 13*, 274–306.

Chung, R., & Bemak, F. (2002). Revisiting the California Southeast Asian mental health needs assessment data: An examination of refugee ethnic and gender differences. *Journal of Counseling & Development, 80*, 111–119.

Coward, H., Davis, L. A., Gold, C. H., et al. (2006). *Rural women's health: Mental, behavioral and physical issues.* New York: Springer Publishing Company, Inc.

de Beauvoir, S. (1952). *The second sex.* New York: Vintage Press.

Dickens, C. (1859). *A tale of two cities.* London: Penguin Books.

Figert, A. E. (1996). *Women and the ownership of PMS: The structuring of a psychiatric disorder.* Hawthorne, NY: Aldine DeGruyter.

Frackiewicz, E., Sramek, J. J., & Herrera, J. M. (1999). Review of neuroleptic dosage in different ethnic groups. In J. M. Herrera (Ed.), *Cross cultural psychiatry* (pp. 107–130). Chichester, England: John Wiley and Sons.

Friedan, B. (1963). *The feminine mystique.* New York: W.W. Norton and Company, Inc.

Fukuyama, M. A., & Sevig, T. D. (1999). *Integrating spirituality into multicultural counseling.* Thousand Oaks, CA: Sage.

Geller, J. L., & Harris, M. (1994). *Women of the asylum: Voices from behind the walls, 1840–1945.* New York: Anchor Books.

Gilligan, C. (1982). *In a different voice.* Cambridge, MA: Harvard University Press.

Glazer, W. M., Morgenstern, H., Doucette, J., et al. (1994). Race and tardive dyskinesia among outpatients at a CMHC. *Hospital Community Psychiatry, 45*(1), 38–42.

Hall, R. E., & Livingston, J. N. (2006). Mental health practice with Arab families: The implications of spirituality vis-à-vis Islam. *American Journal of Family Therapy, 34*(2), 139–150.

Hamilton, J. A., & Yonkers, K. A. (1996). Sex differences in pharmacokinetics of psychotropic medications: Part 1: Physiologic basis for effects. In M. F. Jensvold, R. Halbreich, & J. A. Hamilton (Eds.), *Psychopharmacology and women: Sex, gender, and hormones* (pp. 11–42). Washington, DC: American Psychiatric Press, Inc.

Hargraves, M. (2002). Elevating the voices of rural minority women. *American Journal of Public Health, 92*(4), 514–516.

Kleinman, A. (1981). *Patients and healers in the context of culture: An exploration of the borderland between anthropology, medicine, and psychiatry.* Berkeley, CA: University of California Press.

Klinger, R. L. (2002). Lesbian women. In S. G. Kornstein & A. H. Clayton (Eds.), *Women and mental health: A comprehensive textbook* (pp. 555–567). New York: Guilford Press.

Lawson, W. B. (1996). Clinical issues in the pharmacotherapy of African-Americans. *Psychopharmacology Bulletin, 32*(2), 275–281.

Lim, R. F., & Lu, F. (2005). Clinical aspects of culture in the practice of psychiatry: Assessment and treatment of culturally diverse patients. *Medscape2005.* Retrieved July 29, 2006, from *www.medscape.com/viewprogram/4258_pnt.*

Lin, K-M, Smith, M. W., & Lin, M. T. (2003). Psychopharmacology: Ethnic and cultural perspectives. In A. Tasman, J. Kay, & J. A. Lieberman (Eds.), *Psychiatry therapeutics* (2nd ed., pp. 217–229). West Sussex: John Wiley & Sons, Ltd.

Lin, K. M., & Poland, R. E. (1989). Pharmacotherapy with Asian psychiatric patients. *Psychiatric Annals, 19*(12), 659–663.

Making the grade on women's health: A national and state-by-state report card 2004. Prepared by the National Women's Law Center and Oregon Health & Science University. Retrieved August 2, 2006, from *www.nwlc.org.*

Maloy, M. (2000). Spiritual approaches. In E. Olshansky (Ed.), *Integrated women's health: Holistic approaches for comprehensive care* (pp. 300–319). Gaithersburg, MD: Aspen.

Mendoza, R., Mendoza R., Smith, M. W., et al. (1991). Ethnic psychopharmacology: The Hispanic and Native American perspective. *Psychopharmacology Bulletin, 27*(4), 449–461.

Miller, J. B. (1986). *Toward a new psychology of women* (2nd ed.). Boston: Beacon Press.

Miller, J. B., & Stiver, I. P. (1997). *The healing connection: How women form relationships in therapy and in life.* Boston: Beacon Press.

Millett, K. (1969). *Sexual politics.* New York: Doubleday.

Munoz, C., & Hilgenberg, C. (2005). Ethnopharmacology. *American Journal of Nursing, 105*(8), 40–48.

National Health Care Disparities Report. (2005). NHDR. Retrieved September 1, 2006, from *http://www.ahrq.gov/gual/nhdr05/nhdr05.pdf.*

Primm, A. B., Cabot, D., Pettis, J., et al. (2002). The acceptability of a culturally tailored depression education videotape to African Americans. *Journal of the National Medical Association, 94*, 1007–1016.

Robinson, G. E. (2002). Women and psychopharmacology. *Medscape General Medicine, 4*(1). Retrieved July 18, 2006, from *www.medscape.com/viewarticle/423938.*

Roe, C. M., McNamara, A. M., & Motheral, B. R. (2002). Gender- and age-related prescription drug use patterns. *Annals of Pharmacotherapy, 36*, 30–39.

Ruiz, S., Chu, P., Sramek, J., et al. (1996). Neuroleptic dosing in Asian and Hispanic out-patients with schizophrenia. *Mount Sinai Journal of Medicine, 63*(5, 6), 306–309.

Showalter, E. (1985). *The female malady: Women, madness and English culture, 1830–1980.* New York: Pantheon.

Smith, D. I., & Spraggins, R. E. (2001). *Gender: 2000.* Census 2000 Brief. Washington, DC: U.S. Census Bureau, September, 2001. Retrieved July 19, 2006, from *http://www.census.gov/prod/2001pubs/c2kbr01-9.pdf.*

Solarz, A. L. (Ed.). (1999). *Lesbian health: Current assessment and directions for the future.* Washington, DC: National Academy Press.

Steinmetz, E. (2006). *Americans with disabilities: 2002.* Current Population Reports, P70-107. Washington, DC: U.S. Census Bureau. Retrieved August 2, 2006, from *http://www.census.gov/prod/2006pubs/p70-107.pdf.*

Strickland, T. L., Ranganath, V., Lin, K. M., et al. (1991). Psychopharmacologic considerations in the treatment of black American population. *Psychopharmacology Bulletin, 27*, 441–448.

Tomes, N. (1990). Historical perspectives on women and mental illness. In R. D. Apple (Ed.), *Women, health, and medicine in America* (pp. 143–171). New York: Garland Publishing, Inc.

Trans, P. V., Lawson, W. B., Anderson, S., et al. (1999). Treatment of the African-American patient with novel antipsychotic agents. In J. M. Herrera (Ed.), *Cross cultural psychiatry* (pp. 131–138). Chichester, England: John Wiley and Sons.

Trice, P. D., & Bjorck, J. P. (2006). Pentecostal perspectives on causes and cures for depression. *Professional Psychology: Research and Practice, 37*(3), 283–294.

U.S. Census Bureau. (2000) *Profile of general demographic characteristics: 2000.* Table DP-1. Retrieved August 2, 2006, from *www.census.gov/Press-Release/www%2001khus.pdf.*

U.S. Census Bureau. (2002). *Foreign-born population of the United States current population.* Detailed Tables (PPL-162), Table 1.1 (March, 2002 Current Population Survey) (population for 2002 of females all ages). Retrieved August 2, 2006, from *http://www.bayareacensus.org/counties/SanFranciscoCounty.pdf.*

U.S. Department of Health and Human Services. (1999). *Mental health: A report of the surgeon general.* Rockville, MD: Author.

U.S. Department of Health and Human Services. (2001). *Mental health: Culture, race, and ethnicity. A supplement to mental health: A report of the surgeon general.* Rockville, MD: Author.

Wade-Gayles, G. (1995). Introduction. In G. Wade-Gayles (Ed.), *My soul is a witness: African American women's spirituality* (pp. 1–8). Boston: Beacon Press.

Wang, P. S., Lane, M., Olfson, M., et al. (2005). Twelve-month use of mental health services in the United States. *Archives of General Psychiatry, 62,* 626–640.

Webster, R. A., McDonald, R., Lewin, T. J., et al. (1995). Effects of a natural disaster on immigrants and host population. *Journal of Nervous and Mental Disease, 183,* 390–397.

Wisner, K. L. (2004). Mental health is fundamental to health. *Journal of the American Medical Women's Association, 59*(2), 75–76.

Woodwell, D. A., & Cherry, D. K. (2004). *National ambulatory medical care survey: 2002 summary.* Advanced Data No. 346. Hyattsville, MD: National Center for Health Statistics, August 26.

Joan C. Urbancic

chapter 2

Depressive Disorders

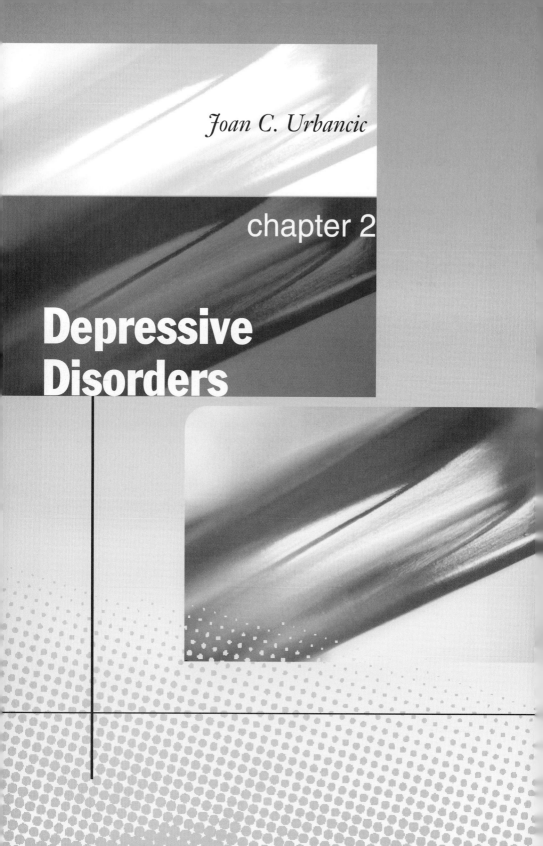

Depression is a major public health problem, with approximately one in six adults in the United States experiencing a depressive episode in his or her lifetime. It is second only to hypertension as the most commonly encountered primary care health problem. The World Health Organization (WHO) ranked depression as the fourth most disabling illness, but for women it ranks as number one (Kornstein, Steiner, Miranda, et al., 2006).

Depression is a common disorder that can be chronic and severely debilitating, but it is highly treatable when diagnosed. However, in primary care, of the approximately 14 percent of patients seeking care who are clinically depressed, only one in three depressed patients are accurately diagnosed (Oquendo and Leibowitz, 2005). The incidence of depression is typically higher among poor urban populations. Because 65 to 70 percent of patients with depression begin treatment for their depression with a primary care provider (PCP), the primary care network has become the primary care mental health network, with the majority of antidepressants being prescribed by family physicians (Robinson, Geske, Prest, et al., 2005). Thus, the treatment of uncomplicated depression has become the domain of primary care.

Experts estimate that depressed employees cost businesses $44 billion per year because of absenteeism and lost productivity as opposed to costs of $13 million for employees without depression. The diminished productivity amounts to approximately 4 months lost out of each year. The cost of treating depression has also increased by approximately 31 percent in recent years because of the greater number of patients who are being diagnosed (Oquendo and Leibowitz, 2005).

For many patients, depression is a recurring, lifelong disorder. Patients with a chronic illness are at increased risk for depression, and conversely, depression exacerbates chronic illness. Often, these patients seek primary care treatment for their somatic complaints and do not recognize that they are depressed and/or they are not diagnosed as such. Without appropriate treatment, depression can become a chronic and relapsing neurodegenerative disease that becomes progressively worse over time (see Chapter 9).

According to the National Comorbidity Survey Replication (Kessler, Chiu, Demler, et al., 2005), about 50 percent of Americans will qualify for a *Diagnostic and Statistical Manual of Mental Disorders* (*DSM-IV*) disorder at sometime in their life. The highest prevalence is for anxiety disorders (28.8 percent) and secondarily for mood disorders (20.8 percent). Women are more likely to experience anxiety and mood disorders, while men are at higher risk for impulse control and substance abuse disorders. Among the individuals identified in the survey as depressed, 57 percent received some type of treatment, although only one in five received adequate treatment for their depression (*adequate* is defined as four outpatient visits and 30 days of antidepressant therapy or eight psychotherapy sessions; Kessler et al., 2005).

In diagnosing depression, it is important that the PCP consider cultural influences. Culture affects the way people exhibit and describe their illnesses, how they cope with the illnesses, and whom they will see for their treatment. Conversely, the culture of the provider may determine the way patients are diagnosed or misdiagnosed, how they are treated, and how their health care is funded (Satcher, Ninan, and Masand, 2005).

For some cultures, depression will often get expressed by physical symptoms. For example, people from Eastern cultures tend to present more heavily with somatic complaints than Westerners. This may be true especially when the culture stigmatizes depression. In some cultures, words such as *depression* and *anxiety* do not exist, which makes it all the more important to have the person describe his or her feelings and experiences.

Another concern related to culture is the potential for differences among racial and ethnic groups in the pharmacokinetics of antidepressant medications including metabolism, effectiveness, and side effects (see Chapter 1).

In addition to the cultural factors that affect the quality of care that people receive, gender must also be considered. Rates for major depressive disorder (MDD) in women are approximately 20 percent as opposed to 10 percent for men (Newport, 2005). These higher depression rates are reported for women across a variety of cultures, social classes, and ethnic and racial groups. In a WHO study involving 14 countries, Maier, Gansicke, and Gater (1999) reported that the female-to-male ratio of 2 to 1 for lifetime major depression begins in adolescence and continues through the childbearing period and senior years with a decline in difference in the very old. The highest period for depression in women is during the childbearing years. And, although rates for men are higher for bipolar disorder, women have rates as high as 4 to 1 when comparing some subtypes of depression, such as seasonal affective disorder (SAD) and atypical depression.

Clearly, it is important that the PCP recognize depression in patients. Because depression in women is often overlooked, this chapter will focus on the assessment, diagnosis, and treatment of depression in women.

HYPOTHESES FOR GENDER DIFFERENCES IN DEPRESSION

One important barrier to understanding gender differences in depression has been the lack of inclusion of women of childbearing age in research studies until recently. Therefore, the actual research in this area is sparse. Although a variety of hypotheses have been offered to explain the gender differences in depression rates, there is no clear evidence that supports any single hypothesis.

Artifact Hypothesis

The artifact hypothesis suggests that gender differences in depression rates stem from circumstances such as women seeking health care services more often than men as well as women reporting symptoms more frequently. However, the consistency of gender differences across cultures as well as community-based versus clinical studies does not support the artifact theory.

Biopsychosocial Model

Biologic hypotheses maintain that differences in brain structure and function account for the differences in depression rates. The most popular model for explaining gender differences is the synthesizing biopsychosocial model that maintains women have potential vulnerabilities that interact to produce greater risk for depression. These vulnerabilities include genetic predisposition, increased exposure to stressful life events, and fluctuating reproductive hormones that impact neuroendocrine functioning (Box 2.1).

Box 2.1 • Evidence to Support the Biopsychosocial Model

1. The correlation that exists between the onset of menarche and female depression suggests that psychosocial factors of adolescence such as peer pressure, acceptance, and stereotypical socialization expectations interact with neuroendocrine changes to increase risk.
2. The effective *treatment* of severe premenstrual syndrome (PMS) and premenstrual dysphoric disorder (PMDD) with selective serotonin reuptake inhibitors (SSRIs) and serotonin norepinephrine reuptake inhibitors (SNRIs) provides support for neuroendocrine and biologic changes.
3. The biopsychosocial model posits that women with postpartum depression (PPD) experience a complex interaction of social events and stressors that interact with reproductive neurochemical changes that may occur after childbirth. Thus, psychotherapy along with SSRI and SNRI therapy have been very effective in treating PPD. Recently, the hormone estradiol has been showing promise as well.
4. The increased risk for depression in women experiencing perimenopause, menopause, and postmenopausal reproductive changes supports the biopsychosocial theory.

From Fredman, S. J., & Rosenbaum, J. F. (2003).

These vulnerabilities interact with life events and factors such as greater limitations and fewer choices for women. Women are much more likely than men to have incomes below the poverty line, which subsequently increases their exposure to crime and interpersonal violence.

Violence against women is the most common cause of injury in women who seek emergency care. It is also a common cause of depression in women, one that causes the depression to persist as the violence increases in frequency and severity. Posttraumatic stress disorder (PTSD) is often a sequel to violence, and it occurs twice as often in women as men. PTSD correlates highly with depression and other psychiatric disorders.

Researchers report that 50 percent of older women live alone compared with 25 percent of men. These women often face both financial and health-related problems in isolation (Cobbs and Ralapati, 1998). In general, chronic stressful life events have the potential to influence the neurotransmitters, thereby increasing the risk for depression.

GENDER DIFFERENCES IN DIAGNOSTIC CRITERIA

Generally, diagnostic criteria for depression are similar for both men and women, but there are some distinct gender differences in the presentation and course of depression (Kornstein et al., 2006). Women present with atypical depressive symptoms such as anxiety, increased appetite, weight gain, and somatic complaints more frequently than men; men tend to have alcohol and substance abuse problems. Women also present with more comorbid medical disorders. They are more likely to attempt suicide but are less successful than men because they use less lethal means (e.g., drug overdoses) than men (e.g., gunshots or hanging).

Another gender difference relates to onset of depression. Many women report onset of symptoms during their early teens, while men report first symptoms in their early 20s. A second peak for women occurs during the childbearing period. Thus, the peak periods for depression in women occur in early onset (10 to 14 years) and adult onset.

Finally, some research indicates that women have longer and more severe episodes of depression, recover more slowly, and are more likely to have a chronic and recurring course of depression than men (Kornstein et al., 2006; Vollmer, 2005).

RISK FACTORS FOR DEPRESSION IN WOMEN

It is generally agreed that gender role stressors place women at greater risk for MDD than men. Unresolved childhood sexual abuse is a significant risk factor for MDD in women because of higher rates of sexual abuse among girls than boys. Besides gender and gender roles, the following increase the chance of a depressive disorder:

- Family history of mood disorders (MDD is 1.5 to 3.0 times more likely among first-degree biologic relatives with MDD than in the general population [Desai and Jann, 2000])
- Socioeconomic status (rates of MDD typically decline as socioeconomic status improves)
- Marital status (single mothers are three times more likely to have experienced an episode of MDD than married mothers)
- Childhood physical and emotional abuse
- Parental negligence
- Parental death
- Alcoholism

Other conditions and situations are believed to increase the risk for depression in women. Among them are premenstrual dysphoric disorder (PMDD), pregnancy and the postpartum period, menopause, and relational losses.

Premenstrual Dysphoric Disorder

The premenstrual phase of a woman's cycle can be a vulnerable period for women with mood disorders. Some women report poor impulse control during this time and increased severity of depressive symptoms as well as new depressive symptoms. Women are also more likely to be admitted to a psychiatric hospital and make more suicide attempts during this phase of their cycles (Vollmer, 2005). Diagnosis of PMDD requires that the woman keep a journal of her symptoms through a minimum of two menstrual periods. Sometimes, it is difficult to differentiate between PMDD and minor depression, so the journal documentation is very helpful in establishing the cyclical nature and PMDD diagnosis. Typically, physical and psychological symptoms appear at the end of the luteal phase and diminish with the onset of menstruation. Unlike premenstrual syndrome (PMS), in which somatic symptoms dominate, PMDD symptoms are primarily those of mood and anxiety. Women with PMDD respond well to selective serotonin reuptake inhibitors (SSRIs) as opposed to antidepressants that are not serotonin enhancing. For this reason, it is believed that PMDD is related to altered serotonin levels (Kornstein et al., 2006).

Pregnancy

The prevalence rate of depression during pregnancy is not higher than the rate of the general population of women. This suggests that pregnancy itself does not increase the risk of depression. At one time, pregnancy was falsely considered a protection against depression (Dolan, 2005; Kornstein et al., 2006). While most women experience a sense of excitement and enhanced well-being during pregnancy, for women with mood disorders, pregnancy can be a very difficult time. Existing depressive symptoms can become more severe when the women become pregnant, whereas for some women, pregnancy can trigger a new depression. The greatest risks for depression during pregnancy include a prior history of mood disorder either personally or within the family, a history of substance abuse, and minimal social support and financial resources. Other risk factors include younger age of the woman, marital conflict, recent stressful life events, a large number of existing children, and unwanted pregnancy. Medical disorders such as gestational diabetes, thyroid dysfunction, and anemia can increase the risk for depression during pregnancy. A recent study by Cohen, Altshuler, and Harlow (2006) highlighted the high depression relapse rate of pregnant women (43 percent of the women experienced relapse) and emphasized the need for maintaining medication to preserve the individual woman's health.

Women who are depressed during pregnancy require specialized treatment, as there are significant risks to both mother and fetus. The mother is at increased risk for suicide, self-neglect, diminished functioning, and serious morbidity. Major depression during pregnancy is also correlated with preterm labor and small-for-gestational-age babies. Although a meta-analysis (Altshuler, Cohen, and Szuba, 1996) of 2,700 pregnant women on antidepressants did not find an increase of teratogenic risk to the fetus, the Food and Drug Administration (FDA) has not approved any psychotropic medication for pregnant women; therefore, there are no guarantees for safety, and the risks of medication to the fetus must be considered against the risks of the untreated depression to the mother and child.

The FDA (2005) labels SSRIs as pregnancy category C drugs (i.e., drugs that demonstrate adverse effects in animals or studies in humans are lacking) along with venlafaxine (Effexor), mirtazapine (Remeron), and nefazodone (Serzone) because of a slight increase in the risk of premature labor. In 2001, an expert panel (Altshuler, Cohen, and Moline, 2001) recommended a combination of both medication and open-ended psychotherapy for the severely depressed pregnant woman. For women with a history of depression, the panel recommended initiating treatment at the first sign of depression. For depressed women who become psychotic, electroconvulsive therapy (ECT) or a combination of antidepressant and antipsychotic medication may be required (Dolan, 2005; Kornstein et al., 2006; Vollmer, 2005).

However, several published studies have identified multiple increased risks for the fetus when the mother is on antidepressants (Chambers, Hernandez-Diaz, Van Marter, et al., 2006; FDA, 2005; Levinson-Castiel, 2005; Santos and Pergolizzi, 2004). But most recently, Louik, Lin, Werler, et al. (2007) conducted an epidemiologic study ($N = 15{,}000$) on infants with birth defects and maternal use of SSRIs in the first trimester. Their findings did not show significant increased risks for the most common heart and brain defects, but they cautioned that although absolute risk is small, there may be increased risk with SSRIs for some rare, specific defects. Thus, the risks for both mother and fetus must be thoughtfully weighed on a case-by-case basis and all possible treatment modalities considered before prescribing antidepressants for pregnant women.

Postpartum Depression

According to the *DSM-IV-TR*, the onset of postpartum depression (PPD) occurs within 4 weeks of delivery and peaks around 10 weeks. Depression ranges from mild symptoms to major depression and, most severely, to postpartum psychosis. Mild symptoms of depression (the "blues") are quite common and affect approximately 30 to 85 percent of women. These symptoms are time limited and usually abate by the 10th postpartum day with little or no intervention.

The risk of depression during the postpartum period does not seem to significantly differ from other periods in a woman's lifetime. However, a previous history of mood disorder and few resources places a woman at increased risk. One concern is that a woman may be depressed and not recognize her symptoms, or she may feel ashamed because of her lack of energy and interest in her new child, so she may not disclose her symptoms to anyone. Therefore, it is imperative that the health care provider carefully observes and specifically inquires about symptoms of depression in new mothers, as they may have a serious impact on the mother–child relationship and early childhood development.

No clear evidence exists to support a purely biologic basis for PPD. According to the biopsychosocial model, PPD most likely stems from the interaction of drastic changes in hormones, biologic vulnerability, and social factors. Desai and Jann (2000) have commented on the similarities between MDD, PPD, and the normal sequelae of pregnancy and childbirth, such as sleep and appetite disturbances and loss of energy and concentration, that complicate the diagnosis of PPD. These researchers recommend the use of the Edinburgh Postnatal Depressive Scale (EPDS) for diagnosing PPD. This instrument is a simple 10-item, self-rating inventory that has been used in a large community study and has demonstrated specificity of 92.5 percent and sensitivity of 88.0 percent. To access the EPDS, refer to the Resources for Providers section at the end of this chapter.

Treatment of PPD is similar to treatment for MDD and includes both antidepressants and psychotherapy. Women should remain on the initial dose of their antidepressant for 2 weeks before the dose is increased. Research studies support both cognitive and interpersonal therapies for effectiveness in PPD. Spouses should be included in the psychotherapy (as long as the woman believes it will be helpful) and live-in help used until the depressive symptoms resolve. For women with a history of MDD, an antidepressant should be started immediately after delivery to prevent the onset of PPD (Kornstein et al., 2006; Vollmer, 2005).

A few women will become psychotically depressed after they deliver. This type of depression is more severe than major depression. Prevalence rates are approximately 0.1 to 0.2 percent. Psychotic depression may present with manic or severe depressive symptoms along with disorganized behavior and hallucinations and delusions. It is considered a medical emergency and requires hospitalization because of danger to the infant and self-harm to the mother. ECT may be considered to achieve rapid improvement in symptoms (Kornstein et al., 2006; Vollmer, 2005).

Women who are breast-feeding and require an antidepressant need special counseling about the potential hazards of antidepressants and other psychotropic medications. Although antidepressants are excreted in breast milk, drug levels are not detectable in infants (Birnbaum, Cohen, and Bailey, 1999; Kornstein et al., 2006).

Kornstein et al. (2006) reported that research on infant outcomes and use of maternal antidepressants is limited even though 50 studies have been published on the topic. Most research was done on sertraline (Zoloft), fluoxetine (Prozac), and paroxetine (Paxil) with no significant adverse effects to infants reported. Premature infants, though, are at greater risk because of their reduced ability to metabolize drugs. Therefore, infants must be thoroughly examined for any abnormalities before the mother begins the medication and must be subsequently closely observed for any behavioral changes such as increased irritability, sleep pattern disturbances, or appetite change. If changes occur, a choice must be made between discontinuing the breast-feeding or the medication. In contrast to the lack of evidence for toxic effects of breast-feeding by women on antidepressants, it is clear that infants may experience a number of negative effects when their mothers are depressed and not being treated. These outcomes include lack of mother–infant bonding, weight loss, and developmental deficits.

Menopause

Menopause is the cessation of menses for 1 year (e.g., age 50 to 51 years), while perimenopause is the transition period before menopause (e.g., age 45 to 50 years). These time periods can vary significantly. Overall, few studies have focused on menopause and depression, but menopause is not considered a high-risk period for depression in women. However, women with a history of depression are at risk for a recurrence during this time (Vollmer, 2005). In contrast, several studies report increases and even a peak in the prevalence of depression during the perimenopausal period (Cohen, Soares, Vitonis, et al., 2006; Freeman, Sammel, Lin, et al., 2006; Kornstein et al., 2006; Vollmer, 2005). The risk of perimenopausal depression appears greater among women who experience severe vasomotor symptoms. Conversely, it may be the case that depression increases the risk for an early menopause as well for the vasomotor symptoms. Because little evidence has been found linking estrogen depletion of menopause and depression, treatment with hormone replacement therapy (HRT) has not been in the mainstream of practice.

Some women find relief from their hot flashes and sleep disturbances with low doses of SSRIs. However, problems for the depressed menopausal woman usually involve weight gain and loss of libido, and SSRIs usually exacerbate these concerns. Bupropion (Wellbutrin) has been successful as an antidepressant for these problems.

Relational Losses

The loss of a loved one is always traumatic and, for some people, it precipitates depression. Studies indicate that 15 to 30 percent of people who have experienced the loss of a loved one become clinically depressed during the first year after the loss. Because women marry younger and live longer than their husbands, there is a higher prevalence of widowhood among women. Some studies indicate that women who are widows appear to have more difficulty adjusting to the loss of the spouse and are more vulnerable to depression than men in the same circumstances (Umberson, Wortman, and Kessler, 1992). Men also tend to recover from their losses more quickly than women. However, researchers report that elderly widows are three times more likely to live in poverty than older married couples (McGarry and Schoeni, 2005). Thus, the economic situation of elderly widows may be a critical factor for their depression.

More research is needed in this area, because there is disagreement as to whether a woman who loses a spouse is more vulnerable to depression.

ASSESSMENT AND DIAGNOSIS OF DEPRESSION

Diagnosing depression can be a serious challenge because of the multiple related disorders that are listed as depression. The depressive disorders that are addressed in this chapter include adjustment disorder with depressed mood, dysthymic disorder, and MDD. The bipolar disorders, including cyclothymia, are discussed in Chapter 3. Additional diagnostic challenges may arise because complaints of depression can be secondary to other health problems and, conversely, some patients who present with multiple somatic complaints may be experiencing a primary depression that is being expressed somatically. Patients in the primary care setting seldom present themselves as "depressed." More often, they present with complaints that are vague and difficult to diagnose ("I'm so tired"; "I have frequent headaches"; "I can't sleep"). An accurate diagnosis is critical because medications and psychotherapeutic approaches are dependent on diagnosis. Box 2.2 highlights some main distinctions in the differential diagnosis for major depression.

Screening for Depression

The U.S. Preventative Services Task Force (USPSTF, 2002) recommends that adult patients in primary care be screened routinely for depression. According to the USPSTF, good evidence exists that screening improves the diagnosis of depression and decreases clinical morbidity. Although many instruments exist for screening and monitoring depression, some like the Hamilton Depression Scale (HAM-D) are labor intensive and more appropriate for research than primary care. The Zung, the Beck, and the PHQ-9 are self-administered questionnaires

Box 2.2 • Differential Diagnosis for Major Depressive Disorder

Dysthymia—milder but chronic
Grief and bereavement
Adjustment disorder
Alcohol and substance abuse
Secondary depression due to medical illness
Secondary depression due to prescribed medications
Dementia
Comorbid psychiatric disorders

Adapted from Newport, D. J. (2005).

that most patients can complete independently. The Zung and the PHQ-9 are available free of charge online. (Refer to the Resources for Providers section for online access to the Zung Self-Rating Depression Scale and the PHQ-9.) These instruments have good reliability and validity, and they provide a measure of depression that can be monitored over time. The PHQ-9 is particularly helpful in primary care settings because of its brevity and the ease with which patients can self-administer it.

An even shorter instrument that has been recommended by the USPSTF is the two-question screening instrument for primary care (PHQ-2). These two questions address depressed mood and anhedonia, which are the basic features of depression. The *DSM-IV-TR* requires that one of these symptoms must exist for at least 2 weeks to screen positive for major depression. The two questions are:

1. Have you been feeling sad or angry lately?
2. Have you lost interest in or stopped enjoying the things that usually give you pleasure?

Researchers have found that these two questions have a sensitivity of 96 percent (USPSTF, 2002).

Physical Symptoms of Depression

In recent years, researchers and clinicians have become much more aware of the relationship between comorbid medical symptoms and depression. Therefore, the PCP should consider depression in all patients who present with three or more unrelated medical conditions. Major medical illnesses with a high incidence of comorbid depression include coronary artery disease, diabetes, chronic obstructive pulmonary disease and asthma, Parkinson's disease, cancer, HIV, migraine headaches, rheumatoid arthritis, and alcohol or substance abuse.

Furthermore, patients in the primary care setting are more likely to reject the possibility of a depression diagnosis than are patients at the psychiatrist's office. When confronted with a diagnosis of depression, a patient may adamantly insist, "There is nothing wrong with my head; it's my body that is the problem." Our challenge is to assist patients to understand the mind–body connection and the effective role of antidepressants and psychotherapeutic interventions. A growing number of studies indicate that antidepressants with dual neurotransmitter actions, such as venlafaxine (Effexor) and duloxetine (Cymbalta), may be more effective than SSRIs in treating the depressed patient with multiple somatic complaints (Silverstone, 2004; Wohlreich, Brannan, and Mallinckrodt, 2004).

Types of Depressive Disorders

Adjustment Disorder with Depressed Mood

Adjustment disorders are generally viewed as a mild and transient form of depression. They occur in people who have been functioning normally until some critical stressor occurs that causes depression. Although the symptoms of depression in an adjustment disorder do not qualify as major depression, they may progress to such. Many times, a person will be able to overcome the crisis and return to premorbid functioning without intervention. However, treatment can often accelerate the return to normal functioning, minimize the distress, and prevent a worsening of symptoms (Box 2.3).

Dysthymic Disorder

Dysthymic disorder (Box 2.4) is characterized as a chronic and persistent depression but one that is not sufficiently severe to qualify as a major depression or bipolar disorder. Its symptoms, however, are sufficiently serious to cause clinically significant distress in social, occupational, and other areas of functioning (American Psychiatric Association [APA], 2000). Often, dysthymic disorder is complicated by concurrent psychiatric diagnoses, such as personality disorders and/or substance abuse. So, treatment becomes more complex and long term. Sometimes, dysthymic patients are difficult to treat because they may experience a low-grade depression for many years and have no interest or motivation for making changes

Box 2.3 • *DSM-IV-TR* Criteria for Adjustment Disorder with Depressed Mood

A. The development of emotional or behavioral symptoms in response to an identifiable stressor(s) occurring within 3 months of the onset of the stressor(s).

B. These symptoms are clinically significant as evidenced by either of the following:
   1. Marked distress that is in excess of what would be expected from exposure to the stressor
   2. Significant impairment in social or occupational (academic) functioning

C. The stress-related disturbance does not meet the criteria for another specific Axis I disorder and is not merely an exacerbation of preexisting Axis I or Axis II disorder.

D. The symptoms do not represent bereavement.

E. Once the stressor (or its consequences) has terminated, the symptoms do not persist for more than an additional 6 months.

Specify Type:
Acute: If the disturbance lasts less than 6 months
Chronic: If the disturbance lasts for 6 months or longer.

From the American Psychiatric Association (2000).

in their lives. Even with medication and psychotherapy, improvement is slower and less dramatic than with the more seriously ill patient.

Criteria for dysthymic disorder requires the presence of symptoms for at least 2 years and the absence of MDD or manic, hypomanic, cyclothymic, or mixed episodes during that period. Also, dysthymic disorder cannot occur during an exclusive psychotic episode or be caused by direct physiologic effects from drugs or a general medical condition.

Major Depressive Disorder

The *DSM-IV-TR* (APA, 2000) requires that five out of a possible nine symptoms be present for a 2-week period for a diagnosis of MDD. These symptoms must reflect a change from prior functioning and cause significant difficulty in daily

Box 2.4 • *DSM-IV-TR* Criteria for Dysthymic Disorder

A. Depressed mood for most of the day for at least 2 years (subjective account or observation by others).

B. Presence, while depressed, of at least two of the following:
   1. Poor appetite or overeating
   2. Insomnia or hypersomnia
   3. Low energy or fatigue
   4. Low self-esteem
   5. Poor concentration or difficulty making decisions
   6. Feelings of hopelessness

Symptoms in Criteria A and B during the 2-year period have not been absent for more than 2 months.

No major depression during the first 2 years, nor has a manic, mixed, hypomaniac episode or cyclothymic disorder been present. The disturbance has not occurred only with a psychotic episode, or due to a substance, or general medication condition. The symptoms must cause significant distress or impairment in important areas of functioning.

From the American Psychiatric Association (2000).

living. At least one of the symptoms is either a depressed mood or a lost of interest or pleasure in life (anhedonia). The symptoms cannot be caused by drugs, substance abuse, a general medical condition, or the loss of a loved one (APA). Refer to Table 2.1, which lists the nine symptoms of MDD in one column and the symptoms most common to depressive symptoms in women in the second column.

Seasonal Affective Disorder

SAD is a subset of MDD, but it is unique because it typically recurs each year in fall/winter with abatement in spring/summer. Approximately 4 to 6 percent of the general population in the United States has SAD, with another 10 to 20 percent experiencing subsyndromal symptoms. The incidence increases as one progresses from southern to northern states (Jepson, Ernst, and Kelly, 1999). Typical onset is the early 20s, with decreasing risk with increasing age. SAD is four times more

Table 2.1 • A Comparison of *DSM-IV-TR* Criteria and Women's Atypical Symptoms of Major Depressive Disorder

DSM-IV-TR Criteria for Major Depressive Disorder (5 of 9 Required)	Women's Atypical Symptoms of Depression
1. Depressed mood	1. Increased appetite or weight gain
2. Significant decline in interest or pleasure	2. Mood reactivity
3. Change in weight (+ or −) or appetite	3. Hypersomnia
4. Insomnia or hypersomnia nearly every day	4. Leaden paralysis (heavy feelings in arms and legs)
5. Psychomotor agitation or retardation	5. Sensitivity to interpersonal rejection
6. Fatigue or loss of energy nearly every day	6. Absence of melancholic or catatonic features
7. Feelings of worthlessness or excessive or inappropriate guilt	
8. Diminished ability to think or concentrate, or make decisions	
9. Recurrent thoughts of suicide or death	

From the American Psychiatric Association (2000).

common among women than men, although this ratio is challenged by some. The *DSM-IV-TR* criteria require that the depression must have occurred during the last 2 years and cannot be explained by seasonal problems alone.

Jepson et al. reported two types of SAD: fall or winter onset and spring onset. The winter type is characterized by vegetative symptoms, such as hypersomnia, increased appetite and weight gain, increased irritability, and interpersonal problems. Spring SAD occurs less commonly and is characterized by symptoms more similar to typical depression: insomnia, weight loss, and poor appetite.

The etiology of SAD is uncertain, but most researchers favor the serotonin hypothesis, which suggests a decline in the blood levels of this neurotransmitter. Evidence-based treatments for SAD include antidepressants and bright artificial light (phototherapy). Light is the traditional treatment for nonpsychotic SAD, and it is believed to increase serotonin levels. Benefits of light therapy include minimal side effects and more rapid relief than with antidepressant therapy. A light box must be purchased, but some insurance companies may reimburse the cost of the box. While light therapy may typically be the first choice of treatment, for patients who are suicidal, have a severe depression, or have not responded to light therapy in the past, antidepressants may be the best choice. SSRIs have been successfully used in multiple drug trials for SAD. However, bright lights can be combined with pharmacotherapy to optimize treatment for SAD patients (Jepson et al., 1999; Sohn and Lam, 2005).

Other Differential Diagnoses

Patients in their 20s and 30s with a diagnosis of *unipolar depression* should be screened for bipolar disorder. This is necessary even without a previous history of a manic or hypomanic episode. A family history of bipolar disorder lends credence to the diagnosis because of the strong genetic component with the disorder. Two simple questions can be very helpful:

1. "Are you a person who frequently experiences ups and downs in mood?"
2. "Do these mood swings occur without cause?" (Goldberg, Cohen, Jackson, et al., 2005).

A positive response to either or both questions increases the probability of bipolar disorder and should be followed by the Mood Disorder Questionnaire (MDQ). The MDQ is a simple nine-item screening test that is available online free of charge (refer to Resources for Providers). More information on bipolar disorders is provided in Chapter 3.

Grief and bereavement can be difficult to discriminate from major depression. While the grief process is a normal one, if a patient continues to grieve excessively for more than 6 months, depression should be a consideration. The PCP should also question the patient about suicidal thoughts.

Substance abuse can complicate existing depression and/or precipitate a depression episode. For example, alcohol in the short term is mood elevating but over the long term, it is a depressant. Because alcohol is a disinhibitor, a person is always at greater risk for suicide when intoxicated than when sober. Cocaine is another drug that places a person at high risk for depression. It is particularly dangerous when the person is withdrawing from the effects of the cocaine.

It is generally recognized that some medications used for medical conditions can precipitate depression. These include chemotherapeutic drugs, beta-blockers, and the interferons. Common medical conditions often associated with depression include poststroke, postmyocardial infarction, and cancer. Depression is also common in patients with dementia.

TREATMENT OPTIONS FOR DEPRESSION

The first strategy in treating the patient with depression is to maintain the patient on the maximum medication dose for at least 4 weeks. The more severely depressed patient may require a medication trial of 8 to 12 weeks because she is in a deeper depression than the typical patient. Differences of opinion exist on how to "operationalize" severe depression.

Also, one must not confuse severity with chronicity. Chronicity requires at least 2 years of symptoms, but these symptoms are not necessarily severe. Typically, "severe" reflects both an excess of symptoms as well as serious functional impairment. Some clinicians maintain that a diagnosis of severe depression should require seven (rather than five) of the nine of the *DSM-IV-TR* criteria. Generally, research studies have used specific cutoff points on standardized instruments to identify the severely depressed patient. For example, a score of 25 or greater on the HAM-D has been used in many studies. But instruments used in research are not always helpful in clinical situations. Other characteristics of severe depression include psychiatric comorbidity, melancholia, and psychotic features such as hallucinations, executive dysfunction, and role function impairment.

Typically, suicide and suicidal ideation have been assumed to be present in severe depression, although some disagreement exists for this claim as well. Nevertheless, the incidence of suicide among patients with MDD is 4 to 6 percent (Newport, 2005).

Every patient with severe or treatment-resistant depression (TRD) should be assessed for hallucinations and delusions. Patients will often not disclose these symptoms, so it is essential to question about them directly. The presence of psychotic symptoms requires the use of antipsychotic medication in conjunction with an antidepressant.

Referral to a Specialist

Patients who are suicidal or homicidal or who have severe depression, psychotic depression, TRD, bipolar disorder, possible organic brain disease, or substance abuse should be referred to a psychiatrist. Generally, patients who have been on maximum doses of antidepressants without significant improvement should be referred for consultation and/or ongoing treatment. A psychiatrist may elect to add an atypical antipsychotic medication to the regimen because these medications are becoming important adjuncts in the treatment of severe depression and refractory PTSD. ECT may be required, but psychiatrists do not use ECT as first-line treatment except in the most severe cases. A general course of treatment involves pharmacotherapy and, in many cases, psychotherapy.

Pharmacotherapy

The major treatment for depression is antidepressant medication. Antidepressants act by blocking the reuptake of various neurotransmitters. The tricyclic antidepressants (TCAs) block the reuptake of norepinephrine and serotonin as do the SNRIs, venlafaxine, and duloxetine. The SSRIs focus mainly on serotonin.

Minimal research exists on gender differences for antidepressants, and some of the studies are quite contradictory. However, research on gender and pharmacokinetics demonstrates differences between men and women in drug absorption, distribution, metabolism, bioavailability, and elimination. Therefore, in women, plasma levels may be higher, drug half-lives longer, and side effects more prevalent than in men. Hormonal changes may also alter circulating medication levels. Researchers have reported that women have a better response to SSRIs but a poorer response to TCAs than men. These responses are more typical of premenopausal women, whereas the responses of postmenopausal women are more similar to the male response (Khan, Brodhead, Schwartz, et al., 2005; Kornstein et al., 2006; Kornstein, Schatzberg, and Thase, 2000).

Recent studies suggest that patients with untreated, persistent depression have neurodegenerative changes in the cortical and subcortical brain regions (Kanner, 2004; Miguel-Hidalgo and Rajkowska, 2002). The basis for brain cell atrophy is the increased stress that raises cortisol levels and decreases brain-derived neutrophic factor. This would explain the repeated, more severe, and more frequent depressive episodes that are seen in patients with untreated depression. This research provides a strong rationale for early and aggressive treatment of depression with continuation of medication until remission.

Even with remission, patients are at risk for relapse. Therefore, it is critical that they understand the importance of remaining on their antidepressant medication for 6 to 9 months after remission to prevent relapse. Generally, it is best to start treatment at a low dose and gradually titrate to the target dose. By 4 weeks, effects will usually be obvious. However, improvement for patients who have been severely depressed for a long time may take 6 to 8 weeks; improvement for those with comorbid anxiety may take 10 to 12 weeks.

All patients need to be educated about the potential for suicidal ideation with the initiation of antidepressants and the need to contact their health care provider immediately if this should occur. Also, patients receiving antidepressant medications need to be seen (or at least contacted by phone) every week on

Box 2.5 • Helpful Hints in Prescribing Antidepressants

1. Prioritize what patient reports as most problematic symptom, and target that symptom first.
2. Consider the antidepressant the patient has previously taken. If it worked, use it!
3. Ask if there is a family history of successful treatment with an antidepressant.
4. Match side effects to patient needs (e.g., weight, sexual functioning).
5. Be aware of concomitant illnesses and interactions with patient's other medications.
6. Be responsive to patient preferences.
7. Consider cost.

initiation of the antidepressant. Once the patient is stabilized, contact should be every month. The medication needs to be continued for approximately 6 to 8 months after recovery.

Medications commonly prescribed for depression appear in Table 2.2, and prescribing tips appear in Box 2.5.

Monoamine Oxidase Inhibitors

The earliest antidepressants were the monoamine oxidase inhibitors (MAOIs). They were initially manufactured to treat tuberculosis and, accidentally, were found to be effective in treating depression. The two most commonly used MAOIs in the United States are phenelzine (Nardil) and tranylcypromine (Parnate) (Table 2.2). These drugs are seldom used today because of their severe interaction potential in foods with high tyramine content and medications such as other antidepressants. For instance, case studies with life-threatening hypertensive crisis have been reported when patients have taken pseudoephedrine (Sudafed) with an MAOI. Another potentially lethal mix is an MAOI and meperidine (Demerol). Nevertheless, psychiatrists may use MAOIs for treatment-resistant patients. Most recently, a new transdermal form of the MAOI, selegiline, was approved by the FDA. This new system bypasses the gut, which therefore reduces the opportunity for the hypertensive reaction that is commonly feared with oral forms of the MAOIs (Nemeroff, DeVane, and Lydiard, 2007).

Tricyclic Antidepressants

The TCAs were the second group of antidepressants to gain acceptance in the United States. This is a large group of medications that is still widely used but generally considered second-line therapy because of the newer SSRIs that have fewer side effects (Table 2.2). TCAs block both norepinephrine and serotonin as well as other drug receptor sites. Because they do target multiple receptor sites, their side effects are often a serious problem.

Anticholinergic side effects—dry mouth, constipation, blurred vision, urinary retention, orthostatic hypotension, and confusion in the elderly—have been especially problematic with TCAs, causing many patients to discontinue them. Moreover, a patient with a month's supply of a TCA has on hand a lethal dose of the medication; this is not the case with SSRIs.

Selective Serotonin Reuptake Inhibitors

SSRIs have now become the first-line treatment choice for depression (Table 2.2). Because of their improved side-effect profile, many more people are being prescribed these antidepressants than in the past. Usually, the side effects, which include nausea, headache, insomnia, anxiety, agitation, and sedation, are time limited and controlled by beginning with a low dose and gradually increasing the dose to the therapeutic level. However, weight gain and sexual dysfunction can be long-term effects, and serotonin syndrome is always a possibility for patients on high doses of SSRIs. Serotonin syndrome occurs because of a buildup of serotonin to toxic levels. Symptoms include mental status changes, rigidity, autonomic instability, fever, tachycardia, diarrhea, and flushing. On rare occasions, serotonin syndrome has resulted in death. Besides treating depression, SSRIs are effective for treating anxiety disorders including PTSD. Patients with anxiety disorders usually need to start on lower doses but also require higher doses for maintenance.

Fluoxetine (Prozac) was the first SSRI to be prescribed in the United States. Since its appearance in 1988, a multitude of SSRIs have become available. Despite the improved side-effects profile of SSRIs, the National Institute of Mental Health (2001) estimates that 10 to 15 percent of patients stop taking their medications after the first week. Of those who do continue on their medications, 20 percent do not respond (less than 50 percent improvement). Even with responders (more than 50 percent improvement), most patients do not achieve remission.

Atypical Antidepressants

The latest group of antidepressants are categorized as "unique" or "atypical." This group, or drug class, is known as the serotonin norepinephrine reuptake inhibitors (SNRIs). Current SNRIs are mirtazapine (Remeron), venlafaxine

Text continues on page 47.

Table 2.2 • Antidepressant Medications

Generic & (Trade Name)	Drug Class	Start Dose	Dose Range	Sedation	Weight Gain	Sexual Side Effects	GI Side Effects	Comments
citalopram (Celexa)	SSRI	20 mg/d; incr. qwk	20–60 mg/d	+	+	++	++	Low drug–drug interactions; avoid with olanzapine and fluoxetine
escitalopram (Lexapro)	SSRI	10 mg/d	Max: 20 mg/d	+/−	+/−	++	+	Low drug–drug interactions; monitor blood glucose level; most selective of SSRIs; Rx: generalized anxiety disorder (GAD); caution with elderly
fluoxetine (Prozac)	SSRI	20 mg/d; incr. after 2–4 wk prn	20–40 mg/d; can be bid; Max: 80 mg	+/−	+/−	++	+	Rx: obsessive-compulsive disorder (OCD); bulimia nervosa; begin at 10 mg for panic disorder; long half-life; approved for adolescent depression; anorexia in elderly
fluvoxamine (Luvox)	SSRI	50 mg; incr. by 50 mg q4–7d	50–150 mg bid; Max: 300 mg					Rx: Limited to OCD; to discontinue (D/C),taper dose gradually; drug–drug interactions
paroxetine (Paxil)	SSRI	20 mg q AM; incr. weekly by 10 mg	20–50 mg qd; Max: 50 mg	+	++	++	+	Rx: Anxiety disorders including PTSD; PMDD; short half-life; greater risk for discontinuation syndrome than other SSRIs; more drug–drug interactions
paroxetine (Paxil-CR)	SSRI	25 mg q AM; incr. 12.5 mg/d qwk	25–62.5 mg; Max: 62.5 mg	+	++	++	+	Same as above

(Continued)

Table 2.2 • (Continued)

Generic & (Trade Name)	Drug Class	Start Dose	Dose Range	Sedation	Weight Gain	Sexual Side Effects	GI Side Effects	Comments
sertraline (Zoloft)	SSRI	50 mg	50–200 mg	+	+	++	++	Short half-life and greater risk for discontinuation syndrome; low drug–drug interactions; Rx: anxiety disorders including PTSD
duloxetine (Cymbalta)	SNRI	40 mg/I d–bid	40–80 mg/d; Max: 80 mg	++	+/−	+	++	Monitor BP; caution with hypertension (HTN); Rx: diabetes mellitus (DM) neuropathy and chronic pain; taper gradually to D/C; obtain baseline liver enzyme levels; avoid in alcoholics
mirtazapine (Remeron)	SNRI	15 mg qhs	15–45 mg qhs	++	++	−	+/−	Potent antihistamine; vivid dreams; craving for carbohydrates (CHO); few drug interactions
venlafaxine (Effexor)	SNRI	37.5 mg bid; incr. q4d	37.5–75 mg bid; Max: 375 mg	+	+	+	+	Rx: chronic pain, anxiety disorders; take w/ food; caution with HTN; NE action at doses above 250 mg
venlafaxine (Effexor XR)	SNRI	37.5–75 mg qd; incr. 75 mg/d q4–7d	75 mg qd; Max: 225 mg	+	+	+	+	Same as above
bupropion (Wellbutrin)	Unique	100 mg bid	Incr. after 3 d; max: 150 mg tid	−	+/−	−	−	Rx: smoking cessation; ineffective for anxiety disorders; blocks NE and dopamine; avoid with bulimic patient; dose-dependent seizure risk; used to augment SSRIs

bupropion (Wellbutrin SR) bupropion (Wellbutrin XL)	Unique	150 mg q AM	Max: 400 mg May incr. to 300 mg 4d; max: 450 mg	+	+	++	++	Sustained release forms better tolerated than immediate release; take in AM to avoid insomnia; smoking cessation Rx: 150 mg qd × 3d; then 150 mg bid for 7–12 wks
amitriptyline (Elavil no longer available in U.S.; only generic available)	TCA	50–150 mg qhs	Incr. 25–50 mg/d q2–3d; max: 300 mg	++++	++	++	–	Low cost; Rx for pain and sleep in low doses (25–150 mg). Highly anticholinergic; may give in divided doses
clomipramine (Anafranil)	TCA	Start 25 mg/d; incr. 25 mg/d q4–7d	150–250 mg; max: 100 mg/d first 2 wk; 250 mg/d maint.	+++	++	++	–	Limited to OCD
desipramine (Norpramin)	TCA	25–75MG qd	100–200 mg; max: 300 mg	++	++	++	–	Metabolite of imipramine; may give in divided doses; can do blood levels; anticholinergic
imipramine (Tofranil)	TCA	25–75 mg qhs	100–300 mg qhs; max: 300 mg	+++	++	++	–	Used for chronic pain; titrate slowly; Rx: anxiety and bedwetting

(Continued)

Table 2.2 • (Continued)

Generic & (Trade Name)	Drug Class	Start Dose	Dose Range	Sedation	Weight Gain	Sexual Side Effects	GI Side Effects	Comments
nortriptyline (Pamelor)	TCA	25–50 mg qhs, incr. 25–50 mg/d q2–3d	50–150 mg qhs; max: 150 mg	+++	++	++	–	Metabolite of amitriptyline
trazodone (Desyrel)	TCA	25–50 mg bid; incr. 50 mg/d q3–4d.	50–100 mg bid or tid; max: 400 mg	+++	++	++	–	Prescribed for sleep in low doses: 25–150 mg qhs; used as adjunct to SSRIs
phenelzine (Nardil)	MAOI	15 mg tid; incr. to 60–90 mg/d	45–90 mg/d divided tid or qid	+	+	+++	–	Although effective, seldom used because of serious interactions with multiple agents; hypertensive crisis
Tranylcypromine (Parnate)	MAOI	10 mg tid	May incr. 10 mg/d q1–3 wk; max: 60 mg	+/–	+	+++	–	Although effective, seldom used because of serious interactions with multiple agents; hypertensive crisis

(Effexor), and duloxetine (Cymbalta) (Table 2.2). Besides addressing depression, the SNRIs are effective in decreasing pain and increasing alertness. However, chronic side effects include the potential for hypertension, sexual dysfunction, weight gain, and serotonin syndrome.

Bupropion (Wellbutrin), another atypical antidepressant, blocks norepinephrine and dopamine rather than serotonin. Bupropion, known by the trade name Zyban, is also used for smoking cessation. It is the only antidepressant that does not cause sexual dysfunction and weight gain. However, it may cause agitation, irritability, insomnia, and even psychosis. It is not a good choice for patients with anxiety disorders, eating disorders, alcoholism, or hypertension.

Strategies for Treating Antidepressant Side Effects and Related Problems

Various side effects and other problems typically stem from pharmacotherapeutic interventions. Some of the common ones are insomnia, sexual dysfunction, discontinuation syndrome, TRD, and partial responses to medication.

Insomnia

Insomnia is a common side effect of antidepressants. But one must first determine if insomnia is a component of the patient's depression or an actual side effect of therapy. If the insomnia is due to the depression, it may gradually subside as the antidepressant begins to take effect. Because many SSRIs do cause insomnia, they should be taken early in the day rather than at bedtime. If insomnia persists, a switch to a more sedating antidepressant can be made or a small dose of a sedating antidepressant can be added. Trazodone (Desyrel) and amitriptyline (Elavil) are used effectively for this purpose. Sleep agents such as zolpidem (Ambien) or zaleplon (Sonata) can also be used. If the patient has insomnia because of anxiety, buspirone (Buspar) can be effective. But beyond the sedation from another antidepressant, patients need to be educated on basic sleep hygiene and insomnia.

Sexual Dysfunction

Another serious side effect of antidepressants is sexual dysfunction. Most of the SSRIs have a negative effect on sexual functioning, as do venlafaxine and duloxetine to a lesser degree. As with insomnia, it is not always clear if the sexual dysfunction is caused by the antidepressant or the depression. Therefore, a history of sexual functioning is important before beginning treatment. Furthermore, the provider must openly inquire about sexual functioning, because many patients will discontinue their medications and drop out of treatment without ever disclosing this problem.

When the depression begins to subside, the patient may experience a spontaneous recovery of sexual functioning because of improvement in energy, mood, and sleep; watchful waiting is warranted. If that is not the case, once the patient is stabilized, she may take "drug holidays," decrease the antidepressant dosage, and/or change the time of the dose. For men, sildenafil (Viagra) 50 to 100 mg can be prescribed, but it does not seem to be helpful for women. Low doses of buspirone, bupropion, or ginkgo biloba have been useful for some patients.

However, it often becomes clear that sexual functioning is a central issue in some patients' lives and, therefore, an antidepressant that does not interfere with it will be critical from the start (Table 2.2).

In recent years, a group of clinicians, sex therapists, and social scientists have begun resisting the "medicalization" of sexuality in clinical settings (Hicks, 2004). These experts claim that there is a danger of failing to address basic human problems in sexuality if the focus is only on the biomedical and pharmaceutical approaches to sexuality problems. This group has named their approach the "New View" in treating women with sexual problems. The foundation for this approach is the integration of the relational and sociocultural factors that contribute to female sexuality and its problems. An online website is cited in the Resources for Providers section for more information on this integrated approach to women's sexuality.

Discontinuation Syndrome

When discontinuing an antidepressant, it is crucial to slowly decrease the dosage (taper) to avoid discontinuation syndrome (flulike symptoms, nausea, sleep problems, dizziness, hyperarousal, agitation, and lightheadedness; Shelton, 2006). Tapering involves a 20 percent decrease in the dose every 1 to 2 weeks. The key to avoiding these symptoms is the half-life of the antidepressant. For example, discontinuation from fluoxetine rarely triggers discontinuation symptoms because of its long half-life ranging between 1 and 4 days. Venlafaxine has the shortest half-life: 5 hours.

Discontinuation syndrome occurs in approximately 20 percent of patients who abruptly stop taking their antidepressants, and it may last up to 2 weeks depending on the half-life of the antidepressant and how long the patient was taking it. Therefore, a crucial part of patient education is to discuss the importance of remaining on the medication and working with the provider to slowly wean off the medication (Box 2.6).

In recent years, much more attention has been given to the discontinuation syndrome and its interchangeable use with the concept of "withdrawal." Shelton

Box 2.6 • General Precautions When Prescribing Antidepressants

1. Monitor for increased depression and suicidality in early months of treatment.
2. Use caution and decreased doses in patients with renal or hepatic impairment.
3. Taper dosage slowly when discontinuing antidepressants.
4. Check for drug interactions before prescribing. All antidepressants have potential for triggering mania in bipolar patients.
5. For patients with anxiety disorders, begin with smaller doses and increase gradually.
6. Prescribe lower doses with elderly patients.

(2006) emphasizes that the two concepts are not synonymous. Patients who have abruptly discontinued their antidepressant do not have the drug craving that is common in withdrawal nor do they exhibit the typical drug-seeking behavior. Discontinuation syndrome is similar to other physiologic responses due to discontinuation of general medications and is managed more easily than withdrawal in drug addiction. If these concepts are considered synonymous, patients may believe that their antidepressants are addictive and resist taking them. A great deal of research is beginning on discontinuation syndrome, and instruments are being developed to identify it (Fava, 2006; Shelton, 2006).

Treatment-Resistant Depression

TRD is defined as failure to achieve a therapeutic response with one or more adequate trials of antidepressant medication or two or more acute treatment trials or failure to respond to four different antidepressant therapies including augmentation, combination, and ECT (Fava and Cosino, 2007). While the goal of treatment is *remission* of depressive symptoms, <50 percent of depressed patients treated in primary care settings achieve remission (Shelton, 2003). Remission is defined as minimal or no symptoms on standardized depression scales such as the HAM-D and a full return to functioning in all aspects of life. In contrast, *response* is operationalized as a 50 percent or greater improvement on a standardized rating scale. Typically, this is the definition used in drug clinical trials. Thus, response is "improvement" while remission is "getting well."

It is commonly recognized that remission not only provides a superior quality of life but also significantly impacts the recurrence of future depressive episodes. Relapse of MDD after 15 months for patients who achieved remission was 20 percent as opposed to responders, who had an 80 percent relapse rate. Emerging evidence suggests that dual uptake inhibitors such as venlafaxine and duloxetine may be more effective in achieving remission than specific SSRIs (Newport, 2005).

Unfortunately, when the patient achieves only a *response* (also referred to as a *partial response*), neither the patient nor health care provider may question the inadequacy of the response or realize that there is a need for additional treatment to achieve remission. Because patients may feel significantly better, they may be satisfied with their outcome.

Reasons for response rather than remission include inadequate dosing, failure to recognize residual symptoms, and/or continuing psychosocial and environmental stressors. Another reason for a partial response is that some patients independently discontinue their antidepressant medication because of side effects or their belief that they are gaining little benefit from the treatment. Such action may result in a greater risk of suicide for the patients.

One intervention to assist in monitoring treatment effectiveness is the use of a standard instrument at regular intervals. Despite failure to reach remission for significant numbers of patients, the STAR*D studies (Fava, Rush, Wisniewski, et al., 2006) emphasized the need to continue trying different regimens and/or combinations of therapies for treatment-resistant patients. In the STAR*D study (the nation's largest depression treatment study), patients were continued in subsequent trials until they reached remission. The STAR*D results indicated that 67 percent of patients who continued through the necessary treatment trials reached remission. However, as patients progressed through the trials, the percentage of those reaching remission declined with each successive trial (Fava et al.). Clearly, more research is necessary to help those most resistant to treatment.

Partial Response: Augmenting or Switching Antidepressants

For patients who achieve only a partial response rather than remission after optimal doses of an antidepressant, two options exist: augmenting or switching medications. Advantages of *augmentation* include maintaining the antidepressant that induced the partial response (which minimizes the probability of relapse) and adding a complementary antidepressant that may produce a synergistic effect.

The disadvantages of augmentation include a more complex treatment regimen, increased potential for side effects and drug interactions, and increased potential for noncompliance by the patient. Augmentation can be quite complex.

The most common strategy used in primary care is augmentation of therapy with another antidepressant. A variety of augmenting medications include mood stabilizers (lithium or lamotrigine), thyroid hormones (T3, not T4), stimulants such as methylphenidate, or the beta-blocker pindolol, which is also a serotonin 1A antagonist. However, one concern about combining antidepressants is the possibility of serotonin syndrome. Other possibilities include adding an anxiolytic or an antipsychotic drug (Newport, 2005).

Switching involves a choice of remaining within the same drug class or using an antidepressant that is outside the class. While the tendency is to switch to an antidepressant outside the class, evidence exists that suggests using another antidepressant in the same class before going outside (Newport, 2005). Remaining within the same class may be effective because of subtle differences in secondary effects.

Psychotherapy

Numerous researchers have reported on the effectiveness of psychotherapy for depression and other psychiatric disorders. In particular, psychotherapy was the mainstay of treatment for mild to moderate depression before the MAOIs and TCAs were used. In recent years, repeated studies indicate that combining medication and psychotherapy for depression rather than using either as a single approach results in improved outcomes for patients. However, managed care barriers and other financial constraints have seriously hampered the use of psychotherapy for many patients who could benefit from it. Recent research suggests that the traditional form of psychotherapy, which is based on a psychoanalytic approach, may not be effective in treating depression. However, research into cognitive behavioral therapy (CBT), in particular, and interpersonal therapy (IPT) strongly supports their effectiveness (Goldapple, Segal, and Garson, 2004; Olfson, Marcus, Druss, et al., 2002; Pies and Rogers, 2005). PCPs need to be trained in these modalities before attempting to use them. However, providers who participate in workshops on CBT have found them very helpful in their practice and find that they are able to apply the principles effectively (Goldapple et al.; Olfson et al.; Pies and Rogers).

Cognitive Behavioral Therapy

Multiple studies provide evidence that CBT is effective in preventing relapse in depressed patients and increasing the numbers of patients who achieve remission (Fava, Rafanelli, Grandi, Conti, et al., 1998; Jarrett, Kraft, Doyle, et al., 2001; Paykel, Scott, and Teasdale, 1999). Some studies indicate that CBT is comparable and sometimes superior to medications for severe depression (DeRubeis, Gelfand, Tang, et al., 1999; Pies and Rogers, 2005).

CBT evolved from the theory that depression emerges from negative thoughts that subsequently result in negative feelings and behaviors. These negative thoughts are usually internalized, long-standing global patterns that are fixed and based on distorted perceptions of the person's beliefs of self, the environment, and the future. The goal of therapy is to change the person's distorted perceptions and beliefs through a systematic examination of them over time.

Interpersonal Therapy

IPT is a brief, highly structured form of therapy that shares many commonalities with CBT. However, IPT focuses on identifying interpersonal problems and addressing them by improving communication skills and interpersonal functioning, while CBT focuses on correcting distorted thoughts. Proponents of IPT claim that depression results from the interaction of symptom formation and deficits in personality and social functioning. IPT is derived from Bowlby's theories on attachment and Sullivan's theories of personifications. Researchers have found IPT to be effective for patients with severe depression, particularly when combined with medication.

Electroconvulsive Therapy

ECT is used as a treatment of choice for severely depressed patients who have not responded to other treatments and particularly for those who are actively suicidal. Some researchers have found that ECT has been effective with patients for whom multiple trials of antidepressants have been unsuccessful. Typically, the patient will receive 6 to 12 sessions of ECT every other day. Side effects such as posttreatment confusion and mild amnesia are minimal and short-lived. On rare occasions, more serious cognitive changes may result.

New research is currently being conducted with several types of brain stimulation that are not based on inducing generalized convulsions as seen in ECT. Two new therapies in particular hold promise: transcranial magnetic stimulation and vagus nerve stimulation.

Complementary and Alternative Therapies

Many over-the-counter medications and herbals exist that patients often take without informing their PCP. Some interact with antidepressants and/or other medications that a patient may be taking. For example, St. John's wort is incompatible with MAOIs, and dangerous results can occur when combined. St. John's wort is a mild SSRI; thus, patients must be cautious about combining it with their prescribed SSRI, because serotonin syndrome can result (Oquendo and Liebowitz, 2005). Thus, PCPs must ask patients specifically if they are taking any such preparations.

Complementary and alternative medicine therapies (CAMT) also include myriad treatments such as yoga, exercise, massage, light therapy, and diet. Chapter 16 details the most commonly used forms of CAMT in primary care.

CONCLUSION

MDD is a major public health problem second only to hypertension as the most commonly encountered problem in primary care. Women are twice as vulnerable to MDD as men, and while many theories exist that attempt to account for these differences, more research is needed to explain depression etiology. Although many similarities in MDD signs and symptoms exist for women as well as men, there are also significant differences; for instance, women have more atypical presentations. Again, reasons for the differences are unclear.

Because most patients with depression are diagnosed and treated by PCPs, it is imperative to be knowledgeable about the diagnosis and treatment of MDD to avoid long-term and more severe neurodegenerative changes for patients. That entails being current on the latest antidepressants and adjunctive medications as well as psychosocial interventions for all depressed patients. Furthermore, PCPs must use mental health professionals for consultation and referral whenever necessary.

Recent research demonstrates that antidepressants in a particular drug class are not equivalent, and therefore switching between them along with augmenting them with other drugs can be productive in achieving remission. Close communication with the patient will be necessary to monitor progress, identify side effects, and prevent the patient from discontinuing the medication for a variety of reasons. PCPs are uniquely positioned to identify and effectively treat many depressed patients who are undiagnosed in primary care. Such interventions can be life changing for these depressed patients.

Resources for Providers

American Psychiatric Association's Practice Guidelines: *www.psych.org/psych_pract/treatg/pg/prac_guide.cfm*

Depression and Bipolar Support Alliance: *http://ndmda.org*

Edinburgh Postnatal Depression Scale (EPDS): *http://health.utah.gov/rhp/pdf/EPDS.pdf*

International Foundation for Research and Education on Depression (iFred): *www.ifred.org*

Medscape's Depression Resource Center for Professionals: *www.medscape.com/pages/editorial/resourcecenters/public/depression/re-depression.ov*

MDQ: The Mood Disorder Questionnaire: *http://www.dballiance.org/pdfs/MDQ.pdf*

National Depressive and Manic-Depressive Association: *http://NDMDA.org*

National Institute of Mental Health: *http://nimh.nih.gov/publicat/index.cfm*

National Library of Medicine: *www.nim.nih.gov*

National Mental Health Association: *www.nmha.org*

New View Approach to Sexuality: *www.medscape.com/viewprogram/3437_pnt*

PHQ9 (Copyright © Pfizer Inc): *www.pfizer.com/phq-9*

Psychology Information Online: *www.psychologyinfo.com/depression*

Zung Self-Rating Depression Scale: *http://healthnet.umassmed.edu/mhealth/ZungSelfRatedDepressionScale.pdf*

Resources for Patients

Depression and Bipolar Support Alliance: *www.dbsalliance.org*

Medscape Patient Depression Education Center: *http://doctor.medscape.com/resource/depression*

National Alliance on Mental Illness (NAMI): *www.nami.org*

Web links were active at time of publication.

References

Altshuler, L. L., Cohen, L. S., Moline, M. L., et al. (2001). The Expert Consensus Guideline Series: Treatment of depression in women. *Postgraduate Medicine,* 1–116.

Altshuler, L. L, Cohen, L. S., & Szuba, M. P. (1996). Pharmacologic management of psychiatric illness during pregnancy: Dilemmas and guidelines. *American Journal of Psychiatry, 153,* 592–606.

American Psychiatric Association (APA). (2000). *Diagnostic and statistical manual of mental disorders* (Revised 4th ed.). Washington, DC: Author.

Birnbaum, C. S., Cohen, L. S., & Bailey, J. W. (1999). Serum concentrations of antidepressants and benzodiazepines in nursing infants: A case series. *Pediatrics, 104,* e11.

Chambers, C. D., Hernandez-Diaz S., Van Marter L. J., et al. (2006). Selective serotonin-reuptake inhibitors and risk of persistent pulmonary hypertension of the newborn. *New England Journal of Medicine, 354,* 579–587.

Cobbs, E. L., & Ralapati, A. N. (1998). Health of older women. *Medical Clinics of North America, 82,* 127–144.

Cohen, L. S., Altshuler, L. L., & Harlow, B. L. (2006). Relapse of major depression during pregnancy in women who maintain or discontinue antidepressant treatment. *Journal of the American Medical Association, 295,* 499–507.

Cohen, L. S., Soares, C. N., Vitonis, A. F., et al. (2006). Risk for new onset of depression during the menopausal transition: The Harvard study of moods and cycles. *Archives of General Psychiatry, 63*, 385–390.

DeRubeis, R. J., Gelfand, L. A., Tang, T. Z., et al. (1999). Medication versus cognitive behavioral therapy for severely depressed outpatients: Mega-analysis of four randomized comparisons. *American Journal of Psychiatry, 156*, 1007–1013.

Desai, H. D., & Jann, M. W. (2000). Major depression in women: A review of the literature. *Journal of American Pharmacy Association, 40*, 525–537.

Fava, M. (2006). Prospective studies of adverse events related to antidepressant discontinuation. *Journal of Clinical Psychiatry, 67*(Suppl 4), 14–21.

Fava, G. A., Rafanelli, C., Grandi, S., et al. (1998). Prevention of recurrent depression with cognitive behavioral therapy: Preliminary findings. *Archives of General Psychiatry, 55*, 816–820.

Fava, M., & Cosino, J. M. (2007). *Augmentation/combination therapy in the STAR* trial. Pharmacologic management of treatment-refractory depression*. Retrieved September 6, 2007, from *www.medscape.com/viewprogram/73333_pnt.*

Fava, M., Rush, A. J., Wisniewski, S. R., et al. (2006). A comparison of mirtazapine and nortriptyline following two consecutive failed medication treatments in depressed outpatients: A STAR*D report. *American Journal of Psychiatry, 163*, 1161–1172.

Fredman, S. J., & Rosenbaum, J. F. (2003). *Mood disorders and their treatment in women across the reproductive life cycle*. Medscape conference coverage of the American Psychiatric Association's 156th annual meeting. Retrieved January 21, 2005, from *www.medscape.com/viewprogram/2470_pnt.*

Freeman, E. W., Sammel, M. D., Lin, H., et al. (2006). Associations of hormones and menopause status with depressed mood in women with no history of depression. *Archives of General Psychiatry, 63*, 375–382.

Goldapple, K, Segal, Z., & Garson, C. (2004). Modulation of cortical-limbic pathways in major depression: Treatment-specific effects of cognitive therapy. *Archives of General Psychiatry, 61*, 34–41.

Goldberg, J. F., Cohen, L. J., Jackson, W. C., et al. (2005). 10 new multidisciplinary ways to look at bipolar disorder (BD). *Consultant*(Suppl), 1–5.

Hicks, K. M. (2004). Women's sexual problems—A guide to integrating the "New View" approach. *Medscape*. Retrieved August 18, 2006, from *www.medscape.com/viewprogram/3437–pnt.*

Jarrett, R. B., Kraft, D., Doyle, J., et al. (2001). Preventing recurrent depression using cognitive therapy with and without a continuation phase. *Archives of General Psychiatry, 58*, 381–388.

Jepson, T. L., Ernst, M. E., & Kelly, M. W. (1999). Current perspectives on the management of seasonal affective disorder. *Journal of American Pharmaceutical Association, 39*, 822–829.

Kanner, A. M. (2004). Is major depression a neurologic disorder with psychiatric symptoms? *Epilepsy Behavior, 5*, 636–644.

Kessler, R. C., Chiu, W. T., Demler, O., et al. (2005). Prevalence, severity and comorbidity of 12 month DSM-IV disorders in the National Comorbidity Survey Replication. *Archives of General Psychiatry, 62*, 617–627.

Khan, A., Brodhead, A. E., Schwartz, K. A., et al. (2005). Sex differences in antidepressant response in recent antidepressant clinical trials. *Journal of Clinical Psychopharmacology, 25*, 318–324.

Kornstein, S. G., Schatzberg, A. F., & Thase, M. E. (2000). Gender differences in chronic major and double depression. *Journal of Affective Disorders, 60,* 1–11.

Kornstein, S. G., Steiner, H., Miranda, J., et al. (2006). *Achieving remission in depression: Managing women and men in the primary care setting.* CME Round Table Discussion sponsored by University of Minnesota and SynerMed Communications on January 5, 2005. Reference ID: DL-06-119. Retrieved April 29, 2006, from *www.medscape.com/viewprogram/5134_pnt.*

Levinson-Castiel, R. (2005). Selective serotonin reuptake inhibitors in pregnant women and neonatal withdrawal syndrome. *Lancet, 365,* 482–487.

Louik, C., Lin, A. F., & Werler, M. M., et al. (2007). First-trimester use of selective serotonin-reuptake inhibitors and the risk of birth defects. *New England Journal of Medicine, 356,* 2675–2683.

Maier, W., Gansicke, M., & Gater, R. (1999). Gender differences in the prevalence of depression: A survey in primary care. *Journal of Affective Disorders, 53,* 241–252.

McGarry, K., & Schoeni, R. F. (2005). Widow(er) poverty and out-of-pocket medical expenditures near the end of life. *Journal of Gerontology: Psychological Sciences and Social Sciences, 60,* S160–S168.

Miguel-Hidalgo, J. J., & Rajkowska, G. (2002). Morphological brain changes in depression: Can antidepressants reverse them? *CNS Drugs, 16,* 361–372.

National Institute of Mental Health. (2001). *Depression in women and men: What's the difference?* Bethesda, MD: Author.

Nemeroff, C., DeVane, C. L., & Lydiard, R. B. (2007). *Emerging trends for monoamine oxidase inhibition in the management of depression: A patient-focused, interactive program.* Office of Continuing Medical Education of South Carolina (MUSC). Retrieved July 7, 2007, from *www.medscape.com/viewprogram/6769_pnt.*

Newport, D. J. (2005). *Family medicine and primary care: Working toward the 3 "Rs" for managing depression.* Symposium held at North Carolina Academy of Family Physicians annual meeting in Atlanta, GA. Retrieved March 25, 2005, from *www.medscape.com/viewprogram/3795_pnt.*

Olfson, M., Marcus, S. C., Druss, B. G., et al. (2002). National trends in the outpatient treatment of depression. *Journal of the American Medical Association, 287,* 203–209.

Oquendo, M. A., & Leibowitz, M. (2005). *Diagnosis and treatment of major depression in primary care. An evidenced-based approach.* A CME/CE offering by Medscape and Columbia University, College of Physicians and Surgeons. Retrieved May 1, 2006, from *www.medscape.com/viewprogram/4571_pnt.*

Paykel, E. S., Scott, J., & Teasdale, J. D. (1999). Prevention of relapse in residual depression by cognitive therapy. *Archives of General Psychiatry, 56,* 829–835.

Pies, R., & Rogers, D. (2005). The recognition and treatment of depression: A review for the primary care clinician. *Medscape CME/CE.* Retrieved October 11, 2005, from *www.medscape.com/viewprogram/4572_pnt.*

Robinson, W. D., Geske, J. A., Prest, L. A., et al. (2005). Depression treatment in primary care. *Journal of American Board of Family Practice, 18,* 79–86.

Santos, R. P., & Pergolizzi, J. J. (2004). Transient neonatal jitteriness due to maternal use of sertraline (Zoloft). *Journal of Perinatology, 24,* 392–394.

Satcher, D., Ninan, P. T., & Masand, S. (2005). A surgeon general's perspective on cultural competency: What is it and how does it affect diagnosis and treatment of major depressive disorder? *Medscape CME*. Retrieved May 21, 2006, from *www.medscape.com/viewprogram/4489_pnt*.

Shelton, R. C. (2003). Treatment-resistant depression. *Medscape*. Retrieved March 6, 2005, from *www.medscape.com/viewprogram/2205_pmt*.

Shelton, R. C. (2006). The nature of discontinuation syndrome associated with antidepressant drugs. *Journal of Clinical Psychiatry, 67*(Suppl 4), 3–7.

Silverstone, P. H. (2004). *Somatic and psychological symptoms of depression*. The Mind, Brain, Body Connection: Treating People with Depression in the 21st Century symposium held in Sidney, Australia. Retrieved February 11, 2004, from *www.medscape/viewprogram/3548_pnt*.

Sohn, C. H., & Lam, R. W. (2005). Treatment of seasonal affective disorder: Unipolar versus bipolar differences. *Current Psychiatry Report, 6*, 478–485.

Umberson, D., Wortman, C. B., & Kessler, R. C. (1992). Widowhood and depression: Explaining long-term gender differences in vulnerability. *Journal of Health and Social Behavior, 33*, 10–24.

U.S. Preventive Services Task Force of the Agency for Healthcare Research and Quality (USPSTF). (2002). *Screening for depression. Recommendations and rationale*. Rockville, MD: Author.

Vollmer, S. (2005). Depression in women: Gender-related differences in occurrence and treatment. *Family Practice Recertification, 27*, 44–64.

Wohlreich, M. M., Brannan, S. K., & Mallinckrodt, C. H. (2004). Onset of improvement in emotional and painful physical symptoms of depression with duloxetine treatment. *World Journal of Biological Psychiatry, 5*(Suppl 1), 91.

M. Linda Hoes

chapter 3

Bipolar Disorder

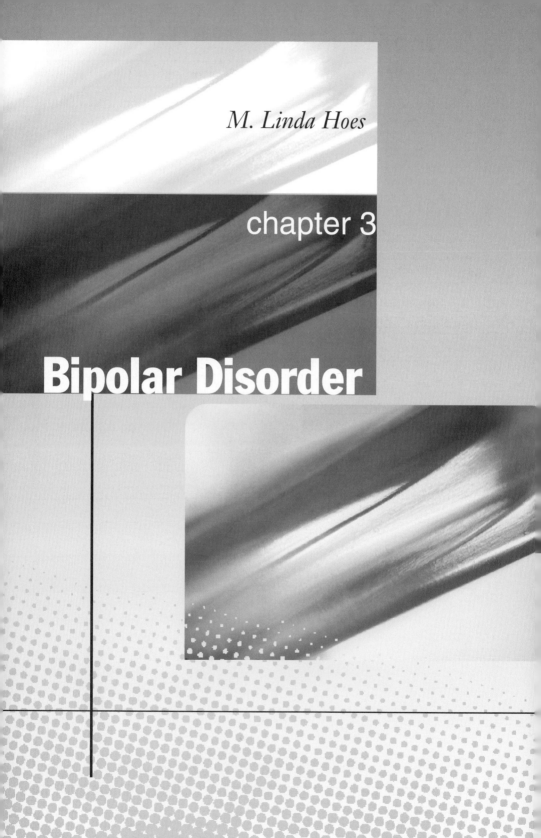

Primary care providers (PCPs) spend an estimated 12.1 hours per week providing direct treatment for psychiatric conditions. One of the most challenging psychiatric conditions is bipolar (BP) disorder, previously known as manic depression. Although current literature indicates an equal prevalence of the disorder among women and men, there is increasing evidence of gender differences in the form, presentation, lifetime course, treatment, and outcome. This chapter will present an overview of BP disorder and recent findings relevant to the epidemiology, diagnosis, clinical course, and treatment of BP disorder in women. Because of the complexities encountered in BP disorders, initial diagnoses and treatment should be done by a psychiatrist or advanced practice psychiatric practitioner. Maintenance treatment and ongoing observation can be accomplished through a collaborative arrangement with primary care practitioners and psychiatric practitioners.

DIAGNOSIS OF BIPOLAR DISORDER

The extremes of BP disorder's mood cycles range from the depths of despondency to elation. Symptom clusters characterized by episodes of depression and mania, hypomania, and mixed states are varied, mild to severe, and frequently changing. BP disorder constitutes a cyclical, recurrent, and relapsing lifelong condition that may take years to accurately diagnose. The course of the illness over a lifetime can be debilitating with increasing risk for suicide, frequent hospitalizations, comorbid medical and psychiatric disorders, and significant disability.

A spectrum of BP symptom categories exists, and specific diagnostic guidelines are outlined in the *Diagnostic and Statistical Manual of Mental Disorders* (*DSM-IV-TR*; American Psychiatric Association [APA], 2000). There are three officially designated subtypes: Bipolar I, Bipolar II (BP I, BP II), and Cyclothymia. By definition, a diagnosis of BP I requires at least one lifetime episode of mania. Although not required for the diagnosis, multiple episodes of severe depression are common. BP II includes both depressive and hypomanic episodes but never a full manic episode. Cyclothymic disorder describes frequent mood cycles that do not meet severity and duration criteria of BP I or II. A fourth classification, bipolar disorder not otherwise specified, allows for myriad atypical presentations. *Rapid cycling* is a modifier formally denoting four or more distinct episodes a year; however, many clinicians use the term to describe mood switches occurring more frequently. Mixed states occur in which symptoms of both mania and depression occur simultaneously for at least 1 week. A mania occurring in the context of substance abuse, medical illness, and certain medications is considered secondary and classified separately.

BP I disorder usually emerges around 18 years of age, and BP II slightly later, at around age 22. The National Comorbidity Survey (NCS-R; Kessler, Bergland, Demler, et al., 2005) reports typical onset of both between the ages of 18 and 44. Epidemiologic studies vary slightly in the estimation of lifetime prevalence rates ranging from 1 to 1.6 percent of the population. Newer data that include a broader diagnostic spectrum report rates of occurrence up to 5 percent (Power, 2004). There are suggestions that BP II may be more common in women than men. Likewise, there is evidence that women are more likely to experience rapid cycling and that mixed and depressive symptoms may be more common in women as well.

Symptom Presentations

Depression

Persons in a state of major depression lose interest in life and pleasurable activities. They feel sad, guilty, worthless, and hopeless. Decision making and concentration are difficult, and delusional ideation may be present. Agitation or lethargy and inertia may occur along with social withdrawal and isolation. Physical symptoms such as fatigue, pain, constipation, and decreased libido as well as appetite, weight, and sleep changes are common. Thoughts of death and dying along with suicidal ideation and attempts often accompany this mood state. A considerable decrease in multiple areas of functioning is apparent.

Mania

Although euphoria is associated with mania, irritability, anger, and hostility are quite common. Unrealistically optimistic and grandiose ideas, racing thoughts, and distractibility cloud thinking and alter judgment. Significant loss of sleep without fatigue and flamboyant, loud, intrusive, and hyperactive behavior accompanied by engagement in multiple projects or reckless and risk-taking activities may occur. Delusions and hallucinations may be present. While full-blown mania is a psychiatric emergency and requires hospitalization, it is more likely that a hypomania will be observed in the BP population seen in the clinic.

Hypomania

The boundary between mania and hypomania is determined by evaluation of severity of functional disturbance, total symptom picture, and symptom duration (Table 3.1). Common manifestations of hypomania include increases in energy

Table 3.1 • Comparison of *DSM-IV-TR* Criteria for Manic and Hypomanic Episodes

Manic Episode	Hypomanic Episode
A. A distinct period of abnormally and persistently elevated, expansive, or irritable mood, *lasting at least 1 week* (or any duration if hospitalization is necessary).	A. A distinct period of persistently elevated, expansive, or irritable mood, *lasting throughout for at least 4 days*, that is clearly different from the usual nondepressed mood.
B. During the period of mood disturbance, three (or more) of the following symptoms have persisted (four if the mood is only irritable) and have been present to a significant degree: (1) Inflated self-esteem or grandiosity (2) Decreased need for sleep (e.g., feels rested after only 3 hours of sleep) (3) More talkative than usual or pressure to keep talking (4) Flight of ideas or subjective experience that thoughts are racing[SF31] (5) Distractibility (i.e., attention too easily drawn to unimportant or irrelevant external stimuli) (6) Increase in goal-directed activity (either socially, at work or school, or sexually) or psychomotor agitation (7) Excessive involvement in pleasurable activities that have a high potential for painful consequences (e.g., engaging in unrestrained buying sprees, sexual indiscretions, or foolish business investments)	
C. The symptoms do not meet criteria for a Mixed Episode.	C. The episode is associated with an unequivocal change in functioning that is uncharacteristic of the person when not symptomatic.
D. The mood disturbance is sufficiently severe to cause marked impairment in occupational functioning or in usual social activities or relationships with others, or to necessitate hospitalization to prevent harm to self or others, or there are psychotic features.	D. The disturbance in mood and the change in functioning are observable by others.
E. The symptoms are not due to the direct physiologic effects of a substance (e.g., a drug of abuse, a medication, or other treatment) or a general medical condition (e.g., hyperthyroidism).	E. The episode is not severe enough to cause marked impairment in social or occupational functioning, or to necessitate hospitalization, and there are no psychotic features.

(*Continued*)

Table 3.1 • (Continued)

Manic Episode	Hypomanic Episode
Note: Maniclike episodes that are clearly caused by somatic antidepressant treatment (e.g., medication, electroconvulsive therapy, light therapy) should not count toward a diagnosis of bipolar I disorder.	
	F. The symptoms are not due to the direct physiologic effects of a substance (e.g., a drug of abuse, a medication, or other treatment) or a general medical condition (e.g., hyperthyroidism.) Note: Hypomaniclike episodes that are clearly caused by somatic antidepressant treatment (e.g., medication, electroconvulsive therapy, light therapy) should not count toward a diagnosis of bipolar II disorder.

Adapted from the American Psychiatric Association (APA) (2000).

and self-confidence; those involved in work, social plans, and activities include spending more money, feeling less shy and inhibited and more optimistic, becoming more talkative, laughing more, and an increased interest in sex. Greater consumption of coffee, cigarettes, and alcohol may be present. Hypomanic episodes are not severe enough to cause marked impairment in social or occupational functioning.

Cyclothymia

In cyclothymic disorder, there are many periods of hypomanic symptoms and many periods of depressive symptoms alternating in individual specific rhythms. The condition is chronic for at least 2 years without reaching criteria sufficient in severity, number, or pervasiveness of symptoms for a diagnosis of BP I or II. Women who initially present with cyclothymia often go on to BP I and II. Criteria for a major depressive episode are shown in Chapter 2.

GENDER DIFFERENCES IN BIPOLAR DISORDER

Few systematic prospective studies exist that have evaluated gender-specific issues in BP disorder. Often, there is a lack of agreement among researchers in many cases where differences are found. However, there is increasing evidence for gender differences in epidemiology, clinical presentation and course, comorbidity, and treatment issues. Increasingly, differences between women and men in the pharmacokinetics and pharmacodynamics of medications used in BP disorder are being reported, along with observations of the impact of the female reproductive cycle on the course and treatment of the disorders.

Epidemiology and Illness Characteristics

While the lifetime prevalence is considered equal between women and men, the consensus is that BP II is more common in women, with lifetime rates ranging from 5.0 to 10.0 percent for women as compared with the overall rate of occurrence, which is about 0.5 percent (Weissman, 1996). If it is true that women also have a higher percentage of major depressive episodes over the course of the illness than men, this would be consistent with the data that women are almost twice as likely to develop unipolar major depression as men, although the association remains unknown.

Men are likely to report the first episode as manic, while the first episode in women is more frequently depression. This is important because research reports that women are more likely to be prescribed antidepressants than men, and treatment with antidepressants is associated with an increase in rapid cycling in women (Power, 2004). Depressive episodes in women are longer in duration and tend to be more treatment resistant. In men, a switch from mania to depression is more common, while in women, a manic or hypomanic episode is most often preceded by a depressive state. The average time from onset of symptoms to treatment is 8 years, yet men with BP I typically begin treatment after 6 years, while women with BP II wait an average of 11 years for such treatment (Power). Treatment delay is associated with poorer social functioning, more hospital admissions, and more suicide attempts.

Mixed States

Women are reported to comprise between 60 and 90 percent of cases of mixed manic and depressive states (Arnold, McElroy, and Keck, 2000). The true occurrence is confounded, however, by inconsistencies in the definition of mixed states among investigators. Young women with an early onset of illness and those with alcohol and substance abuse histories appear to be at the greatest risk for developing mixed episodes. It is unknown why women may be more susceptible to this form of the illness, but the main theories hypothesize involvement of the hypothalamic-pituitary-adrenal axis and thyroid axis (Curtis, 2005).

Rapid Cycling

There is variance in the prevalence of rapid cycling across different studies over the last 30 years, ranging from 13 to 56 percent. Because rapid cycling is a specifier of BP disorders, it can occur in both BP I and II. Three consistent characteristics have been identified as risk factors for rapid cycling: (1) BP II subtype, (2) female gender, and (3) a younger age of onset. Rapid cycling is associated with treatment resistance, poor long-term prognosis, and higher risk for suicide (Schneck, 2006). Persistent rapid cycling usually begins with depression followed by mania; therefore, women seem to be more vulnerable to this severe form of the illness. Although rapid cycling occurs in 15 to 20 percent of all patients with BP disorder, women account for between 70 and 90 percent of rapid cyclers (Calabrese, Muzina, Kemp, et al., 2006). Etiology of the rapid cycling phenomenon and the explanation for gender differences is not clear. Proposed factors are hypothyroidism (also more prevalent in women), effects of gonadal steroids, and greater use of antidepressant medication in women.

Comorbidity

The presence of comorbid physical and psychological disorders in BP disorder is more common than not. Comorbid psychiatric disorders in individuals with BP disorder are associated with poorer outcome and poorer treatment response. Women are twice as likely to have a comorbid diagnosis as men. The National Comorbidity Study Replication Study (Kessler et al., 2005) found that over 50 percent of individuals with a BP diagnosis will have an active concurrent alcohol or substance abuse problem and up to a 90-percent prevalence over the course of their lifetime. Alcohol and marijuana are most frequently used, with alcohol use higher in women. Although studies show that men with BP disorder have a greater prevalence of alcoholism than women, women with BP disorder have a much greater risk for alcoholism than women in the general population (Frye, Altshuler, McElroy, et al., 2003). Comorbidity of substance abuse may mask proper diagnosis, especially in women who are too frequently not asked about their use of substances. Drugs of abuse, especially with chronic use, can mimic depression and mania. Alternatively, the clinician may attribute mood volatility to substance use and miss signs of hypomania or depression. It is important to ask about affective symptoms predating the use of substances and if they persist during abstinence.

Anxiety disorders with panic, generalized anxiety, social anxiety, obsessive-compulsive, and posttraumatic stress states occur in 40 to 65 percent of individuals with BP disorder and worsen the course of the illness. Women have higher rates than men, particularly of panic disorder (21 percent) and social phobia (47 percent). Eating disorders, especially bulimia (65 percent), and posttraumatic stress disorder (38 percent) are also more common in women with BP disorder than in men (Keller, 2006; McElroy, 2004).

An extensive literature review discovered not only high rates of non–mood disorder primary psychiatric diagnosis but also high rates of personality disorder (36 percent). Studies of the relationships between personality and BP disorder show higher rates of borderline personality disorder, which is also more commonly seen in women. The relationship between mood disorders and personality is complex and deserves further study.

Many children diagnosed with attention deficit disorder eventually develop manic and depressive symptoms. Almost one third of adults identify BP symptoms occurring before age 13, and an estimated half of severely depressed prepubescent children may eventually develop mania or hypomania (Goldberg and Ernst, 2002). Attention deficit hyperactivity can exist along with BP symptoms in adult women and complicate diagnoses and treatment.

Other frequently seen co-occurrences are migraine (28 percent), type 2 diabetes (10 percent), hypothyroidism (9 percent), and overweight and obesity (79 percent). Obesity (body mass index equal to or greater than 30) is associated with significant increases in lifetime diagnosis of BP disorder (Krishnan, 2005; Simon, Von Korff, Saunders, et al., 2006). Ongoing research is attempting to determine the direction of causal relationships in this highly comorbid group. The role of social and cultural factors, biologic factors, and medications are being investigated. The high incidence of obesity in women with BP disorders along with the use of atypical antipsychotic and mood-stabilizing medications put women at risk for the metabolic syndrome, which is a major risk factor for heart disease, stroke, and diabetes. Careful diagnostic assessment and attention to the primary care needs of women with BP disorder is indicated; clinical care may demand simultaneous management of several concurrent problems.

Racial and Sociocultural Issues

BP disorder has not been associated with sociodemographic factors. No association between race or ethnicity or socioeconomic status has been identified, nor is there a difference seen in rural versus urban populations. However, possible differences in symptom experience and reporting may affect the way the illness is recognized and diagnosed among minorities. Women from various cultural backgrounds may view symptoms in different ways. Such factors should be considered when working with women from special populations. Cultural competence and sensitivity to stigma are especially important in treating women with psychiatric disorders.

Suicide and Suicide Attempts

Individuals with BP disorder have a rate of suicide 15 percent higher than that of the general population. Lifetime risk of completed suicide for both BP I and BP II may be as high as 26 percent. However, completed suicides and suicide attempt rates are much higher in those with BP II and may represent 44 percent of all suicides. In comparison, unipolar major depression accounts for 54 percent of all suicides. No gender differences have been found for completed suicides between women and men with BP diagnoses, unlike rates in the general population where men are three to four times as likely to die from suicide (Baldassano, 2006). Women with a rapid cycling course have been found to have a higher risk for suicide compared with those who do not have this feature.

Inquiry about suicide ideation should always be made on initial interviews and when mood switches are observed. Suicide ideation often occurs during switches from depression to mania, but the risk is highest during depression. Women in mixed states are especially at risk. Careful observation for suicide risk should be made after beginning antidepressant medications.

Assessment and Differential Diagnosis

The differential diagnosis of BP disorder is quite extensive and complex. As previously noted, BP disorder may take years to accurately diagnose. Mixed mood states can be mistaken for many other conditions, including anxiety disorders and personality disorders. Borderline personality disorder with labile mood may be confused with cyclothymia. Mania can mimic schizophrenia, and hypomania is usually denied or considered productive or positive, often described as a "type

A" personality. Reckless and impulsive or antisocial behaviors are seen in substance abuse, personality disorders, and attention deficit hyperactivity disorders as well as manic presentations.

Hypomania can present a mood that is often charming and infectious and may be conducive to creativity or productive endeavors. Symptoms like those seen in a hypomanic episode may accompany intoxication or withdrawal from drugs of abuse. Women with BP II may simply remove themselves from social situations when in a depressed state or minimize one or both of the mood states.

The evaluation of a woman for BP disorder includes a neuropsychiatric assessment with a detailed history and physical examination. Corroborating information should be sought from family, friends, or prior treatment facilities. Screening instruments are helpful in eliciting manic symptoms and differentiating episodic symptoms from chronic symptoms. The Mood Disorder Questionnaire (Hirschfeld, Williams, Spitzer, et al., 2000) is a useful and easy tool to administer in primary care. Seven positive answers out of 13 and endorsement of functional or social impairment associated with the symptom cluster calls for a full psychiatric evaluation. A mood chart allows women to record important information so that a graphic illustration of their illness characteristics and treatment effects can be observed over a month's time. Recording of mood states, medication levels, menstrual cycle, important life events, and stressors helps them and their clinicians to recognize patterns and triggers of symptoms.

Several styles of daily rating forms and prospective live charting forms are available to assist clinicians. The Daily Record of Severity of Problems Form (Endicott and Harrison, 1990) allows women to record observations of physical, emotional, and social aspects of functional symptoms. A comprehensive psychiatric diagnostic assessment tool developed for use in primary care is the PRIME-MD (Spitzer, Williams, Kroenk, et al., 1994). Refer to the Resources for Providers section for additional tools.

A systematic approach to screening for BP disorders is listed in Box 3.1. Initial assessment interviews that include questions about the topics listed will provide needed information for making diagnostic, treatment, and referral decisions.

Common triggers of mood switches include hypothyroidism and conditions that disrupt sleep, such as untreated sleep apnea or travel across time zones. Phototherapy as well as many medications and hormones can trigger affective instability. Consider any biological or substance triggers that may explain symptoms. Some medical conditions that may cause secondary mania include cerebrovascular disease and stroke, head trauma, brain neoplasms, HIV infection, epilepsy, endocrine disorders, neurosyphilis, and, in the elderly, B_{12} deficiency

Box 3.1 • Systematic Diagnostic Considerations in the Assessment of Bipolar Disorders

- Family history—first-degree relatives with known BP disorder, recurrent unipolar depression, schizoaffective disorder, suicide, or panic disorder
- Personal history—periods of accelerated rate of thinking, speech, activity; cognitive disturbances such as distractibility and inattentiveness
- Periods of diminished sleep without fatigue and reports of mood change effects from sleep deprivation, time zone changes, seasonal mood changes, and postpartum affective disturbances
- Comorbid disorders—alcohol or drug abuse, severe anxiety states, a previous diagnosis of a personality disorder
- Prepubescent age of onset of symptoms
- Depressive symptoms—recurrent, brief, frequent episodes, atypical features, evidence of psychotic features
- Medication history—evidence for antidepressant-induced mania, hypomania, or cycling; diminishing effects of antidepressants in the past may indicate cycling; a positive response to mood stabilizing drugs in the past may be consistent with a bipolar diagnosis (but not always)

and influenza. Table 3.2 lists substances and medications that may trigger mania or depression in vulnerable women. Psychosocial triggers such as conflict with others, grief, or loss of social support systems should also be considered. Positive life changes, such as job promotion or marriage, may also produce sufficient stress to activate affective shifts.

There are no biological or laboratory tests to confirm a clinical diagnosis of BP disorder. Laboratory tests are used on a case-by-case basis to determine if symptoms are of a secondary mania, such as substance induced, or due to an underlying medical condition. Suggested diagnostic studies are listed in Box 3.2. Correction of the underlying medical condition may effectively reverse secondary mania or make it easy to treat. Current or past hypothyroidism or laboratory evidence of mild thyroid hypofunction may be associated with rapid cycling (see p. 427, *DSM-IV-TR*; APA, 2000).

Women who present with the first episode of mania late in life are likely to have a negative family history of a mood disorder. Irritability is often the presenting symptom. Psychosis or early dementia-like cognitive dysfunction is more common than in early primary mania. If age of onset for the first episode of mania is past the

Table 3.2 • Substances as Potential Causes of Secondary Mania and Depression

Mania	Deprssion
Substance Intoxication	**Substance Intoxication**
Amphetamines Anticholinergics Barbiturates Benzodiazepines Cocaine Hallucinogens Opiates Phencyclidine	Alcohol Barbiturates Benzodiazepines Cannabis
Withdrawal	**Withdrawal**
Alcohol Barbiturates Benzodiazepines	Amphetamines Cocaine
Medications	**Medications**
Baleen Bromide Bromocriptine Bronchodialators Calcium replacement Captopril Cimetidine Corticosteroids Cyclosporine Decongestants Disulfiram Hydralazine Isoniazid Levodopa Methylphenidate Metoclopramide Metrizamide Procarbazine Procyclidine Yohimbine	Acetazolamide Amantadine Anticholinesterases Azathioprine Baciofen Barbiturates Benzodiazepines Bleomycin Bromocriptine Butyrophenones Carbamazepine Chloral hydrate Cimetidine Clonidine Clotrimazole Corticosteroids Cycloserine Danazol Dapsone Digitalis Disulfiram Fenfluramine Gresofulvine Guanethidine Hydralazine Ibuprofen

(Continued)

Table 3.2 • (Continued)

Mania	Deprssion
	Indomethacin Levodopa/Methyldopa Lidocaine Meclizine Metoclopramide Methsuximide Mithramycin Nitrofurantoin Opiates Oral contraceptives Phenacetin Phenothiazines Phenylbutazone Phenytoin Prazosin Procainamide Propranolol Reserpine Streptomycin Sulfonamides Tetracycline Triamcinolone Vincristine

Box 3.2 • Suggested Laboratory Tests

- Thyroid panel (TSH, T3, T4)
- Urine or blood toxicology
- Serum chemistries
- Complete blood count (CBC)
- Erythrocyte sedimentation rate (ESR)
- Liver panel
- Renal studies
- Pregnancy test
- Electrocardiogram (ECG)
- Electroencephalogram (EEG)

age of 40 years, the clinician should be alerted to the possibility that the symptoms are due to a secondary mania, general medical condition, or substance abuse.

Additional information that should be acquired is a history of response to antidepressant medication, history of family members' response to antidepressant medication, and mood changes during menstrual cycles, pregnancies, postpartum, perimenopause, and menopause.

Major Depression versus Bipolar Disorder

The most common and difficult confounder of accurate diagnosis is unipolar depression. BP disorder should always be considered in the differential diagnosis of women with depression. Overall, depression is the most commonly occurring pole of symptoms experienced by persons with BP. As noted, women most often present with depression as the index episode, and up to 40 percent eventually convert to a course of BP II, usually within 2 to 11 years. BP depression is often misdiagnosed as unipolar depression, and hypomania in BP II is often overlooked, leading to a missed diagnosis. Initiation of antidepressant medication at first episode, especially the selective serotonin reuptake inhibitors (SSRIs), is believed to precipitate not only a switch to hypomania but also a mixed state or rapid cycling pattern in these women. Although this association has not been found in all studies, it is prudent to be cautious in the use of antidepressants in women with BP disorders. Mood lability and energy–activity are two factors most predictive of BP II depression. As an aid to differential diagnosis, Box 3.3 shows clinical features more likely to be seen in women with BP depression.

Box 3.3 • Clinical Features Occurring More Frequently in Bipolar Depression Than in Unipolar Depression

- Family history of manic depression
- Earlier age of onset
- High number of depressive episodes
- Greater portion of time ill
- Hypersomnia
- Lack of weight loss or weight gain
- Psychomotor retardation
- Postpartum episodes
- Greater degree of anxiety and less sadness

Effects of the Female Reproductive Cycle on the Course of Bipolar Disorder

Special treatment considerations for BP disorder in women are hypothesized to involve interactions between the illness and the female reproductive cycle. Despite a recent increase in interest in gender-specific relationships to BP disorder, published data in this area remain scarce. Changes along the reproductive cycle are observed, but little consistent prospective data exist to guide the clinician.

The Menstrual Cycle

It has been determined that gonadal steroids can modulate the activity of serotonin, noradrenalin, and gamma-amino-butyric acid (GABA) in women, all of which play a part in mood regulation. Fluctuations in estrogen and progesterone are implicated in symptom expression in women with premenstrual dysphoric disorder. Overrepresentation of women in rapid cycling and mixed states of BP disorder has led to the supposition that a dysregulation of reproductive hormones is responsible. Some studies have found an increase in suicide, suicide intent, and hospitalizations in women with BP disorder during the premenstrual and menstrual phases of their menstrual cycle (Barnes and Mitchell, 2005). Menstrual dysfunction prior to onset of BP illness has been reported by women with an eventual BP diagnosis (Joffe, Kim, Foris, et al., 2006). Other prospective studies, however, have found no relationship between the menstrual phase and mood symptoms in women, even in a sample of women with rapid cycling BP disorder. There are insufficient prospective studies to clarify the effect of exogenous estrogens and progesterone on the course of BP disorders, although oral contraceptives (OCs) have been used to stabilize women through menstrual cycle mood shifts.

Pregnancy

In the past, it was thought that pregnancy is a time when women are less likely to experience episodes of affective illness, but there are limited data on the course of illness during pregnancy. The rates of recurrence in the first 40 weeks were similar in pregnant and nonpregnant women in one study (Viguera, Cohen, Bouffard, et al., 2002), but many women with BP disorders experienced postpartum exacerbation. Abrupt rather than slow discontinuation of lithium treatment in pregnancy appears to be a factor. Another group of investigators found that 40 to 50 percent of women in their study experienced an exacerbation of symptoms during pregnancy (Freeman, Wosnitzer-Smith, Freeman, et al., 2002). It is unclear whether pregnancy itself is a risk factor for symptomatic relapse or emergence of an episode of depression, mania or hypomania, but what appears to predict the greatest risk is stopping medication. Women who remain well during pregnancy are less likely to have a postpartum relapse. Conversely, becoming ill during pregnancy is the strongest predictor for becoming ill postpartum (Viguera, Nonacs, Cohen, et al., 2000).

A risk of fetal malformation does exist when some of the mood-stabilizing agents are used during pregnancy. Careful management is needed to reduce the risks to the fetus and possible neurobehavioral problems in the infant as well as effectively managing BP symptoms in the mother. The risks of treatment versus no treatment should be discussed with the mother. When possible, decisions regarding the use of psychotropics should be made before a woman conceives.

There is strong evidence for heritability of mood disorders. Genetic counseling is advised for women considering pregnancy if they have a strong positive family history of mood disorders. Information is available at *www.womensmentalhealth.org/* to help guide women in the decision to become pregnant, on the reproductive safety of various medications, the risk of relapse if medication is stopped, and the dangers of untreated illness. A list of approved drugs for the treatment of BP disorders can be found in Table 3.3, along with comments on their potential teratogenicity and pregnancy class. For women who require treatment during pregnancy, the first-line treatment is lithium. The highest reported risks in pregnancy are with valproate (Depakote), and the greatest concern during breast-feeding is with lithium use (Freeman and Gelenberg, 2005).

Postpartum

It is well accepted that the postpartum period is a time of high risk for the emergence of affective disorders and psychosis. This is particularly true for women with preexisting BP disorder. Reports of rates of occurrence for postpartum relapse in women with previous episodes of BP events vary significantly in the literature. Much of the empirical evidence reported in a dearth of studies over the last 40 years estimated an average occurrence at about 50 percent. Recent evidence indicates higher rates of relapse within 3 to 6 months postpartum, variously between 67 and 82 percent (Freeman et al., 2002; Viguera et al., 2000). Mixed states and depression are the most common presentation.

An estimated 20 to 30 percent of women with BP disorders are at risk for a postpartum psychotic episode. Postpartum psychosis is actually rare in the general population, occurring in only 1 in 1,000 women (Viguera, 2005). Postpartum psychosis in women with BP disorder, which is basically a manic episode, presents with a rapid onset of symptoms within 48 to 72 hours of delivery. Auditory, visual, and tactile hallucinations are often present. Hospitalization is necessary in the case of acute postpartum psychosis.

Table 3.3 • Approved Treatments for Bipolar Disorder and Their Relationship to Reproductive Issues*

Drug	Indication	Pregnancy Category	Reproductive Issues
Lithium	• Treatment of manic episodes • Maintenance therapy preventing or diminishing intensity of subsequent episodes in patients with history of mania	Considered D	• Ebstein's anomaly Risk = 1 in 1,000 (0.1%) • Breast milk excretion
Valproate	• Treatment of manic episodes • Effectiveness for long-term use in mania (<3 wk) has not been systematically evaluated in RCT	D Boxed Warning	• Neural tube defects (1%–2%) • Craniofacial, cardiovascular malformation, limb and genital defects, hydrocephalus reported • Polycystic ovary with potential impact on cycle • Breast milk excretion
Olanzapine	• Short-term treatment of acute manic episodes in BP I • Effectiveness for long-term use in mania (>4 wk) has not been systematically evaluated in RCT	C	• Limited pregnancy registry data • Hyperprolactinemia • Amenorrhea, frequent AE
Lamotrigine	• Maintenance treatment of BP I disorder to delay the time to occurrence of mood episodes (depression, mania, hypomania, mixed episodes) in patients treated for acute mood episodes with standard therapy • Effectiveness in the acute treatment of mood episodes has not been established	C	• Rate of malformations during first-trimester monotherapy is 2.9% in ongoing pregnancy registry • Breast milk excretion

(Continued)

Table 3.3 • (Continued)

Drug	Indication	Pregnancy Category	Reproductive Issues
Olanzapine/ fluoxetine combination	• Treatment of depressive episodes • Effectiveness beyond 8 weeks has not been established in RCT	C	• No adequate studies in pregnant women
Quetiapine	• Short-term treatment of manic episodes in BP I as either monotherapy or adjunct therapy to lithium or valproate • Effectiveness for long-term use in mania (>3 wk) has not been systematically evaluated in RCT	C	• No adequate studies in pregnant women
Risperidone	• Short-term treatment of acute manic or mixed episodes in BP I as either monotherapy or adjunct therapy to lithium or valproic acid • Effectiveness for long-term (>3 wk) or prophylactic use in mania has not been systematically evaluated in RCT	C	• No adequate and well-controlled studies in pregnant women • One report of a case of agenesis of the corpus callosum in an infant exposed to risperidone in utero
Carbamazepine (extended release)	• Acute mania	D	• Neural tube defects • Same as valproate • Drug interactions • Breast milk excretion

RCT, randomized controlled clinical trial.
*Review latest version of package insert and current literature.
Adapted from Hilty, Leamon, Lim, et al. (2006).

A family history of puerperal psychosis is a strong indicator of risk. Additional risk factors to be aware of include prepartum psychosis, primiparity, and psychophysiological stressors such as preterm delivery, cesarean section, and difficult labor. Suicide risk increases significantly during the first year after childbirth in women with severe postpartum psychiatric episodes.

One episode of postpartum psychosis increases subsequent risk by 50 to 90 percent. Recent expert practice is to restart women on mood-stabilizing medications long before delivery, at 36 weeks gestation, or right after the first trimester to prevent postpartum relapse (Viguera, 2005). Lithium is the most studied and most often used agent in the prophylactic treatment of pregnant and postpartum women.

Women with BP disorder should be informed about the high risk for relapse in the postpartum period. Ask new mothers with depressive symptoms if they feel unusually happy, irritable, or highly energetic at times. The Edinburgh Postnatal Depression Scale (Cox, Holden, and Sagovsky, 1987), a 10-item self-report screening tool that takes about 5 minutes to complete, can help identify postpartum depression. Early referral of vulnerable women to experts in psychiatry and women's reproductive health for management and counseling is important and may greatly reduce the risk of infanticide associated with postpartum psychosis.

Perimenopause and Menopause

There is little information on the effect of menopause on BP disorder. Some women report improvement, some report increased depression or a switch to cycling without periods of euthymia in the perimenopause phase of hormone flux, and some experience no change in their usual mood patterns. Interestingly, women not using hormone replacement therapy (HRT) are significantly more likely to report perimenopausal and menopausal worsening of mood (Freeman et al., 2002), but to date, there are no studies assessing the effects of HRT on BP depression or on the course of BP illness.

TREATMENT INTERVENTIONS FOR WOMEN WITH BIPOLAR DISORDER

Much like other chronic illnesses such as hypertension and diabetes, the goals of treatment for BP disorder include the symptomatic control of acute episodes, the elimination of residual symptoms between episodes, and psychosocial management to increase and maintain functioning of the individual. Increasingly, attention is being paid to relapse and recurrence prevention and the involvement of the patient and family in a collaborative management partnership.

The PCP can have a significant impact on early recognition, intervention, and health maintenance practices of women with BP disorder. First episodes are often seen in the primary care or women's health clinic. Once diagnosed, even when referrals are made, ongoing primary medical care is the norm. Monitoring psychiatric status is an ongoing process and necessary for early detection of recurrence. Assisting a woman in identifying common and individual specific signs and symptoms of emerging episodes empowers her to become an active participant in long-term illness management. A therapeutic alliance with the practitioner encourages acceptance of the diagnosis and active participation in and adherence to the treatment plan. Developing collaborative alliances among interdisciplinary members of the medical/psychiatric treatment team will help the practitioner increase a woman's sense of stability when negotiating an often fragmented health care system.

Women with a serious mental illness often face shame, isolation, self-blame, and doubt. Offering education about the illness and supporting attendance at peer support groups can help her work through stigma issues, fears, denial, and a feeling of isolation and promote a better sense of personal control. Assistance with management of stressors and maintenance of regular patterns of activity, wakefulness, and diet can help her improve mood and stability. Encourage family participation when possible. Explore social and religious support systems available to women as well as community assistance agencies that may be of use for ongoing education, support, and service provision. Maintain regular contact, even if you are not the primary caregiver. Sometimes, the presence of one trusted pivotal practitioner makes the difference between health maintenance and repeated relapse or recurrence.

Biologic Treatment Considerations

Possible gender differences in pharmacokinetics and pharmacodynamics that have been identified between women and men include drug distribution, absorption, metabolism, elimination, and response. Women can experience fluctuations in hepatic metabolic rates related to cyclic changes in reproductive hormones. Because of these differences, it has been proposed that women with BP disorder may show different plasma drug levels, especially in the follicular phase of the menstrual cycle. Decreased secretion of gastric acid and progesterone and fluid retention in the luteal phase affect gastric emptying, reduce absorption, and may affect serum drug concentrations. Longer half-lives of drugs such as lithium may occur in women because of slower renal elimination. Women are, therefore, more likely to experience more side effects as a consequence and be at greater risk for toxicity than men.

Unfortunately, studies that have been done to evaluate the reproductive cycle effects on women with mood disorders are still preliminary, often confounded by methodologic problems, and findings have been mixed or contradictory. Most of the studies focused on unipolar depression, so little evidence with clinical utility exists on women with BP disorder.

OCs reduce the activity of some hepatic cytochrome P450 enzymes, which may lead to higher concentrations of some of the atypical antipsychotics used to treat BP disorder, such as olanzapine (Zyprexa). Several anticonvulsants used to treat mood swings lower the efficacy of OCs; carbamazepine (Tegretol), oxcarbazepine (Trileptal), and topiramate (Topamax) accelerate the clearance of OCs, thereby reducing their effectiveness (Baldassano, Guille, Truman, et al., 2002).

Clinical Considerations

Drug interactions are possible, especially with the combination drug regimens often prescribed for complicated cases like rapid cycling disorder, mixed states, and BP depression. Clinicians should stress the importance of the patient maintaining an up-to-date list of all currently prescribed, over-the-counter, and alternative or contemporary substances and sharing the list with all health care providers (Box 3.4).

Treating Bipolar Depression

Depressive symptoms contribute more to the psychosocial disability associated with BP disorder than mania or hypomania. BP depression is actually a more

Box 3.4 • General Tips for Advising Women with Bipolar Disorder

- Regularly review the patient's medications with her. You may be the first to discover serious or life-threatening drug or drug–food combinations.
- Advise women that abruptly stopping many psychotherapeutic medications can result in an unpleasant withdrawal-like syndrome.
- Keep in mind that women who have a diagnosis of BP disorder are, above all, women. Consider the effect a diagnosis of a lifelong chronic, recurrent illness has on their life and sense of self. Allow them to talk about fears and concerns. All aspects of a woman's life may be affected, such as sexuality and intimate relationships, parenting, work aspirations, and life goals. Take care not to view patients as a diagnosis or an anomaly.

significant problem than elevated mood states. Significantly more time is spent in a depressed state than in hypomanic or manic state in all BP diagnostic categories, and it takes longer to recover from a depressive episode. Effective management of depressive episodes is the greater clinical challenge (Thase, 2006). The bulk of research on BP medication treatments has centered on management of mania, and only recently has BP depression been actively addressed.

There is a growing concern that many women who seek treatment for depression may be misidentified as having unipolar depression when they actually are in a state of BP depression. Early introduction of antidepressants and delay in adding mood stabilizers may induce cycling and worsen the course of the illness (Goldberg and Ernst, 2002). Along with this concern is the lack of supportive evidence for efficacy and safety of traditional antidepressants in BP depression. In the recent Systematic Treatment Enhancement Program for Bipolar Disorder (STEP-BP) trials, the highest rates of mood switching were associated with SSRIs (Ostacher, 2006). Treatment guidelines recommend adding antidepressants late in therapy for treatment-resistant depression and then only in conjunction with a mood stabilizer. The only combination approved for use in the United States is olanzapine and fluoxetine (Prozac) (Tohen, Vieta, Calabrese, et al., 2003).

Lamotrigine, an antiepileptic, has been found to be effective in patients with BP I depression and has been approved for this indication (Keck, Perlis, Otto, et al., 2004). Most clinicians will start with either lithium or lamotrigine. Electroconvulsive therapy (ECT) is considered especially if there is a serious risk of suicide. ECT is effective, works rapidly, and is the safest treatment in the first trimester of pregnancy (Hirschfeld, Bowden, Gitlin, et al., 2002; Pearson, Nonacs, and Cohen, 2002).

Medication Guidelines

The Expert Consensus Guideline Series (Keck et al., 2004) and the APA (Hirschfeld et al., 2002) have published practice guidelines for the treatment of BP disorder, citing the most current evidence-based research on medications approved for treating BP disorder. Recent publications based on early results of the STEP-BP clinical trial add additional data for clinical practice management of acute manic and mixed episodes in a systematic manner (Sachs, 2006). The STEP-BP guidelines allow for customized treatment strategies in alternative pathways. Rather than designate a particular drug, classes of medications are indicated, and choices can be individualized to improve effectiveness and reduce adverse events.

The medications listed in Table 3.4 have received Food and Drug Administration approval for the indications listed. Treatment selections are based on

Table 3.4 • Guidelines for Treatment of Mood Episodes in Bipolar Disorder

Episode Type	American Psychiatric Association*	Consensus Guideline**
Mania—euphoric	Lithium	Lithium or valproate
Mania—mild or moderate	Lithium or valproate	Lithium or valproate
Mania—severe	Valproate or lithium with AAP	Valproate and AAP
Mania—mixed	Valproate	Lithium Valproate and AAP
Rapid cycling—depression	Mood stabilizer	Lamotrigine or lamotrigine/lithium
Rapid cycling—mania	Mood stabilizer	Valproate or valproate/AAP
Depression—mild or moderate	Optimize mood stabilizer	Not addressed
Depression—severe	Mood stabilizer and SSRI Mood stabilizer or ECT	Not addressed

AAP, atypical antipsychotic; SSRI, selective serotonin reuptake inhibitor; ECT, electroconvulsive therapy.
*From the American Psychiatric Association (APA) (2002).
**From Keck, P., Perlis, R., Otto, M., et al. (2004).

efficacy data; tolerability varies. Skilled clinical management involves balancing known efficacy and tolerability to optimize treatment outcomes. Factors that influence the selection of medication are target symptoms, side effects, ease of adherence, cost and access to medications, and patient or family history of response. Often, combination strategies with off-label use of mood-stabilizing and atypical antipsychotic agents are implemented, but clinical practice precedes the research database in this area.

Lithium Lithium (lithium carbonate, Lithobid) is the oldest mood stabilizer and perhaps still the most effective for mania and suicide prevention. Blood levels must be kept in a therapeutic range and checked periodically to avoid toxicity and maintain effectiveness. Thyroid and kidney functions must be monitored. Side effects include nausea, vomiting and diarrhea, tremors, concentration and memory problems, sexual function changes, and increased thirst and urination.

Weight gain, hair loss, and thyroid deficiency may be of special concern when treating women. Annual serum electrolytes, thyroid-stimulating hormone, and calcium levels are recommended as well as electrocardiography for women over the age of 40 years or those with heart disease.

Valproate Valproate (Depakote, Depakene) is a widely used mood stabilizer and the first antiepileptic with indication for BP disorder. Side effects include nausea, diarrhea, drowsiness, tremors, rarely leucopenia, thrombocytopenia, pancreatitis, and hepatotoxity. Tolerance may develop.

Weight gain, alopecia, fluid retention, menstrual abnormalities, and potential polycystic ovaries may be of special concern for women. Laboratory monitoring includes serum drug levels to ensure adequate dosing, baseline and regular liver function tests, and complete blood count at 3, 6, and 12 months, then yearly.

Lamotrigine Lamotrigine (Lamictal) has a relatively low side-effect profile; most common is headache, nausea, and dry skin. A serious and potentially fatal drug rash, Stevens-Johnson syndrome occurs in 1 of 1,000 adults. Therefore, the drug must be started at a low dose and slowly titrated up over 6 weeks to reduce the risk. No laboratory data are required or helpful. Gender differences have not been studied.

Antipsychotics Atypical antipsychotics, including olanzapine (Zyprexa), quetiapine (Seroquel), risperidone (Risperdal), are approved for mania and are used in BP depression for psychosis and insomnia. Side effects are sedation, akathisia, dry mouth, headache, and a low incidence of tardive dyskinesia. Extrapyramidal side effects and hyperprolactinemia (and associated menstrual dysfunction) may occur with Risperidone.

Abnormalities in glucose regulation have been suggested in persons with BP disorder. Risk for weight gain, diabetes, and hyperlipidemia is linked with atypical antipsychotics. Women are especially vulnerable to the metabolic syndrome, which is a major health risk for heart disease, stroke, and type 2 diabetes. The American Diabetes Association and APA encourage practitioners to monitor persons taking antipsychotic drugs and to watch for signs of insulin resistance. Metabolic effects can be monitored by assessing weight, body mass index, glucose, cholesterol, and high-density lipoprotein (HDL) levels. The set of health risks for women includes at least three of the following: (1) a waist larger than 35 inches, (2) HDL cholesterol under 50 mg/dL, (3) triglycerides above 150 mg/dL, (4) blood pressure above 130/85, and (5) fasting blood glucose level higher than 110 mg/dL (or use of medication for diabetes).

Psychotherapeutic Considerations

The addition of psychotherapeutic treatments as an adjunct to medication is clinically beneficial, improving outcomes and adherence to long-term treatment plans. Brief evidence-based therapies contribute to significant improvements in the quality of life of individuals with BP disorder and their families. Cognitive behavioral, interpersonal, and social rhythm therapy; family-focused psychoeducation; and group therapies are the empirically tested recommendations for BP disorders (Johnson and Leahy, 2004).

Consumer advocacy and self-help organizations complement the mental health system and offer social support; a meaningful sense of belonging and self-efficacy; and an accepting, destigmatizing environment for women. Clinicians are well advised to refer women and their significant others for psychotherapy as part of a comprehensive treatment plan.

CONCLUSION

Only recently have investigators begun to consider the important gender differences that impact the diagnosis and treatment of BP disorder in women. Reports that include data specific to women are few and sometimes contradictory. Yet, the trend is toward more depth of investigation into the etiology, course, and treatment specific to women with BP disorder.

It appears that women are at risk for the most severe and debilitating forms of BP disorder. Symptoms are unrecognized and remain untreated for a longer period of time in women than men. The fact that women most often present with depression in the first episode may explain this finding. This observation and the increased propensity for women to develop mixed states and a rapid cycling pattern point to the importance of a routine in-depth history and psychiatric evaluation prior to initiation of antidepressant medications.

Monitoring for mood shifts and substance use should be part of ongoing care. Educating women in signs, symptoms, and features of BP disorder and engaging them in mood charting, especially in relation to the menstrual cycle, will assist in developing a collaborative partnership in the monitoring and maintenance of stability. When evidence for BP return is found, women should be referred to a psychiatric practitioner for further evaluation. Establishing a collaborative connection with a psychiatric practitioner will assist the primary care or woman's health practitioner with handling difficult diagnostic and treatment issues in the women they care for.

Clinicians can improve their diagnostic assessment skills by becoming familiar with the *DSM-IV-TR* criteria for manic, hypomanic, and major depressive episodes. Remember that mania and hypomania consist of clusters of signs and symptoms. Mood swings alone are relatively nonspecific for a diagnosis, much like chest pain in the absence of other signs does not differentiate angina from other possible causes.

Skillful and comprehensive interview techniques are necessary to elicit important, often missed information. Ask about hypomania preceding or following a depression, particularly if it is a first episode or in a young woman. Interview the family if possible to obtain information the woman may avoid reporting or is unaware of. Family history of mania or manic-like symptoms is a good predictor of BP II.

There is increasing evidence for gender differences in a number of reproductive-related events that may have relevance for management, but research in this area is lacking. There are still many uncertainties, including the impact of menopause on BP mood shifts, the effects of HRT, and the relationship of gender to the side effects of medications being used in treatment. Further research is needed before there is sufficient evidence to inform clinical practice.

A wide range of pharmacotherapy options now exist for managing BP disorder. BP illness in women may include manic, hypomanic, mixed states, and major depression as well as psychosis, coexisting anxiety disorders, substance abuse, attention deficit disorder, and comorbid medical conditions, not to mention multiple medications, adverse side effects, and problems with adherence. When the varied and often complicated course of the illness is considered, it is evident that management of severe BP illness is best referred to the experts. Once a treatment is established and the woman is stable, medication management may be continued or overseen by the primary care practitioner in consultation with a psychiatrist.

PCPs are in a position to identify vulnerable women and catch signs of depression and hypomania early, especially because they may see women over the course of their lives and can monitor changes in a woman's psychological and physiologic state. A woman's relationship with her PCP has the potential to improve adherence to ongoing collaborative treatment management and improve ultimate outcomes. It is hoped that information gleaned here will assist clinicians in this task.

Resources for Providers

American Psychiatric Association's Practice Guidelines: *www.psych.org/psych_pract/treatg/pg/prac_guide.cfm*

Edinburgh Postnatal Depression Scale: *www.drgrelling.com/Downloads.htm*
http://health.utah.gov/rhp/pdf/EPDS.pdf

Massachusetts General Hospital Bipolar Clinical and Research Program:
www.manicdepressive.org

Bipolar Disorder Resource Center, Medscape *www.medscape.com*

Mood and Anxiety Disorders Institute: *www.mghmadi.org*

Systematic Treatment Enhancement Program for Bipolar Disorder: *www.stepbd.org*

References

American Psychiatric Association (APA). (2000). *Diagnostic and statistical manual of mental disorders* (Revised 4th ed.). Washington, DC: Author.

Arnold, L. M., McElroy, S. L., & Keck, P. E. (2000). The role of gender in mixed mania. *Comprehensive Psychiatry, 153*, 163–173.

Baldassano, C. F. (2006). Illness course, comorbidity, gender, and suicidality in patients with bipolar disorder. *Journal of Clinical Psychiatry, 67*(Suppl 11), 8–11.

Baldassano, C. F., Guille, C., Truman, C. J., et al. (2002). Gender differences in bipolar mood disorder and implications for treatment. In D. H. Pearson, S. B. Sonawalla, & J. F. Rosenbaum (Eds.), *Women's Health and Psychiatry* (pp. 57–65). Philadelphia: Lippincott Williams & Wilkins.

Barnes, C., & Mitchell, P. (2005). Considerations in the management of bipolar disorder in women. *Australian and New Zealand Journal of Psychiatry, 39*, 662.

Calabrese, J. R., Muzina, D. J., Kemp, D. E., et al. (2006). Predictors of bipolar disorder risk among patients currently treated for major depression. *Medscape General Medicine*. Retrieved August 15, 2006, from *www.medscape.com*.

Cox, J. L., Holden, J. M., & Sagovske, R. (1987). Detection of postnatal depression: Development of the 10-item Edinburgh Postnatal Depression Scale. *British Journal of Psychiatry, 150*, 782–786.

Curtis, V. (2005). Women are not the same as men: Specific clinical issues for female patients with bipolar disorder. *Bipolar Disorder*, 7(Suppl 1), 16–24.

Endicott, J., & Harrison, W. (1990). *Daily Record of Severity of Problems form*. New York: Department of Research Assessment and Training, New York State Psychiatric Institute.

Freeman, M. P., & Gelenberg, A. J. (2005). Bipolar disorder in women: Reproductive events and treatment considerations. *Acta Psychiatrica Scandinavica, 112*(2), 88–96.

Freeman, M. P., Wosnitzer-Smith, K., Freeman, S., et al. (2002). The impact of reproductive events on the course of bipolar disorder in women. *Journal of Clinical Psychiatry, 63*, 284–287.

Frye, M. A., Altshuler, L. I., McElroy, S. L., et al. (2003). Gender differences in prevalence, risk, and clinical correlates of alcoholism co-morbidity in bipolar disorder. *American Journal of Psychiatry, 160*, 883–889.

Goldberg, J. F, & Ernst, C. L. (2002). Features associated with the delayed initiation of mood stabilizers at illness onset in bipolar disorder. *Journal of Clinical Psychiatry, 63*(11), 958–991.

Hilty, D. M., Leamon, M. L., Lim, R. F., et al. (2006). Diagnosis and treatment of bipolar disorder in the primary care setting. *Primary Psychiatry, 13*(7), 77–85.

Hirschfeld, R. M. A., Bowden, C. L., Gitlin, M. J., et al. (2002). Practice guidelines for the treatment of patients with bipolar disorder (revision). *American Journal of Psychiatry, 159*(Suppl), 1–35.

Hirschfeld, R. M., Williams, J. B., Spitzer, R. L., et al. (2000). Development and validation of a screening instrument for bipolar spectrum disorder: The Mood Disorder Questionnaire. *American Journal of Psychiatry, 157*, 1873–1875.

Joffe, H., Kim, D. R., Foris, J. M., et al. (2006). Menstrual dysfunction prior to onset of psychiatric illness is reported more commonly by women with bipolar disorder than by women with unipolar depression and healthy controls. *Journal of Clinical Psychiatry, 67*(2), 297–304.

Johnson, S. L., & Leahy, R. L. (Eds.). (2004). *Psychological treatment of bipolar disorder.* New York: Guilford Press.

Keck, P. E., Perlis, R., Otto, M., et al. (2004). The Expert Consensus Guidelines series: Medication treatment of bipolar disorder. *Postgraduate Medicine Special Report,* 1–120. Retrieved August 15, 2006, from *www.psychguides.com.*

Keller, M. B. (2006). Prevalence and impact of comorbid anxiety and bipolar disorder. *Journal of Clinical Psychiatry, 67*(Suppl 1), 5–7.

Kessler, R. C., Bergland, P., Demler, O., et al. (2005). Lifetime prevalence and age-of-onset distributions of *DSM-IV* disorders in the National Comorbidity Survey Replication. *Archives of General Psychiatry, 62*, 593–602.

Krishnan, K. R. R. (2005). Psychiatric and medical comorbidities of bipolar disorder. *Psychosomatic Medicine, 67*, 1–8.

McElroy, S. L. (2004). Bipolar disorders: Special diagnostic and treatment considerations in women. *CNS Spectrums, 9*(8 Suppl 7), 5–18.

Ostacher, M. J. (2006). The evidence for antidepressant use in bipolar depression. *Journal of Clinical Psychiatry, 67*(Suppl 11), 18–21.

Pearson, K. H., Nonacs, R., & Cohen, L. S. (2002). Practical guidelines for the treatment of psychiatric disorders during pregnancy. In K. H. Pearson, S. B. Sonawalla, & J. F. Rosenbaum (Eds.), *Women's health and psychiatry*. Philadelphia: Lippincott Williams & Wilkins.

Power, M. (Ed.). (2004). *Mood disorders a handbook of science and practice.* Hoboken, NJ: John Wiley & Sons, Ltd.

Sachs, G. S. (2006). Implementing evidence-based treatment of manic and mixed episodes. *Journal of Clinical Psychiatry, 67*(Suppl 11), 112–117.

Schneck, C. D. (2006). Treatment of rapid-cycling bipolar disorder. *Journal of Clinical Psychiatry, 67*(Suppl 11), 22–27.

Simon, G. E., Von Korff, M., Saunders, K., et al. (2006). Association between obesity and psychiatric disorders in the US adult population. *Archives of General Psychiatry, 63*, 824–830.

Spitzer, R. L., Williams, J. B. W., Kroenke, K., et al. (1994). Utility of a new procedure for diagnosing mental disorders in primary care. The PRIME-MD 1000 Study. *Journal of the American Medical Association, 272*, 1749–1756.

Thase, M. E. (2006). Antidepressants and bipolar I affective disorder. *Medscape Psychiatry & Mental Health 11*(1) © 2006 Medscape. Retrieved April 10, 2006, from *www.medscape.com/nurses.*

Tohen, M., Vieta, E., Calabrese, J., et al. (2003). Efficacy of olanzapine and olanzapine-fluoxetine combination in the treatment of bipolar I depression. *Archives of General Psychiatry, 60*(11), 1079–1088.

Viguera, A. C. (2005). Bipolar disorders and women: Special considerations. An expert interview with Adele Casals Viguera, MD. *Medscape Psychiatry & Mental Health, 8(1)*. Retrieved July 18, 2005, from *www.medscape.com/viewarticol/506804.*

Viguera, A. C., Cohen, L. S., Bouffard B. A., et. al. (2002). Reproductive decisions by women with bipolar disorder after pregnancy psychiatric consultation. *The American Journal of Psychiatry, 159*, 2102–2104.

Viguera, A. C., Nonacs, R., Cohen, L. S., et al. (2000). Risk of recurrence of bipolar disorder in pregnant and non-pregnant women after discontinuation lithium maintenance. *American Journal of Psychiatry, 157*, 179–184.

Weissman, M. M. (1996). Cross-national epidemiology of major depression and bipolar disorders: Comparison of women and men. *Journal of the American Medical Association, 76*, 293–299.

Joan C. Urbancic
Sharon Moser

chapter 4

Anxiety Disorders

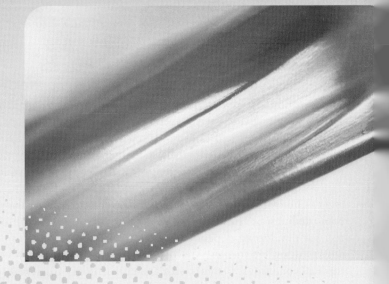

Anxiety disorders are the most common psychiatric disorder seen in primary care practice. Approximately 25 percent of the U.S. population will have an anxiety disorder during their lifetime, and a majority of this group will have a concurrent anxiety disorder or other comorbidity, such as depression. On a yearly basis, 30 million Americans will have an anxiety disorder. Women tend to have twice the rate of anxiety disorders of men. Pollock and Kuo (2004) reported that 6 percent of men and 13 percent of women will have an anxiety disorder within a 6-month period. Most significantly, only about 30 percent of these individuals will seek treatment for their disorders. Children are not exempt: about 13 percent of them also suffer from anxiety disorders each year (Satcher, Delgado, and Masand, 2005). The estimated yearly cost of anxiety disorders is $40 billion, and this cost does not take into account the diminished quality of life and loss of personal and professional growth and development.

This chapter covers the anxiety disorders most commonly seen in primary care settings. These include panic disorders (with and without agoraphobia), phobias, social anxiety disorder (SAD), obsessive-compulsive disorder (OCD), acute stress disorder (ASD), posttraumatic stress disorder (PTSD), and generalized anxiety disorder (GAD). Table 4.1 contains a list of medications most commonly prescribed for the treatment of some of these disorders.

ANXIETY DISORDERS

Anxiety disorders are described as conditions with pathologic levels of fear that cause great distress to the sufferer. As with depression, the anxious patient seen in primary care settings does not often realize that she is anxious; instead, the anxiety is expressed on a somatic level that may involve cardiovascular, respiratory, muscular, gastrointestinal, and genitourinary symptoms. Anxiety often precedes depression, and when it is a comorbidity, the depression is usually more severe and disabling. Suicide is an important consideration, particularly in patients with comorbidities. Because of the distress, patients with anxiety disorders are at great risk for developing dependencies on alcohol or other substances. In general, anxiety disorders increase the risk for a wide variety of psychopathologies and medical conditions. Patients with anxiety disorders are at risk for hypertension, arthritis, asthma, irritable bowel, migraines, and eating disorders.

Because of multiple comorbidities, anxiety disorders may be overlooked or misdiagnosed. Satcher et al. (2005) emphasized that anxiety disorders are often presented differently in primary care settings than in a psychiatrist office; that is, they are often subsyndromal, with symptoms not sufficiently severe to warrant a

Table 4.1 • Therapeutic Profile of Common Medications for Anxiety Disorders

Drug	Panic Disorder	SAD	OCD	PTSD	GAD	Major Depression
SSRIs	++++*	++++*	++++	++++*	++++*	++++
Venlafaxine	++++	++++	+++	++	+++	++++
Tricyclics	++++	++++	++++**,*** NE	+++	++++	++++
Buspirone	NE	++++	+	+	++++	++
Mirtazapine	+++	++	+/NE	+++	++	++++
Bupropion	++	?	?	NE	?	++++
Duloxetine	?	?	?	?	?	++++

++++, FDA approved; +++, efficacy in >1 placebo-controlled trials; ++, many open trials; +, few cases reported; NE, not effective; ?, no data.
*Desipramine not effective.
**Not all SSRIs FDA approved.
***Clomipramine effective.
From Satcher, D., Delgado, P. L., & Masand, P. S. (2005); American Psychiatric Association (APA), *www.psych.org/cme*.

Diagnostic and Statistical Manual of Mental Disorders (*DSM-IV-TR*) diagnosis. Nevertheless, the symptoms are often emotionally crippling and have a significant effect on morbidity. Also, anxiety disorders occur commonly across all cultures and ethnic groups, so the primary care provider (PCP) needs to consider a diagnosis of anxiety disorders and/or depression in patients that present with multiple unexplained somatic symptoms. The greater the number of these symptoms, the more likely an anxiety disorder, depression, or both are present.

Etiology

Anxiety disorders are based on the complex interaction of multiple factors including genetics, biology, life experiences, resiliency, support systems, and coping strategies and skills. While genetic vulnerabilities are important, an environmental trigger seems to be necessary for the anxiety disorder to develop (Satcher et al., 2005). According to Starcevic (2006), it is not clear if anxiety disorders are several distinct diagnostic entities or one broader syndrome with loose boundaries among the various disorders.

Distinguishing Between Anxiety and Depression

Anxiety disorders and depression are a serious challenge to the PCP, and these disorders often occur together (40 percent of patients with anxiety disorders also have depression). Their symptoms tend to overlap, and both present with somatic complaints and simulate medical conditions. Both depression and anxiety are frequently chronic and have great stigma, comorbidity, and subsyndromal disorders. They also may require higher doses of medication in combination with psychotherapy, but patients might still not achieve remission (Susman, 2005).

Because of their overlapping symptoms, anxiety states and depression may be difficult to distinguish; however, there are a few distinguishing characteristics that can be seen in each disorder. Depression occurs in late adolescence or early adulthood and usually develops into a chronic, recurring episodic condition. Conversely, anxiety occurs in childhood and early adulthood, and once it is established, it becomes persistent and continuous. People with depression are rarely disturbed by the hypervigilance that is characteristic of anxiety disorders, while the anxious patient will typically not have the depressed mood, sense of hopelessness, and guilt common in depression (Culpepper, 2004). However, when depression and anxiety are comorbid, patients will have more severe symptoms, increased use of health care services, poorer response to treatment, a more chronic course, and a greater threat of suicide. Table 4.2 identifies the most

Table 4.2 • Distinguishing Characteristics of Depression and Anxiety Disorders

Depression	Anxiety Disorders	Depression and Anxiety
Depressed mood	Hypervigilance	Apprehension/fear
Hopelessness	Helplessness	Somatic symptoms
Weight gain	Phobias	Worrying (unrealistic)
Loss of interest/pleasure	Rituals	Agitation & irritability
Guilt		Poor concentration
		Insomnia
		Fatigue
		Suicide risk

Adapted from Culpepper, L. (2004).

Box 4.1 • Common Conditions to Rule Out When Diagnosing Anxiety and Depression

Substance abuse: Amphetamines, cocaine, alcohol

Prescription medications: Beta-adrenergics, anticholinergics, SSRIs, steroids

OTC medications: Ephedrine, caffeine, anabolic steroids

Herbal remedies: Ephedra (Ma Huang)

From Susman, J. L. (2005).

important distinguishing characteristics between depression and anxiety states as well as their overlapping features.

Anxiety and depression must not be a diagnosis of exclusion. Susman (2005) emphasized the need to aggressively treat anxiety and depression if the patient meets the criteria rather than trying to exclude every possible medical condition first; one can continue to search for possible medical comorbidities while treating the anxiety and depression. Box 4.1 identifies common possibilities to rule out in the diagnosis of anxiety and depression (Susman, 2005).

Risk of Suicide

Individuals with anxiety disorders are at increased risk for suicide. Susman (2005) reported that a person with PTSD, GAD, or panic disorder has a risk odds ratio of 6 to 1. For uncomplicated depression, the risk for suicide is 8 percent. But when anxiety and depression are both present, the risk for suicide increases to approximately 20 percent (Susman). The comorbidity of depression and anxiety increases the chronicity of the disorders, the severity of symptoms, impairment, and the response to treatment.

Ethnicity and Culture

In general, culture exerts a significant role in the treatment of anxiety disorders for both the patient and the provider. For the provider, culture influences the way patients are diagnosed and treated as well as how services are organized and financed. Because patients with anxiety disorders have distorted or exaggerated perceptions of reality, one must be able to communicate effectively to address these beliefs and help them with their problems.

Another important aspect of ethnicity is pharmacotherapeutics of treatment. Some ethnic groups view medication for mental health problems as stigmatizing, which may influence the patient's decision about accepting medication. Another consideration is the polymorphisms in hepatic cytochrome enzymes (CYP) among various ethnic groups. Because psychotropic medications are metabolized chiefly through the CYP system, a range of effects can occur across different ethnic groups. These factors are important considerations when developing treatment plans for patients (American Psychiatric Association [APA], 2004).

PANIC DISORDER AND PANIC ATTACKS

Panic disorder is a common anxiety disorder that affects approximately 3 to 8 percent of the world's population (Feusner, Cameron, and Bystritsky, 2005). It can be devastating and crippling to the affected. The disorder occurs more frequently among women than men, and the average age group in which it occurs is early adulthood, although it may occur in late adolescence. Like depression, panic disorder is most commonly diagnosed in primary care settings, with patient complaints focusing on physical symptoms such as chest pain, tachycardia, and dyspnea. Because of their many somatic complaints, patients with panic disorder seek treatment but are often undiagnosed. Typically, the undiagnosed anxiety disorder causes the medical problems to worsen.

Panic Attacks

Panic attacks are discrete events that are characterized by intense fear and a variety of somatic symptoms. People experiencing a panic attack may have a sense of impending doom, believe they are dying, or losing all control. A panic attack will occur without warning and without any obvious danger under a variety of medical, substance abuse, and mental health conditions. It will typically last 10 minutes or less but in rare cases can continue in waves for 2 hours. The *DSM-IV-TR* (APA, 2000) requires at least 4 of 13 somatic or cognitive symptoms to be present for the diagnosis (Box 4.2). Attacks that do not meet the criteria are commonly labeled as limited-symptom attacks.

The *DSM-IV-TR* (APA, 2000) identifies three types of panic attacks: unexpected (uncued), situationally bound, and situationally predisposed. With the unexpected panic attack, the person is not able to make any connection between internal or external triggers and is caught by surprise. (The unexpected panic attack is a requirement for the diagnosis of panic disorder.) The situationally

Box 4.2 • *DSM-IV-TR* Criteria for Panic Attacks

A discrete period of intense fear or discomfort, in which *four (or more)* of the following symptoms developed abruptly and reached a peak within 10 minutes.

1. Palpitations, pounding heart, or accelerated heart rate
2. Sweating
3. Trembling or shaking
4. Sensations of shortness of breath or smothering
5. Feeling of choking
6. Chest pain or discomfort
7. Nausea or abdominal distress
8. Feeling dizzy, unsteady, lightheadedness, or faint
9. Derealization (feelings of unreality) or depersonalization
10. Fear of losing control or going crazy
11. Fear of dying
12. Paresthesias (numbness or tingling sensations)
13. Chills or hot flushes

Adapted from the American Psychiatric Association (APA) (2000).

bound attack is the opposite in that the person expects to have an attack when exposed to the causative trigger and almost always does so. The situationally predisposed panic attack is similar to the situationally bound attack in that the person anticipates the attack after being exposed to the trigger, but the attack does not invariably occur.

Panic Disorder

Panic disorder consists of repeated, unexpected panic attacks. It is further characterized by persistent fear about having these attacks such that the fear of future attacks becomes an extremely disabling factor in the lives of those with the disorder. According to *DSM-IV-TR* criteria for panic disorder, after the unexpected panic attack, the person must have *at least 1 month* of persistent anxiety and fear

Table 4.3 • Distinguishing Between Panic Attacks and Panic Disorder

Panic Attacks	Panic Disorder
Discrete	Uncued & unpredictable
Intense	Persistent concern
Fear or discomfort	Worry about consequences
Clear peak within 10 minutes	Change in behavior

From Susman, J. L. (2005).

about the prospect of having another attack or demonstrate significant behavioral change because of it. A diagnosis of panic disorder cannot be made if the panic attacks are the result of a medical condition or induced by a substance. With antidepressants, behavioral therapy, or both, patients can recover in 4 to 8 weeks. Keller (2005) has noted that among the anxiety disorders, panic disorder has the most rapid time to recovery and the lowest rate of becoming chronic. However, it also has the highest probability of recurrence. Table 4.3 distinguishes panic attacks and panic disorder.

From a theoretical perspective, Feusner et al. (2005) identified three components of panic disorders: an increase in the alarm reaction, misperceptions in information processing with the outcome of catastrophic thinking, and a pattern of ineffective coping strategies characterized by avoidance behaviors that become ritualistic. These three components represent a sequential process that later may become "wired" neurologically in specific brain structures (Feusner et al., 2005).

Panic disorders have a high incidence of multiple comorbidities, including depression and all of the other anxiety disorders. They are also associated with high incidence of alcohol and substance use disorders as well as use of prescription and nonprescription medications (e.g., antiasthmatics may stimulate panic attacks; Feusner et al., 2005). The presence of comorbidities increases the severity of symptoms and the potential for suicidal behavior.

Panic Disorder with Agoraphobia

Agoraphobia is a common comorbidity of panic disorder. It occurs in approximately 50 percent of patients with panic disorder and is more common in women. The patient with agoraphobia may present with a variety of symptoms such as fear of crowds, public places, or confined spaces from which escape might be difficult. The symptoms experienced when the patient does leave the house alone or goes to public places involves tremors, palpitations, diaphoresis, sometimes chest pain or tightness, air hunger, choking sensations, nausea, dizziness, fear of "going crazy," fear of fainting, and even a fear of death (Hayward, Killen, and Taylor, 2003). Patients may also fear being alone because of the possibility of a panic attack with nobody there to support them. Fear of embarrassment is another significant problem, particularly for women. The agoraphobia combined with the panic disorder results in patients who are reluctant to leave their homes and, thus, they become quite homebound. If they do leave their homes, they must be accompanied by a supportive person and will only tolerate a short period of absence from the safety of their home. Feusner et al. (2005) reported that approximately 25 percent of patients with panic disorder are on disability or welfare.

Assessment of Panic Disorder

In a review of the research on panic disorder, Katon (2006) reported that patients typically undergo multiple medical tests before being diagnosed with panic disorder. However, he emphasized that panic disorder is highly diagnosable and treatable. A patient who presents with severe anxiety and multiple somatic complaints requires a complete assessment to determine the basis for the complaints. A thorough history and physical exam along with laboratory tests and electrocardiogram are necessary to rule out medical conditions that may cause severe anxiety and panic attacks. The patient's medications must also be evaluated for the possibility of causing panic attacks. Table 4.4 describes the differential diagnosis of the most common medical and psychiatric conditions that can mimic panic disorder.

Treatment of Panic Disorder

For patients with panic disorders, high-intensity exercise is more effective than low-intensity. Patients also need to be aware of the association between smoking and panic disorders. Breslau, Novak, and Kessler (2004) reported that smoking cessation could prevent panic disorder and agoraphobia. Cannabis use is also associated with panic attacks and panic disorder and should be avoided (Cloos, 2005).

Pharmacotherapy

Treatment of panic disorder consists of pharmacotherapy, psychotherapy, and psychoeducation. The selective serotonin reuptake inhibitors (SSRIs) are the first-line treatment for panic disorders because of their effectiveness, safety, low

Table 4.4 • Differential Diagnosis of Panic Disorder

Medical Conditions	Psychiatric Conditions
Cardiac conditions 1. Arrhythmias 2. Supraventricular tachycardia 3. Mitral valve prolapse	**Affective disorders** 1. Major depression 2. Bipolar disorder
Endocrine disorders 1. Thyroid abnormalities 2. Hyperparathyroidism 3. Pheochromocytoma 4. Hypoglycemia	**Other anxiety disorders** 1. Acute stress disorder 2. Obsessive-compulsive disorder 3. Posttraumatic stress disorder 4. Social phobia 5. Specific phobia
Vestibular dysfunctions	**Psychotic disorders**
Seizure disorders	**Substance abuse & dependence**
1. Temporal lobe epilepsy	1. Withdrawal from CNS depressants including alcohol, BZDs, & barbiturates
Asthma	2. Stimulants including cocaine, amphetamines, & caffeine

Adapted from Feusner, J., Cameron, M., & Bystritsky, A. (2005).

incidence of side effects, and ability to treat comorbid conditions such as depression and/or other anxiety disorders. These medications do not cause physical dependence (Table 4.1). Although tricyclic antidepressants (TCAs) are also effective, their side-effect profile is higher than the SSRIs. In recent clinical trials, selective serotonin norepinephrine reuptake inhibitors (SNRIs) and mirtazapine (Remeron) have been identified as effective for panic disorder, but only venlafaxine (Effexor) is currently approved by the Food and Drug Administration (FDA). Bupropion (Wellbutrin) was not effective in clinical trials for panic disorder. SSRIs with FDA approval for panic disorder are sertraline (Zoloft), fluoxetine (Prozac), and paroxetine (Paxil); however, fluvoxamine (Luvox), citalopram (Celexa), and escitalopram (Lexapro) have been reported as equally effective (Feusner et al., 2005).

Despite their effectiveness, antidepressants have some drawbacks in the treatment of anxiety disorders. These include serious side effects such as gastrointestinal symptoms, sexual dysfunctions, and agitation as well as a prolonged period of time before the medication becomes effective. Because of the high incidence of increased anxiety and agitation when anxious patients begin treatment with SSRIs, it is critical to start with low doses and gradually titrate to the target dose. High-potency benzodiazepines (BZDs), including clonazepam (Klonopin), alprazolam (Xanax), and lorazepam (Ativan), can be used as an initial supplement to the antidepressant in panic disorder. The BZDs have been found to be effective in panic disorder because they take effect quickly, are well tolerated, and can calm the initial agitation from the SSRIs. However, the BZDs present other problems such as dependence, rebound anxiety, sedation, cognitive impairment, and withdrawal problems. Therefore, BZDs are considered second-line treatment (Cloos, 2005; Starcevic, 2006).

Cognitive Behavioral Therapy

Multiple studies exist that support the effectiveness of cognitive behavioral therapy (CBT) for both acute and long-term treatment of panic disorder. Cloos (2005) reported on the effectiveness of group therapy CBT, virtual reality CBT, and video conferencing with CBT in the treatment of panic disorder.

The goal of CBT for panic disorder is to change the catastrophic thinking of the person in response to bodily sensations. The first steps are to educate the patient about panic disorder and the physiologic mechanisms of anxiety. Next, deep breathing and relaxation exercises are taught and practiced as homework. The patient is also instructed to begin monitoring her thoughts to identify triggers and learn cognitive restructuring. Finally, the patient is exposed to bodily sensations that evoke fear, and gradually the exposure results in habituation and loss of fear to the stimulus. Although panic disorders tend to wax and wane, some patients will attain complete remission while approximately 20 percent of patients will not benefit from any or all treatments (Feusner et al., 2005).

SPECIFIC PHOBIAS

Specific phobia (formerly known as simple phobia) is a persistent, irrational fear of particular objects or situations that the patient understands to be irrational. For a diagnosis of specific phobia, the fear must be sufficiently severe to interfere with the person's functioning (Albucher, 2005). Specific phobias are the most common psychiatric diagnosis among women of all ages. The female-to-male ratio is 2:1, although this varies depending on the specific phobia.

Etiology

It is not always clear how specific phobias originate. Some can be traced to a traumatic life event, but often they coexist with a GAD or panic disorder. It is most likely a combination of factors, including genetic predisposition and traumatic life events. Sometimes, it is the child's modeling behavior of a parental fear. Several theories have been formulated to support a biologic basis for phobic disorders, most determining the cause to be a dysregulation of endogenous biogenic amines. Genetic (twin studies) have shown a repeatedly strong causation in both social phobia and specific phobia, especially blood-injection-injury fear, where two thirds to three fourths of patients have at least one affected first-degree relative (Albucher, 2005).

Types

There are many specific phobias, but the most common ones include a fear of animals (which usually originates in childhood), environmental fears (water, high places, thunderstorms), fear of blood or injections (which tend to run in families), situational phobias (flying, driving, tight spaces) and miscellaneous phobias such as fear of vomiting, choking, and getting sick. Phobias become a problem when they interfere with functions of daily living. Most of the specific phobias start in childhood and are usually outgrown by adulthood. Adult phobias usually date from early childhood (average age 5 years) and continue for many years. A smaller number of specific phobias start in adult life after a very stressful experience. However, if they persist well into the 20s, they do not usually subside without treatment.

Assessment

Phobias are expressed as both a psychological and physical reaction to the object of fear. Patients have feelings of dread or horror when encountering the object or even thinking about it. They understand that their fear of the object is irrational and overblown. They have somatic reactions to the feared object due to sympathetic nervous system activation, with rapid heart rate and palpitations, dyspnea, a tremor, and an urge to flee ("fight or flight" response) that is uncontrollable and overwhelming. Often, the phobic object will trigger a feeling of panic or a full-blown panic attack. Therefore, patients will avoid the object at all costs.

The emotional distress of phobias may lead to other anxiety disorders, major depressive disorders, and substance-related disorders, especially alcohol use disorder. The presence of other disorders should be probed during a thorough psychiatric history. Box 4.3 provides the diagnostic criteria for specific phobias.

Box 4.3 • *DSM-IV-TR* Criteria for Specific Phobia DSM

A. Marked and persistent fear that is excessive or unreasonable, cued by the presence or anticipation of a specific object or situation (e.g., flying, heights, animals, receiving an injection, seeing blood).
B. Exposure to the phobic stimulus almost invariably provokes an immediate anxiety response, which may take the form of a situationally bound or situationally predisposed panic attack.
C. The person recognizes that the fear is excessive or unreasonable.
D. The phobic situation(s) is avoided or else is endured with intense anxiety or distress.
E. The avoidance, anxious anticipation, or distress in the feared situation(s) interferes significantly with the person's normal routine, occupational (or academic) functioning, or social activities or relationships, or there is marked distress about having the phobia.
F. In individuals under age 18 years, the duration is at least 6 months.
G. The anxiety, panic attacks, or phobic avoidance associated with the specific object or situation are not better accounted for by another mental disorder.

Adapted from the American Psychiatric Association (APA) (2000).

Treatment

Phobias are very treatable, and most people successfully overcome their fears with professional help. Therefore, referral to a mental health professional is usually required. Simple phobias are often treated through behavior therapy such as progressive desensitization. With this approach, people with specific phobias are gradually exposed to the anxiety-provoking stimulus until they no longer experience the anxiety. CBT is also important to correct the distorted beliefs that the person may have about the feared stimulus. Medication is sometimes used at the initial stage of confrontation when the anxiety is too high to proceed with the therapy, but it is gradually withdrawn as the patient gains control over her fear and fear reactions. An SSRI antidepressant or a BZP is most frequently utilized.

SOCIAL ANXIETY DISORDER

SAD, also known as social phobia, is the third most common psychiatric disorder in the community after major depression and substance abuse disorders. The lifetime prevalence for SAD is 3 to 13 percent; the age of onset is mid-teens but may occur in childhood (APA, 2000). In community samples, the prevalence is greater in women than men with a ratio of 3 to 2. However, in clinical samples, there is no difference between the sexes in prevalence. A familial pattern seems to exist because people with first-degree biological relatives with SAD are more likely to have the disorder than those in the general population. Individuals with SAD usually do not seek treatment, and when they do, it is not for their SAD but for the secondary problems resulting from SAD, such as panic attacks, depression, and substance abuse (Belzer, McKee, and Liebowitz, 2005). Therefore, because SAD is debilitating and often linked to several other psychiatric problems, it is particularly important for the PCP to recognize and treat this condition with the latest evidence-based interventions. Some researchers have argued that SAD should be viewed as a spectrum, with the most severe cases represented by SAD and/or avoidant personality disorder and the mildest cases encompassing subsyndromal manifestations such as shyness and behavioral inhibition (Schneier, Blanco, Antia, et al., 2002).

Assessment

According to the *DSM-IV-TR*, SAD is characterized by a strong and persistent fear of social or performance situations in which persons fear they will embarrass themselves. Persons with anxiety disorder fear that they will look or sound "stupid" or that people will see them trembling and think they are "weird or sick." When exposed to such situations, the person becomes very anxious and may experience a panic attack. The diagnosis of SAD is only made if the anxiety is sufficiently severe to become disabling and constraining in daily functioning. Typically, the anxiety is accompanied by autonomic symptoms such as sweating, diarrhea, tremors, blushing, muscle tension, and confusion.

If an individual's fears become generalized to most social situations, it is given the subtype diagnosis of "generalized." Most of the people in community samples have the generalized subtype, which is more impairing than a more specific SAD (Belzer et al., 2005). This generalized subtype is highly comorbid with avoidant personality disorder.

Some diagnoses that need to be differentiated from SAD include panic disorder with and without agoraphobia, avoidant personality disorder, and schizoid personality disorder. The 12-item self-report instrument entitled the Brief Fear of Negative Evaluation Scale (BFNE) can be helpful in screening patients with SAD (Collins, Westra, Dozois, et al., 2005). It has validity and reliability in nonclinical samples as well as clinical samples. The items are focused on assessing the person's thoughts related to expectations of being judged harshly in social situations and embarrassing themselves.

However, the simplest screening is the use of two questions recommended by the International Consensus Group on Depression and Anxiety (Susman, 2005):

1. "Are you uncomfortable or embarrassed at being the center of attention?"
2. "Do you find it hard to interact with people?"

Box 4.4 describes the *DSM-IV-TR* diagnostic criteria for SAD/social phobia.

Box 4.4 • *DSM-IV-TR* Criteria for Seasonal Affective Disorder/Social Phobia DSM

A. A marked and consistent fear of a social and/or a performance situation in which the person fears being severely embarrassed or humiliated.

B. Experiencing the social situation leads to anxiety and/or panic attacks.

C. The person realizes that the fear is unrealistic.

D. The person avoids the feared situation or endures it with great distress.

E. The avoidance interferes with the person's daily functioning.

F. In persons under age 18 years, the fear endures for at least 6 months.

G. The fear is not due to direct physiological effects of a medical or another mental condition.

H. If another mental or medical disorder exists, the fear is unrelated to that disorder.

Adapted from the American Psychiatric Association (APA) (2000).

Treatment

Although the severity of SAD can vary depending on life situations, the course of SAD is usually chronic and persistent because these individuals avoid seeking treatment. Consequently, they often progress through life with increasing difficulty and are highly vulnerable to substance abuse, depression, and other anxiety disorders. Treatment consists of both medication and psychotherapy, particularly for patients with the generalized subtype of SAD.

Pharmacotherapy

The first medication to show significant effectiveness was phenelzine (Nardil), a monoamine oxidase inhibitor (MAOI). In four double-blind placebo-controlled studies, phenelzine demonstrated improvement in SAD from 64 to 91 percent. Two other MAOIs were also found to be effective, but because of their serious side effects, the use of MAOIs has been minimal. TCAs, beta-blockers, and buspirone have not shown effectiveness in clinical trials (Keller, 2005). Clinical guidelines recommend the use of SSRIs and SNRIs as first-line treatment for SAD (Belzer et al., 2005). Although all the SSRIs have been effective in double-blind placebo-controlled studies, only sertraline (Zoloft), paroxetine (Paxil), and the SNRI venlafaxine XR (Effexor XR) have FDA approval as first-line treatment for generalized SAD. Currently, escitalopram (Lexapro) is under review for approval by the FDA (Table 4.1).

Generally, a trial of 8 to 12 weeks with a gradual titration to the therapeutic dose is required. The patient should remain on the medication for 6 months to stabilize the clinical improvement. For those patients who do not respond to SSRIs or SNRIs, a medication from another class should be tried. For partial responders, clonazepam (Klonopin) can be used for augmentation.

Two BZDs have also been studied for use in SAD. Alprazolam (Xanax) was compared with phenelzine (Nardil) in a controlled study, but only 38 percent of patients were responders to the alprazolam as compared with 69 percent of the patients receiving the phenelzine. Much better study results were demonstrated with clonazepam (Klonopin), which had a 78 percent response rate as compared with 20 percent receiving the placebo. Traditionally, providers have hesitated to prescribe BZDs because of concerns about abuse potential, sedation, and cognitive and physical impairment as well as the potential for severe problems on discontinuation. However, BZDs are effective because of their rapid onset of action, good tolerability, flexibility in dosing, and safety. Belzer et al. (2005) have emphasized that clinicians will need to assess the benefits of BZDs on an individual basis, as there are no clinical guidelines that favor BZDs over SSRIs for SAD.

Another medication sometimes used for specific SAD is the beta-blocker (e.g., propranolol). It is specifically recommended for use when a person has extreme physiologic arousal to a discrete public event at which they must perform. Two anticonvulsants are also being researched for effectiveness with generalized SAD. Both gabapentin (Neurontin) and pregabalin (Lyrica) have demonstrated superior effectiveness in clinical trials, but both need more research before they can be recommended (Belzer et al., 2005).

Cognitive Behavioral Therapies

A variety of CBTs have been effective in clinical trials in the treatment of SAD. This usually requires referral to an experienced therapist, but many PCPs have taken workshops on the basic principles of CBT and are able to use them effectively. Relaxation, deep breathing, and imagery are used for the severe anxiety and physiologic arousal of SAD. Social skills training for confidence and competency have been effective, as has systematic exposure (a gradual progression to the full anxiety-producing situation). From the cognitive perspective, individuals with SAD have distorted perceptions and expectations of how people will respond to them in the anxiety-provoking situation. It is these beliefs that generate their anxious feelings, so the focus requires cognitive restructuring, a form of CBT, to correct their distorted thinking.

Combining Medication and Psychotherapy

Evidence is mixed for superiority of the combination treatment in comparison to either treatment alone, but many clinicians are optimistic about the combined approach. Large-scale controlled studies that examine various combinations and sequencing are needed before definitive statements can be made.

OBSESSIVE-COMPULSIVE DISORDER

OCD is a disorder that is characterized by recurrent intense obsessions and/or compulsions that cause discomfort, impair the ability to function on a daily basis, and consume a great deal of time. Obsessions are defined as recurrent and persistent thoughts, impulses, or images that are excessive and cause intense anxiety. Usually, the patient understands that she is irrational and ridiculous but is unable to stop them. Compulsions are behaviors that are repeated or ritualistic (e.g., excessive washing of hands, hoarding, or keeping things excessively orderly) or mental acts (e.g., repeatedly reciting the alphabet or a poem, counting to 1,000).

OCD has been described as a heterogenous disorder, and many investigators have found multiple obsessions to be replicable among studies and various population clusters (Allen and Hollander, 2005; Watson and Wu, 2005). There has been much discussion concerning the low prevalence of OCD in the general population that meets full criteria as listed in the *DSM-IV-TR*; most patients fit a subclinical definition of this syndrome.

Prevalence and Contributing Factors

OCD affects approximately 2.2 American adults (Kessler, Chiu, Demler, et al., 2005), and it is the fourth most common mental disorder in the United States. Although OCD can be effectively treated in primary care, less than half of patients receive treatment. It often first becomes a problem in children, adolescents, or in young adults, and it affects men and women equally. Modal age at onset is between ages 6 and 15 years for males and between ages 20 and 29 years for females (Allen and Hollander, 2005). This disorder most often appears as a comorbid condition. OCD was found to exist along with GAD and panic disorder much more often in women (85.6 percent), while in men it was often a comorbidity with bipolar disorder (69.6 percent) (Angst, Gamma, Endrass, et al., 2005). Childhood-onset OCD is more common in males and more likely to be linked genetically with attention deficit hyperactivity disorder (ADHD) and Tourette's disorder.

Many patients may wait years before they seek treatment. In an effort to hide their symptoms from those closest to them as well as their health care practitioners, patients eliminate any support they might receive because of their shame and embarrassment.

Etiology

The precise pathology of OCD is still under question. The bulk of the research in the field points to the abnormal serotonin transmission at the 5-HT receptor sites as the primary disarrangement. There is also abnormal dopamine transmission that has been studied extensively. This explains the symptom response to both SSRIs and neuroleptic agents.

Assessment

A comprehensive medical history should be taken that includes specific questions about the nature and degree of severity of both the obsessive symptoms and compulsive behaviors. The Yale-Brown Obsessive Compulsive Scale (Y-BOCS) can be given to a patient to rate the severity of the symptoms and to track the response to a particular treatment protocol (Allen and Hollander, 2005). The Y-BOCS can be found online. See the Resources for Providers section for more information.

The PCP should be on the alert for psychiatric comorbidities, such as depression, bipolar disorder, GAD, panic disorder, and substance abuse. Body dysmorphic disorder, trichotillomania (hair pulling), and habit problems (e.g., nail biting) have an obsessive-compulsive component and should be investigated, as should any history of ADHD or Tourette's disorder. The physical examination should be done to rule out medical conditions that could be causing the disorder, focusing especially on the neurologic system. Any focal neurologic symptoms or cognitive impairments should warrant a full workup for delirium, dementia, or other organic causes for OCD such as pervasive developmental disorder and mental retardation.

Some infectious causes for OCD have been studied. Cases have appeared in both children and adults after an acute group A streptococcal infection or herpes viral outbreak. Some women only have OCD during pregnancy or symptoms worsen during pregnancy. Other women experience a worsening during their premenstrual cycle (Allen and Hollander, 2005). Box 4.5 contains diagnostic criteria for OCD.

Differential Diagnosis

OCD has been found to coexist with both bipolar I and II and minor bipolar disorders, GADs, and panic disorder but not with depressive disorders or phobias other than social phobia (Angst et al., 2005). The "fear" component of OCD is often a component in PTSD, panic disorder, and agoraphobia; therefore, they should all be considered and explored in a differential diagnosis. A patient with bipolar disorder would experience a strong affective component, cycling from major depression to hypomania/mania. Some OCD symptomatology may appear during distressful exacerbations, but the affective component is prevalent and meets diagnostic criteria as outlined in Box 4.5 (APA, 2000). GADs have a "free-floating" anxiety component as the prevalent symptom.

Treatment

Psychosocial Interventions

Historically, clinicians have used monotherapies consisting either of CBT with Exposure and Ritual Prevention (EX/RP) or pharmacotherapy. EX/RP is dependent on effective skills of a trained therapist. Multiple studies have

Box 4.5 • *DSM-IV-TR* Criteria for Obsessive-Compulsive Disorder

DSM

A. Either obsessions or compulsions:

Obsessions as defined by (1), (2), (3), & (4):

1. Recurrent and persistent thoughts, impulses, or images that are experienced as intrusive and inappropriate and that cause marked anxiety or distress.
2. These thoughts are not simply excessive worries.
3. The person tries to ignore or suppress such thoughts, impulses, or images.
4. The person recognizes that the obsessional thoughts, impulses, or images are a product of his or her mind (not imposed from without as in thought insertion).

Compulsions as defined by (1) & (2):

1. Repetitive behaviors that the person feels driven to perform in response to an obsession, or according to rules that must be applied rigidly.
2. Behaviors or mental acts are aimed at preventing or reducing distress or preventing some dreaded event or situation.

B. At some point during the course of the disorder, the person has recognized that the obsessions or compulsions are excessive or unreasonable.

C. The obsessions or compulsions cause marked distress, are time-consuming, or significantly interfere with the person's normal routine and functioning.

D. If another Axis I disorder is present, the content of the obsessions or compulsions is not restricted to that disorder.

E. The disturbance is not due to the direct physiologic effects of a substance (e.g., a drug of abuse, a medication) or a general medical condition.

Adapted from the American Psychiatric Association (APA) (2000).

found CBT to be as effective or possibly more effective than medications (Foa, Liebowitz, and Kozak, 2005). Cognitively, the patient learns to correct distorted thinking about the fear of danger concerning the stimulus. Behaviorally, the patient learns to confront the feared stimulus without resorting to compulsive rituals. Thus, the focus is on exposure to the stimulus and prevention of subsequent ritualistic behavior. Once the obsessions and compulsions are overcome and treatment completed, the patient can return for booster sessions.

Psychopharmacotherapy

According to Allen and Hollander (2005), six SSRIs (citalopram [Celexa], fluoxetine [Prozac], fluvoxamine [Luvox], escitalopram [Lexapro], sertraline [Zoloft], and paroxetine [Paxil]) are uniquely effective in OCD. Two SNRIs, venlafaxine (Effexor) and clomipramine (Anafranil), a TCA, and an SNRI are also effective (Table 4.5). Although these medications are highly effective in gaining significant responses (40 to 60 percent), none of them results in remission, nor has any of these medications been more successful than the others, although individual patients may respond better to one than the others. Some research has suggested that clomipramine is more effective than the others, but more studies are needed to support this contention. Also, clomipramine has more adverse effects than the other medications, particularly anticholinergic and adrenergic effects (Allen and Hollander, 2005). In general, time required for a treatment response to OCD is longer, and higher doses of medications are required than with other anxiety disorders.

Table 4.5 • Medications and Dosages for Obsessive-Compulsive Disorder

Generic Name	Brand Name	Lowest Recommended Dose for OCD	Highest FDA-Approved Dose	Comments
Citalopram	Celexa	20 mg/day	60 mg/day	Mild adverse effects
Clomipramine	Anafranil	150 mg/day	250 mg/day	More adverse effects than SSRIs
Escitalopram	Lexapro	10 mg/day	20 mg/day	Least drug–drug effects
Fluoxetine	Prozac	40 mg/day	80 mg/day	Mild adverse effects
Fluvoxamine	Luvox	150 mg/day	300 mg/day	Mild adverse effects
Sertraline	Zoloft	50 mg/day	200 mg/day	Low-level anxiety effects
Paroxetine	Paxil	40 mg/day	60 mg/day	Higher anticholinergic effects & weight gain
Venlafaxine	Effexor	150 mg/day	225mg/day	Risk of blood pressure increase at higher doses

Adapted from Allen, A., & Hollander, E. (2005).

Most patients with OCD present to their PCP for initial treatment. Therefore, it is important for PCPs to have treatment knowledge of this common disorder. However, psychiatric referral may be necessary for the patient with comorbidities as well as for those who do not respond to treatment.

ACUTE AND POSTTRAUMATIC STRESS DISORDERS

Acute Stress Disorder

ASD is a more recent addition to the *DSM-IV-TR* and was included because experts recognized that some people will be severely stressed by a traumatic event, and early diagnosis and treatment can be critical in avoiding the chronicity of PTSD. ASD is similar to PTSD in that it is preceded by an exposure to an extreme traumatic event followed by the development of symptoms within 2 days to 4 weeks after the event. If the symptoms last longer than 4 weeks, the diagnosis is PTSD. As with PTSD, the diagnosis depends on the person's response to the stressor as well as the stressor itself. Because of dissociation, the person may not recall feelings of fear, helplessness, or horror. Box 4.6 describes the *DSM-IV-TR* criteria for ASD.

Posttraumatic Stress Disorder

It was during World War II that posttraumatic stress was recognized. At that time, it was generally referred to as "combat fatigue." After World War II, the diagnosis of PTSD was expanded beyond combat trauma to include individuals who were exposed to an overwhelming environmental stressor that was outside the realm of usual human experience. Currently, the *DSM-IV-TR* no longer requires an overwhelming environmental stressor but merely that a person has been exposed to a traumatic event, with the emphasis now on the person's perception of the traumatic event. It is very likely that the number of people with PTSD will increase in future years because of world and societal violence and wars as well as natural disasters.

Prevalence

Research on the prevalence of ASD is unknown. However, PTSD research indicates a lifetime prevalence of 8 percent in the United States. Women have a lifetime

Box 4.6 • *DSM-IV-TR* Criteria for Acute Stress Disorder

A. The person has been exposed to a traumatic event in which both of the following were present:
   1. The person experienced or witnessed events that involved actual or threatened death or serious injury to self or others.
   2. The person's response was intense fear, helplessness, or horror.

B. Either while or after experiencing the event, the individual has three (or more) of the following dissociative symptoms:
   1. Numbing, detachment, or absence of emotional responsiveness
   2. A reduction in awareness of surroundings (e.g., being in a daze)
   3. Derealization, depersonalization, dissociative amnesia

C. The traumatic event is persistently re-experienced in at least one of the following ways:
   1. Recurrent images, thoughts, dreams, illusions, flashbacks or a sense of reliving the experience
   2. Distress on exposure to reminders of the event

D. Marked avoidance of stimuli that arouse recollections of trauma

E. Marked symptoms of anxiety or increased arousal (e.g., difficulty sleeping, irritability, poor concentration, hypervigilance, exaggerated startle response, and motor restlessness).

F. Clinically significant distress impairs functioning.

G. The disturbance lasts a minimum of 2 days and a maximum of 4 weeks and occurs within 4 weeks of the traumatic event.

H. The disturbance is not due to some other disorder.

Adapted from the American Psychiatric Association (APA) (2000).

prevalence of 10 percent, while men have a prevalence of 5 percent. Women are more likely to be exposed to traumas such as rape and domestic violence, while men are more often exposed to traumas related to combat and physical violence. Some research (APA, 2004) has indicated that women take longer to recover from PTSD than men (48 months vs. 12 months). Although the majority of the U.S. population have experienced severe trauma at some time in their lives, only 25 percent of those will develop ASD or PTSD.

Both ASD and PTSD can occur throughout the life span, including infancy. The age component can be very important in determining treatment interventions because the person's developmental status will affect their perception of and response to the trauma. Earlier traumatic experiences may also impact future traumatic experiences (APA, 2004). ASD usually precedes the development of PTSD, but not always. Sometimes, the PTSD may develop months and years after the traumatic event. Because patients with PTSD present with multiple physical and psychological symptoms and complaints, they are seldom properly diagnosed in primary care settings. Early diagnosis is essential to prevent the stress from becoming chronic PTSD. Because mood disorders, other anxiety disorders, alcohol, and/or other substances frequently accompany PTSD, these comorbidities must be treated concurrently for successful outcomes.

Neurobiologic Basis

Extensive research on the neurobiologic basis for chronic PTSD has demonstrated that stress-related neurotransmitter, neurohormonal, and immune system function are all altered in PTSD, resulting in a dysregulated hypothalamic-adrenal-pituitary (HPA) axis response. Some of these alterations include increased circulating levels of norepinephrine and thyroid hormone along with increased reactivity of alpha 2 adrenergic receptors, increased corticotropin-releasing factor, and low cortisol levels. This chronic increase of stress hormones is pathophysiologic and results in an overly sensitive negative-feedback system. Individuals with PTSD are subjected to persistent hyperarousal, hypervigilance, increased threat appraisal, lower stress tolerance, increased irritability, and an inability to regulate affect and arousal. This inability to "shut down" their systems results in frequent re-enactments, traumatic memories, insomnia, and other types of "reliving" of the PTSD event. These individuals are easily triggered and can experience rapid mood changes: from calmness to anger, anxiety, panic, and feelings of extreme distress. Because of these overwhelming emotions, individuals with PTSD may fear they are "going crazy."

Assessment

The first requirement for a diagnosis of ASD or PTSD is the experiencing of an extreme traumatic event that the person perceives as life threatening or resulting in serious injury. The person feels terrified and helpless when experiencing this event. These events include a wide range of experiences such as military combat, interpersonal violence, automobile or other serious accidents, natural or manmade disasters, and life-threatening illnesses (APA, 2000). As a result of the traumatic event, three clusters of symptoms occur: re-experiencing the symptoms of the traumatic event, increased arousal, and avoidance behaviors. The symptoms must be present for more than 1 month and cause significant problems in all areas of human functioning.

The *DSM-IV-TR* (APA, 2000) makes a distinction between acute and chronic PTSD: the acute disorder has symptoms that last less than 3 months; the chronic course of PTSD has symptoms that are present for 3 months or more. Delayed onset of symptoms may occur at least 6 months after experiencing the traumatic event. Box 4.7 lists the *DSM-IV-TR* criteria for PTSD.

Posttraumatic Stress Disorder Screening Instruments for Use in Primary Care

Brewin (2005) reviewed 13 PTSD screening instruments and reported that instruments with fewer items and simpler responses and scoring methods performed equally well as the longer, more complex instruments. Conner, Foa, and Davidson (2006) described three such short instruments that could be used in primary care to identify individuals at increased risk for developing PTSD. These instruments assume that the individual has been exposed to a severe trauma and are not intended to replace a clinical evaluation. The three instruments are the 10-item Trauma Screening Questionnaire (TSQ) that is based on *DSM- IV* criteria (Brewin, Rose, and Andrews, 2002); the seven-item Breslau scale derived from two structured interviews (Breslau, Peterson, Kessler, et al., 1999); and the four-item SPAN that is derived from the Davidson Trauma Scale (Meltzer-Brody, Churchill, and Davidson, 1999).

Complex Posttraumatic Stress Disorder

PTSD symptoms can range from mild to crippling and disabling. Therefore, the PCP needs to recognize the symptom diversity and the complexity that patients can present. While many will recover from their traumatic experiences, approximately one third of patients with PTSD will have chronic symptoms indefinitely (APA, 2004). Many of these more difficult cases have a prolonged history of childhood sexual and/or physical abuse and neglect and are referred to by some researchers as complex PTSD or as a disorder of extreme stress (Iribarren, Prolo, Neagos, et al., 2005). Military personnel that are exposed to extended threats of warfare are also at risk for complex PTSD. These patients need to be referred to mental health specialists.

Besides the three main clusters of PTSD symptoms (arousal, re-experiencing, and avoidance), individuals with complex PTSD have symptoms of dissociation,

Box 4.7 • *DSM-IV-TR* Criteria for Posttraumatic Stress Disorder

A. The person has been exposed to a traumatic event in which both of the following were present:
   1. The person experienced or witnessed events that involved actual or threatened death or serious injury to self or others.
   2. The person's response was intense fear, helplessness, or horror.

B. The traumatic event is persistently re-experienced in one (or more) of the following ways:
   1. Recurrent recollections of the event
   2. Recurrent distressing dreams, hallucinations, and dissociations of the event
   3. Intense psychological and physiologic distress at exposure to cues that represent the event

C. Persistent avoidance of stimuli associated with the trauma and numbing of general responsiveness as indicated by three (or more) of the following:
   1. Efforts to avoid thoughts, feelings, and activities related to the trauma
   2. Inability to recall an important aspect of the trauma
   3. Diminished interest in significant activities
   4. Feeling of detachment or estrangement from others
   5. Restricted range of affect and sense of foreshortened future

D. Persistent symptoms of increased arousal as indicated by two or more of the following:
   1. Difficulty falling or staying asleep
   2. Irritability and hypervigilance
   3. Difficulty concentrating and exaggerated startle response

E. & F. Duration of symptoms in B, C, D is more than 1 month and causes severe distress

Specify Type:

Acute: Symptoms less than 3 months

Chronic: Symptoms are 3 months or more

Delayed Onset: Symptoms are at least 6 months after stressor

Adapted from the American Psychiatric Association (APA) (2000).

revictimization, multiple somatic complaints, relationship problems, and affect dysregulation. There is disagreement among experts about the role of dissociation in PTSD. Some claim that complex PTSD involves a more complex structural dissociation than simple PTSD, because complex PTSD involves some portion of a person's personality being dissociated from the trauma and able to function, while other portions remain fixated in the traumatic experience (van der Hart, Nijenhuis, and Steele, 2005).

Risk Factors

A wide variety of events and experiences can be risk factors for developing PTSD. A history of mood disorders, anxiety disorders, earlier trauma, and a previous diagnosis of ASD or PTSD all are important risk factors. Female gender, lower economic status, disrupted parental attachments, age between 40 and 60 years, and threatened loss of life or injury to self or close family are other risk factors. The terrorist attack of 9/11 was a man-made disaster of profound proportions that placed thousands at great risk for PTSD. Natural disasters such as Hurricane Katrina, where people lost their homes and all their possessions and were displaced from their neighborhoods, was also a powerful risk factor for the victims (Kablinger, Singh, and Liles, 2006).

Differential Diagnosis

The differential diagnosis of ASD and PTSD includes a long list of both psychiatric and physical disorders. Adjustment disorder may be confused with PTSD. The important difference is that with PTSD, a stressor must be perceived as extremely traumatic to the individual, but there is no such requirement for an adjustment disorder. Many psychiatric disorders are comorbidities of PTSD that complicate the diagnosis even more. In particular, the mood, substance abuse, and anxiety disorders are important to consider in the differential diagnosis. Other considerations are traumatic grief, personality disorders, and eating disorders. Patients with PTSD have many unexplained somatic complaints over the range of body systems. Therefore, the patient who is frequently seen by the health care provider and has multiple complaints, both emotional and physical, needs to be assessed for a history of trauma.

Treatment

PTSD can be a highly complex disorder that will require patient psychoeducation about the disorder, psychotherapy, and medications. The first step in the treatment of patients with ASD and PTSD is to evaluate the potential for self-harm and/or harm to others. When assessing the suicide risk, one must directly inquire about suicidal ideation, intent to act on the ideation, whether a plan exists to carry out the intent, and how lethal the plan. The suicide risk is even more serious if the patient has a previous history of suicidal behavior. Previous behaviors need to be evaluated because some patients with chronic PTSD have a history of self-harming behaviors (e.g., self-cutting) that may escalate over time. If the patient has comorbidities such as depression and/or psychotic features such as paranoid delusions, substance abuse, and panic attacks, the potential for self-harm or harm to others is also increased. These patients must be admitted to an inpatient setting unless they have a responsible caregiver who is able to remain with the patient and monitor her closely until the crisis is over.

In general, patients with severe ASD or PTSD need to be referred to a psychiatric specialist with the reassurance that they will benefit and get relief from their symptoms. Some patients will resist seeking psychiatric care, but many will be more receptive if they understand that the therapist will not force them to disclose traumatic events that are too painful to discuss. Also, providing them with educational resources about PTSD and its symptoms is very important (see the Websites for Organizations section). In most cases, patients should be encouraged to talk about the traumatic event with close members of their support system and discuss the feelings they have about the event. Family members need to understand the patient's need for catharsis and how they can facilitate it. However, this is not always possible with patients who have a history of childhood sexual or physical abuse because the family may deny the events or blame the victim.

Pharmacotherapy

According to a meta-analysis conducted by Stein (2006), SSRIs are the first-line agents in the treatment of PTSD. Davidson (2006) has added the SNRI venlafaxine (Effexor) to the first-line list. In clinical trials, these agents were successful in reducing the core PTSD symptoms of re-experiencing, arousal, and avoidance over the long term.

TCAs and MAOIs have been effective in some studies but are limited by their side effects and low therapeutic index (Table 4.1). However, not all patients with PTSD respond fully to SSRIs, and some researchers question whether women respond better than men in clinical trials (Hamner, 2004). More research is clearly indicated for the treatment of PTSD.

As with all anxiety disorders, clinicians need to start patients at low doses to minimize the anxiogenic effects of antidepressants and slowly increase the dose to maximum tolerated doses. An adequate trial of the antidepressant for anxiety requires at least 8 to 12 weeks at maximum dose. Maximum effects may require 6 to 9 months of treatment. When patients have only a partial response to medication, the clinician will need to add adjunctive agents to the regime or psychotherapy. A variety of choices exists (Davidson, 2006). One may add a second antidepressant, a mood stabilizer, an anticonvulsant, an atypical antipsychotic, and/or antiadrenergics. However, mood stabilizers and anticonvulsants have limited evidence on their effectiveness and safety; therefore, they should be reserved for second- or third-line treatment. For example, the anticonvulsant topiramate (Topamax) has had three small double-blind studies that demonstrated efficacy, but larger clinical trials are now needed (Berlant, 2006). The adrenergic antagonist prazosin (Minipress) has demonstrated significant improvement over several studies in nightmares, sleep problems, and overall PTSD functioning as compared with placebo. Anxiolytics can be helpful in accelerating a therapeutic effect before a prescribed antidepressant begins to work. However, while they can be helpful for promoting sleep and decreasing anxiety, they are not recommended for ASD or early PTSD because of difficulties discontinuing them and the abuse potential, particularly in patients with substance abuse problems. Therefore, trazodone 50 mg (Desyrel) may be more effective for sleep problems (Davidson).

Most recently, atypical antipsychotics have been demonstrating effectiveness in both bipolar and anxiety disorders. They have a mood stabilizing effect on agitated patients and are required if the patient has psychotic symptoms. They are also helpful for the patient with poor impulse control, aggression, or poor response to other medications. However, one must consider the side effects of atypical antipsychotics such as weight gain, postural hypotension, hyperglycemia, and extrapyramidal effects (Davidson, 2006).

An algorithm for the management of PTSD has been developed by the International Psychopharmacology Algorithm Project and is available online (Davidson, Bernik, Conner, et al., 2005; see Resources for Providers). Table 4.6 lists the starting and maximum doses for medications effective for PTSD.

Psychosocial Interventions

Because of the complexity of PTSD, many medications and psychosocial treatments are being studied and used with varying success. The most researched psychosocial intervention is CBT. Foa (2006) described the most commonly used CBTs that have demonstrated effectiveness in multiple studies. These include psychoeducation, anxiety management through deep breathing and relaxation, and exposure therapy. Crisis intervention and group therapy have also been helpful, especially in cases of natural disasters.

Table 4.6 • Evidence-Based First-Line Medications for the Adult Treatment of Posttraumatic Stress Disorder

SSRIs/SNRIs	Initial Dose	Maximum Dose
Citalopram (Celexa)	20 mg	60 mg
Fluoxetine (Prozac)*	10–20 mg	50 mg
Escitalopram (Lexapro)	10 mg	20 mg
Fluvoxamine (Luvox)	50 mg	300 mg
Paroxetine (Paxil)*	10 mg	50 mg
Paroxetine CR (Paxil)*	12.5 mg	75 mg
Sertraline (Zoloft)*	25 mg	200 mg
Venlafaxine (Effexor XR)	37.5 mg	225 mg

*FDA approved for PTSD.
Note: Start at the lowest dose and gradually increase as needed; geriatric patients always require the lowest initial dose.

GENERALIZED ANXIETY DISORDER

GAD, more common in women than men, is found in approximately 4 to 6 percent of the population. People who have a first-degree relative with GAD have a prevalence rate of 20 to 22 percent for the disorder (Schulz, Gotto, and Rapaport, 2005). It tends to be a chronic condition, seen often in family practice clinics instead of psychiatrist offices. These patients present with multiple medical complaints and undergo extensive medical tests attempting to seek relief. Because of their many somatic complaints, the underlying GAD is often missed. Consequently, the identification of GAD in primary care settings is particularly important because it may go undetected indefinitely, and there will be abundant overuse of tests and procedures to no avail.

Patients with GAD frequently have a history of smoking and abuse substances more than the general population (Hettema, Prescott, Myers, et al., 2005).

Assessment

GAD presents with excessive worry that leads to cognitive difficulties and somatic distress. As a result, the patient with GAD demonstrates poor coping strategies. The diagnostic criteria outlined by *DSM-IV-TR* require the excessive worry to have been present for at least 6 months and to have caused functional problems in the patient's life, such as work or school difficulties and relationship problems. It can occur at any time, but the onset of symptoms is usually late teens and early 20s. GAD is often present with other psychiatric conditions, including major depression, dysthymia, panic disorder, and substance abuse. It is also common with OCD, paranoid personality disorder, and avoidant personality disorder.

The evaluation of a patient with generalized excessive worry should begin with a comprehensive history and physical. A thorough medical examination focusing on cardiac, neurologic, and endocrine systems may uncover a patient with hyperthyroidism, pheochromocytoma, Cushing's disease, mitral valve prolapse, or cancer. A history of current medications may reveal drugs that enhance the sympathetic nervous system, including over-the-counter pseudoephedrine, SSRIs for depression, theophylline for asthma, digoxin for congestive heart failure, and various herbals and supplements with psychoactive properties. Box 4.8 presents diagnostic criteria for GAD.

Researchers have recently developed a brief screening tool for GAD (seven items) for use in primary care settings (Spitzer, Kroenke, Williams, et al., 2006). According to the researchers, the tool is designed to assess symptom severity and their change over time. The tool (GAD-7) measures how frequently the seven anxiety symptoms appear within a 2-week period, and most patients are able to complete the test independently. Both reliability and validity were excellent for the GAD-7, but because it is a new tool, more research is needed.

Differential Diagnosis

Patients should be evaluated for major depressive disorder and panic disorder, both as a differential diagnostic consideration and a screen for comorbidity. A persistent condition meeting the criteria for GAD is usually not precipitated by a single stressful occurrence but can be exacerbated by one (a condition referred to as "double anxiety"). Generally, GAD appears before the appearance of a major depressive disorder or panic disorder. In primary care settings, a patient does not often meet the full criteria for any of these diagnoses, as outlined in the *DSM-IV-TR*, appearing instead as subclinical mixed presentations. Other psychiatric disorders to include in the differential diagnosis are anxiety disorder due to a general medical condition, a substance-induced anxiety disorder, obsessive-compulsive disorder, and social phobia.

A substance abuse history must be obtained, as intoxication and withdrawal from these substances may cause a prolonged anxiety state. In the GAD patient

Box 4.8 • *DSM-IV-TR* Criteria for Generalized Anxiety Disorder

A. Excessive anxiety and worry for at least 6 months about a number of events or activities.

B. The person finds it difficult to control the worry.

C. The anxiety and worry are associated with three (or more) of the following six symptoms:
   1. Restlessness or feeling keyed up or on edge
   2. Being easily fatigued
   3. Difficulty concentrating or mind going blank
   4. Irritability
   5. Muscle tension
   6. Sleep disturbance (difficulty falling or staying asleep, or restless unsatisfying sleep)

D. The focus of the anxiety and worry is not confined to features of an Axis I disorder.

E. The anxiety, worry, or physical symptoms cause clinically significant distress or impairment in important areas of functioning.

F. The disturbance is not due to the direct physiologic effects of another disorder.

Adapted from the American Psychiatric Association (APA). (2000).

who presents with primarily somatic complaints with anxiety, a diagnosis of somatization disorder must be considered. This condition is characterized by chronic complaints across various organ systems that do not appear to be related; GAD patients present with a narrower range of symptoms that can be explained by increased sympathetic nervous system activation (palpitations, dizziness, nausea, and gastrointestinal complaints).

Treatment

Pharmacotherapy

Patients with severe anxiety should be treated for at least 6 months, but the optimum duration of treatment has not been established. Sixty to 80 percent of patients relapse within 1 year of discontinuing medication; in many patients, medication may be required indefinitely.

For many years, BZDs had been the first-line treatment of GAD. However, these medications cause sedation, anterograde amnesia, and concentration problems, the latter two developing within weeks, along with tolerance to these effects. Other serious concerns with the use of BZDs include the development of dependence after regular use with difficult withdrawal symptoms. Individuals with substance abuse and alcohol problems are at risk for abusing these drugs. For these reasons, BZDs are no longer first-line treatment and have been replaced by SSRIs, SNRIs, and other medications (Pollock, 2006). It is important to note that individuals without abuse problems do not seem to have this same risk with BZDs (Schulz et al., 2005).

The antidepressants are more desirable because they avoid the pitfalls of the BZDs but also are effective in the treatment of comorbidities, such as depression, which is the most common comorbidity of GAD. The anxiolytic effects of antidepressants occur in 2 to 3 weeks, but this time lag can be very difficult for patients to tolerate, and augmentation with a BZD may be required. While the effects of antidepressants have been effective, few patients with GAD reach remission. However, Pollock (2006) emphasizes that symptom relief may gradually improve over months. Between 8 weeks to 6 months, remission rates with venlafaxine (Effexor) increased from 34 percent to 43 percent. This was particularly evident in the more seriously ill patients.

All the SSRIs are used for GAD along with the SNRI venlafaxine (Effexor) and some tricyclics. However, only escitalopram (Lexapro), paroxetine (Paxil), and venlafaxine (Effexor) have FDA approval for treatment of GAD. The other antidepressants are used because of clinical trials that support their efficacy. All medications need to be started at low doses and gradually increased until they have a beneficial effect. Elderly patients always require lower doses.

The side-effect profile of paroxetine (Paxil) is close to that of the other SSRIs, but paroxetine is associated with higher rates of sedation and constipation, probably because of its anticholinergic activity. Weight gain, drug interactions, and sexual dysfunction tend to be slightly higher with paroxetine than with fluoxetine (Prozac) and sertraline (Zoloft). Side effects for venlafaxine include asthenia, sweating, somnolence, insomnia, and sexual dysfunction. Escitalopram's (Lexapro) most common side effects are reported as insomnia and somnolence.

TCAs have also been used efficaciously to treat GAD, but the side-effect profile is often a problem for patients who experience dizziness, dry mouth, sedation, and weight gain. Imipramine (Tofranil) is the tricyclic approved to treat both GAD and panic disorder.

There are some novel agents being tested that have demonstrated efficacy for GAD but have not been approved by the FDA. A very recent study demonstrated

Table 4.7 • Medication Chart for Generalized Anxiety Disorder

Medication	Starting Dose	Daily Dose Range
Paroxetine (Paxil)	20 mg	10–50 mg
Escitalopram (Lexapro)	10 mg	10–20 mg
Venlafaxine (Effexor)	37.5 mg	75–225 mg
Alprazolam (Xanax)	0.25–0.5 mg qid	0.5–6.0 mg
Chlordiazepoxide (Librium)	5–10 mg tid	15–100 mg
Clonazepam (Klonopin)	0.5–1.0 mg bid	0.5–10.0 mg
Diazepam (Valium)	2–5 mg tid	6–40 mg
Lorazepam (Ativan)	0.5–1.0 mg tid	2–6 mg
Oxazepam (Serax)	15–30 mg tid	30–120 mg

Adapted from Schulz, J., Gotto, J., & Rapaport, M. H. (2005).

that the anticonvulsant pregabalin (Lyrica) is an effective treatment of GAD, with rapid improvements in psychic and somatic anxiety factor scores (Pohl, Feltner, Fieve, et al., 2005). Table 4.7 lists common medications used in the treatment of GAD.

Psychosocial Interventions

As with other anxiety disorders, CBT has been reported in multiple studies to also be effective in the treatment of GAD (Burke, 2006). CBT provides long-term benefits to patients on measures of cognition, mood, and anxiety (Schulz et al., 2005). Progressive relaxation has also been found to be effective.

WHEN TO REFER PATIENTS WITH ANXIETY DISORDERS

Susman (2005) stresses the chronicity of anxiety disorders and the need for long-term care and watchfulness for recurrence of symptoms when patients are in remission and recommends the following guidelines for referring patients to psychiatric specialists with anxiety disorders.

1. Uncertain diagnosis
2. Complex psychiatric or medical comorbidities (e.g., severe substance abuse and rapid cycler)

3. High suicide potential
4. Counseling services otherwise unavailable
5. Electroconvulsive therapy required
6. PCP overwhelmed and needs assistance and reassurance.

CONCLUSION

Despite clear evidence that effective treatments including medications, CBT, and various combinations exist for anxiety disorders, many patients continue to have severe symptoms and remain undiagnosed. The majority of these individuals seek care from their PCPs, so the onus for successful diagnosis and treatment resides with these practitioners. Providers need to become more aware of the severe incapacitation that anxiety disorders can create and the comorbidities associated with them, especially major depression. With this awareness, it is hoped that more effective diagnosis and treatment will follow. Although a great deal of research has been conducted for anxiety disorders, research must continue to search for improved medications, improved CBT methods, and combinations that maximize results for all patients who suffer with anxiety disorders and other mental health problems.

Resources for Providers

International Psychopharmacology Algorithm Project (for management of PTSD): *www.ipap.org.PTSD*

Yale-Brown Obsessive Compulsive Scale (Y-BOCS): *www.atlantapsychiatry.com/forms/YBOCS.pdf*

Resources for Patients

Websites of Organizations

American Psychiatric Association: *www.psych.org*

Center for the Study of Traumatic Stress/Disaster and Terrorism Care Resources: *www.centerforthestudyoftraumaticstress.org*

Centers for Disease Control and Prevention/Trauma and Disaster Mental Health Resources: *www.bt.cdc.gov/mentalhealth*

International Psychopharmacology Algorithm Project (for treatment of PTSD): *www.ipap.org*

National Center for Posttraumatic Stress Disorder (NCPTSD): *www.ncptsd.org*

National Institute of Mental Health: *www.nimh.nih.gov*

The Anxiety Disorders Education Program, National Institute of Mental Health: *www.nimh.nih.gov*

Self-Help Resources

Anxiety Disorders Association of America. A self-help organization with publications, newsletter, and list of anxiety disorder self-help groups in each state. *www.adaa.org*

Anxiety Disorders—NOAH: *www.NOAH-health.org/en/mental/disorders/anxiety.html*

FearFighter. A computer-aided online exposure self-help system for anxiety disorders with brief therapist support by phone helpline. *www.fearfighter.com*

Obsessive-Compulsive Disorder. A quick fact sheet from the National Mental Health Association. *http://nmha.org/infoctr/factsheets/33.cfm*

References

Albucher, R. C. (2005). *Phobic disorders.* Retrieved June 21, 2006, from *www.emedicine.com/med/topic1821.htm.*

Allen, A., & Hollander, E. (2005). Diagnosis and treatment of obsessive compulsive disorder. *Primary Psychiatry, 12,* 34–42.

American Psychiatric Association (APA). (2000). *Diagnostic and statistical manual of mental disorders* (Revised 4th ed.). Washington, DC: Author.

American Psychiatric Association (APA). (2004). *The practice guideline for the treatment of patients with acute stress disorder and posttraumatic stress disorder.* Washington, DC: Author.

Angst, J., Gamma, A., Endrass, J., et al. (2005). Obsessive-compulsive syndromes and disorders. *European Archives of Psychiatry and Clinical Neuroscience, 255,* 65–71.

Belzer, K. D., McKee, M. B., & Liebowitz, M. R. (2005). Social anxiety disorder: Current perspectives on diagnosis and treatment. *Primary Psychiatry, 12,* 35–48.

Berlant, J. (2006). Topiramate as a therapy for chronic posttraumatic stress disorder. *Psychiatry, 3*(3), 40–45.

Breslau, N., Novak, S. P., & Kessler, R. C. (2004). Daily smoking and the subsequent onset of psychiatric disorders. *Psychological Medicine, 34,* 323–333.

Breslau, N., Peterson, E. L., Kessler, R. C., et al. (1999). Short screening scale for DSM IV Posttraumatic Stress Disorder. *American Journal of Psychiatry, 156,* 908–911.

Brewin, C. R. (2005). Systematic review of screening instruments for adults at risk of PTSD. *Journal of Traumatic Stress, 18,* 53–62.

Brewin, C. R., Rose, S., & Andrews, B. (2002). Brief screening instrument for post-traumatic stress disorder. *British Journal of Psychiatry, 181,* 158–162.

Burke, W. (2006). Identifying and treating comorbid generalized anxiety disorder in the primary care setting. Anxiety disorders and medical comorbidities: A focus on diagnosis and treatment. A self-study supplement to *Clinician Reviews,* 4–10.

Cloos, J. M. (2005). The treatment of panic disorder. *Current Opinions in Psychiatry, 18*, 45–50.

Collins, K. A., Westra, H. A., Dozois, D. J., et al. (2005). The validity of the brief version of the Fear of Negative Evaluation Scale. *Journal of Anxiety Disorders, 19*, 345–359.

Conner, K. M., Foa, E. B., & Davidson, J. R. (2006). Practical assessment and evaluation of mental health problems following a mass disaster. *Journal of Clinical Psychiatry, 67*(Suppl 2), 26–33.

Culpepper, L. (2004). Management of comorbid depression and anxiety in the primary care setting. *Clinician Reviews, 14*, 104–110.

Davidson, J. R. T. (2006). Pharmacologic treatment of acute and chronic stress following trauma. *Journal of Clinical Psychiatry, 67*(Suppl 2), 34–39.

Davidson, J., Bernik, M., Connor, K. M., et al. (2005). A new treatment algorithm for the posttraumatic stress disorder. *Psychiatric Annals, 35*, 887–900.

Feusner, J., Cameron, M., & Bystritsky, A. (2005). Pharmacotherapy and psychotherapy for panic disorder. *Primary Psychiatry, 12*, 49–55.

Foa, E. B. (2006). Psychosocial therapy for posttraumatic stress disorder. *Journal of Clinical Psychiatry, 67*(Suppl 2), 40–45.

Foa, E. B., Liebowitz, M. R., & Kozak, M. J. (2005). Randomized, placebo-controlled trial of exposure and ritual prevention, clomipramine, and their combination in the treatment of obsessive-compulsive disorder. *American Journal of Psychiatry, 162*, 151–161.

Hamner, M. B. (2004). Atypical antipsychotics in anxiety and posttraumatic stress disorder. Paper presented at the 2004 American Psychiatric Association's 55th Institute on Psychiatric Services on Broadening the Horizon of Atypical Antipsychotic Applications. Retrieved May 1, 2005, from *www.medscape.com/viewprogram/3137_pnt.*

Hayward, C., Killen, J. D., Taylor, C. B. (2003). The relationship between agoraphobia symptoms and panic disorder in a non-clinical sample of adolescents. *Psychological Medicine, 33*(4), 733–738.

Hettema, J. M., Prescott, C. A., Myers, J. M., et al. (2005). The structure of genetic and environmental risk factors for anxiety disorders in men and women. *Archives of General Psychiatry, 62*(2), 182–189.

Iribarren, J., Prolo, P., Neagos, N., et al. (2005). Post-traumatic stress disorder: Evidence-based research for the third millennium. *Evidence Based Complementary Alternative Medicine, 2*, 503–512.

Kablinger, A. S., Singh, J. K., & Liles, L. T. (2006). Posttraumatic stress disorder in women: A refresher course after the hurricane. *Women's Health in Primary Care*, 36–43.

Katon, W. J. (2006). Clinical practice: Panic disorder. *New England Journal of Medicine, 354*(22), 2360–2367.

Keller, M. B. (2005). *Treating anxiety with and without depression: A look to utilizing antidepressants.* A CME activity provided by the FCG Institute for Continuing Education. Retrieved July 3, 2005, from *www/medscape.com/viewprogram/3793_pnt.*

Kessler, R. C., Chiu, W. T., Demler, O., et al. (2005). Prevalence, severity and comorbidity of 12 month DSM-IV disorders in the National Comorbidity Survey Replication. *Archives of General Psychiatry, 62*, 617–624.

Meltzer-Brody, S., Churchill, E., & Davidson, J. R. (1999). Derivation of the SPAN, a brief diagnostic screening test for posttraumatic stress disorder. *Psychiatry Research, 88*, 63–70.

Pohl, R. B., Feltner, D. E., Fieve, R. R., et al. (2005). Efficacy of pregabalin controlled comparison of bid versus tid dosing. *Journal of Clinical Psychopharmacology, 25*(2), 151–158.

Pollock, M. H. (2006). *Generalized anxiety disorder—Overview and case history.* Medscape CME offering. Retrieved August 24, 2006, from *www.medscape.com/viewprogram/5212_pnt.*

Pollock, R. & Kuo, I. (2004). *Treatment of anxiety disorders: An update.* International Congress of Biological Psychiatry. Medscape CME offering. Retrieved May 1, 2006, from *www.medscape.com/viewprogram/2997_pnt.*

Satcher, D., Delgado, P. L., & Masand, P. S. (2005). *A surgeon general's perspective on the unmet needs of patients with anxiety disorders.* A psychCME series presented by CME Outfitters, L.L.C. Retrieved November 18, 2007, from *www.medscape.com/viewprogram/4650_pnt.*

Schneier, F. R., Blanco, C., Antia, S. X., et al. (2002). The social anxiety spectrum. *Psychiatric Clinics of North America, 25,* 757–774.

Schulz, J., Gotto, J., & Rapaport, M. H. (2005). The diagnosis and treatment of generalized anxiety disorder. *Primary Psychiatry, 12,* 58–67.

Spitzer, R. L., Kroenke, K., Williamsj. B. W., & Lowe, B. (2006). A brief measure for assessing generalized anxiety disorder: The GAD-7. *Archives of Internal Medicine, 166,* 1092–1097.

Starcevic, V. (2006). Anxiety states: A review of conceptual and treatment issues. *Current Opinions in Psychiatry, 19,* 79–83.

Stein, D. J. (2006). Pharmacotherapy for post traumatic stress disorder (PTSD). Cochrane Review abstracts. Retrieved April 1, 2006, from *www.medscape.com/viewarticle/486224_print.*

Susman, J. L. (2005). *Differentiating between depression an anxiety disorders in family practice.* A CME activity provided by the FCG Institute for Continuing Education. Retrieved July 3, 2005, from *www/medscape.com/viewprogram/3793_pnt.*

van der Hart, O., Nijenhuis, E. R., et al. (2005). Dissociation: An insufficiently recognized major feature of complex posttraumatic stress disorder. *Journal of Traumatic Stress, 18,* 413–423.

Watson, D., & Wu, K. D. (2005). Development and validation of the Schedule of Compulsions, Obsessions, and Pathological Impulses (SCOPI). *Assessment, 12,* 50–65.

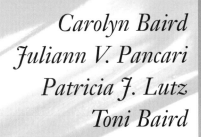

Carolyn Baird
Juliann V. Pancari
Patricia J. Lutz
Toni Baird

chapter 5

Addiction Disorders

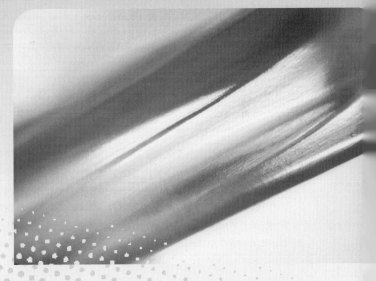

As part of the U.S. Department of Health and Human Services, the Substance Abuse and Mental Health Services Administration (SAMHSA) has confirmed that substance use/abuse continues to challenge the provision of health care in the United States and throughout the world. While significant advances have been achieved in the areas of diagnosis and coordinated service delivery, identifying addiction and recognizing the impact of substance misuse and related activity on the individual and society remains a critical factor in providing affordable, effective health care that results in favorable patient outcomes.

Addiction has taught professionals that not every situation fits into a pre-established mold of an addiction category. Asking the right questions and using reliable tools can bring information to the surface so that addiction can be addressed in the early phases of treatment as well as during the maintenance of recovery.

Addiction and related disorders are chronic conditions. The progression of addiction and concurrent physical and psychologic effects often present in the primary care setting. Of the 2.3 million persons 12 years of age and older who received substance use treatment in 2005, about 254,000 received treatment in a doctor's office (Substance Abuse and Mental Health Services Administration, National Survey on Drug Use and Health [SAMHSA, NSDUH], 2005). Researchers have confirmed that office-based interventions by primary care providers (PCPs) have favorable outcomes and have effectively decreased addictions and associated harmful effects. Further, women tend to seek treatment at mental health or primary care clinics rather than addiction treatment programs (Back, Contini, and Brady, 2007).

An individual whose life is being compromised because of an addiction may present in the primary care setting for many different reasons. Examples of red flags that warrant further assessment include the following:

- Vague physical complaints and requests for medication to improve sleep, energy, anxiety, concentration, indigestion, and others
- Requests for samples of medications or to refill prescriptions earlier than the recommended schedule, with a variety of reasons why the medication is currently not at the patient's disposal
- Unexplained bruises or injuries suggesting falls or other accidents resulting from substance-induced impairment or blackouts
- Increased frequency of visits or calls to the office requesting treatment for self or a family member that may include prescribing a medication that has the potential for abuse
- Unexplained weight loss or symptoms of malnourishment resulting from diminished need for food or the lack of money to buy food

- Decline in oral hygiene resulting from overall neglect of care and other activities of daily living (ADLs) or eating disorders that cause dental damage
- Changes in the menstrual cycle associated with weight loss or gain and other eating disorders
- Skin conditions indicating poor general hygiene, malnourishment, or injection sites
- Overall changes in appearance, presentation, or laboratory values that may include unfavorable response to previously prescribed remedies
- Unexplained tremors, ataxic gait, and poor coordination

Guidelines for PCPs should emphasize the value of including questions about substance use/abuse while discussing the individual's lifestyle. Best practice recommendations further suggest periodic and routine screening of all patients for substance abuse (SAMHSA, TIP 24, 2007). Because an alarming 19% of women with substance abuse problems and 26% with psychiatric conditions remain undetected and untreated (Back et al., 2007), PCPs can play an integral part in early intervention.

The process to link a symptom or behavior to a high-risk behavior that includes addiction begins with early detection and intervention. Statistics available from studies funded through SAMHSA for the year 2005 estimate that 22.5 million Americans 12 years of age or older could be classified as having a substance abuse or dependence problem but that only 2.3 million of them would receive treatment (Snow and Delaney, 2006).

During the 20th century, a double standard developed: While substance-abusing men would be offered treatment, it was more likely that substance-abusing women would be hidden, protected, or abandoned. Most statistics do not identify a male-to-female ratio. However, they do conclude that 4.4 million women abuse or depend on alcohol, meaning that one of every three alcohol-dependent individuals is female and that 2 million women abuse or are dependent on illicit drugs (Doweiko, 2006).

In October 2003, the Center for Substance Abuse Treatment (CSAT) awarded seven national Screening, Brief Intervention, Referral, and Treatment (SBIRT) grants. The center's intention was to partner with various state agencies to develop a continuum that would place the activities of screening, intervention, and referral within medical and community settings that act as entry to treatment. Each of the original seven states—and many states not included in the original project—have developed resources to assist PCPs who wish to increase their effectiveness in screening for misuse and abuse of substances.

Table 5.1 • *DSM-IV-TR* Definition of Terms

Term	Definition
Substance	A drug of abuse, a medication, or a toxin.
Substance-related disorder	Disorders related to the taking of a drug of abuse, including alcohol, to the side effects of a medication, and to toxin exposure.
Substance abuse	A maladaptive pattern of substance use marked by recurrent and significant negative consequences related to the repeated use of substances. This may include harmful effects to a person's life.
Substance dependence	A cluster of cognitive, behavioral, and physiologic symptoms indicating that the individual is continuing use of the substance despite significant substance-related problems. A person experiencing substance dependence shows a pattern of repeated self-administration that usually results in tolerance, withdrawal, and compulsive drug-taking behavior.
Substance intoxication	The development of a reversible substance-specific syndrome the result of the recent ingestion of or exposure to a substance.
Substance withdrawal	The development of a substance-specific maladaptive behavioral change, usually with uncomfortable physiologic and cognitive consequences, that is the result of a cessation of or reduction in heavy and prolonged substance use.

From American Psychiatric Association (2000). *Diagnostic and statistical manual of mental disorders* (Revised 4th ed.). Washington, DC: Author.

This chapter discusses the phenomenon of addiction in women. Assessment and screening tools, diagnostic criteria, current treatment options, and related legal and ethical considerations are presented as well. Table 5.1 may assist the clinician in establishing consistency when applying terms and attempting to draw conclusions from subjective or objective patient information. Clinicians should understand that a 12-step program may substitute the word *process* for *substance* when referring to a type of addiction.

WOMEN AND ADDICTION

Differences in substance usage patterns and predisposition to addiction and addictive behaviors exist between women and men. The 2005 National Survey on Drug Use and Health (SAMHSA, NSDUH, 2005) study revealed that women are more vulnerable to developing addictions because they become substance dependent at a faster rate than men. This survey reported that women advance more quickly than men from initial substance use to regular use to the first treatment episode. Although the time from initial use to problematic use may be shorter than in men, women tend to exhibit more severe symptoms when they enter treatment. Women average more medical, psychiatric, and adverse social consequences of substance use than men (a phenomenon known as "telescoping"). This includes women identifying interpersonal and other lifelong stressors as contributing to substance use as well as to relapse (Back et al., 2007).

Researchers associate the fluctuation in monthly estrogen levels with the ability of a woman's brain to control addictive behaviors. Estrogen can trigger sensitization and cravings similar to the feelings and experiences that result from substances, such as cocaine, or the excitement that results from engaging in addictive behaviors. Neural changes that occur while a woman ingests her drug of choice or engages in addictive behavior may be the result of the impact of estrogen and other reproductive hormones on the brain's ability to inhibit impulse control, leading to an increased risk of addiction (Bouchez, 2006).

The risk of addiction for the woman of childbearing age as well as the pregnant female warrants specific prevention, education, and treatment interventions. Concerns range from smoking during pregnancy to engaging in sexual behaviors such as prostitution as a means of financing an active addiction. The inherited and elected cultural influences associated with nationality, religion, and other beliefs must also be considered to thoroughly understand the individual and the choices she makes.

In 2004, women accounted for 31.5% of the nationwide admissions to treatment, which supports the necessity of providing assessment and treatment specific to women (SAMHSA, NSDUH, 2005). Obtaining a thorough history and conducting an assessment that concludes with the development of an initial recovery plan is critical to individualizing treatment for women in addiction. However, the first step is to understand the types of addictive disorders.

ADDICTIVE DISORDERS

Addiction, which can occur at any time over the life span, can be a lifelong disease with remissions and exacerbations, or it can occur as an isolated episode (Antai-Otong, 2006). Individuals may be addicted to a substance or may be addicted to a particular course of action, known as a process addiction, which may include thoughts, feelings, or behaviors.

Process and Substance Addictions

Process addictions are sometimes more difficult to identify than substance addictions. The validity of their existence has been questioned, but their impact and consequences are serious (Wieland, 2005). These are the "hidden" addictions, those that are not necessarily associated with a diagnosis but nonetheless present the addictive behaviors that are similar to the signs and symptoms associated with known addictions (Freimuth, 2005). Freimuth details the pertinence of listening to the clinical clues about undisclosed addictions and the importance of accurate addiction assessment and diagnosis. Clinical judgment on the part of the health care provider is essential to provide the relevant assessment when the data available to guide diagnosis and treatment are absent (Freimuth). Process addictions can have equally devastating effects as more common drugs of choice such as alcohol and marijuana, but they are often overlooked during the interview and data collection phase of assessing the individual's presentation for services (Freimuth).

Process and substance addictions seek the same result: an alteration of mood. Addictive disorders have in common loss of control, preoccupation with the substance or behavior, secrecy and lies about use or actions, and a continuation of the activity despite negative consequences. Withdrawal symptoms, physiologic or psychologic, occur when the addictive behaviors are stopped (Power, 2005). It is possible to identify interaction between the various addictions. Thus, it is important to look for cross-tolerance, use of one behavior or substance to mediate withdrawal from another behavior or substance, replacement of one behavior or substance with another behavior or substance, and alternating cycles of addictive behavior. Also, some form of ritual may be present. Substances or behaviors may be used to adjust feelings or emotions through masking, intensifying, numbing, inhibiting, or disinhibiting (Power).

PCPs should be alert to repeating patterns of behavior of an impulsive or compulsive nature. Although the *Diagnostic and Statistical Manual of Mental Disorders*, 4th ed., Text Revision (*DSM-IV-TR*) does not have a diagnostic category for process addictions, such as gambling, sex, Internet obsession, shopping/spending, eating (food), or working, the associated behaviors may be described in the category of Impulse Control Disorder, Not Otherwise Specified (Wieland, 2005).

Treatment options for process and substance addictions are similar, consisting of a mix of therapies, usually cognitive behavioral and insight-oriented psychotherapy as well as psychotherapeutic medications. Because of the compulsive nature of addictive behavior, the selective serotonin reuptake inhibitors (SSRIs) have been used to good effect (Power, 2005). Substance disorders may require the specific treatment of associated physiologic disorders. Self-help groups are another part of the treatment process. Many variations on the original 12-step groups have been developed to address the various process addiction behaviors.

Tables 5.2 and 5.3 identify both process and substance addictions and can assist the PCP in recognizing the potential for substance abuse and address the risks associated with addiction identified in the practice. The *DSM-IV-TR* lists specific diagnoses for alcoholism and specific substance addictions. PCPs should refer to the *DSM-IV-TR* to determine the levels of severity and to differentiate and define behaviors such as abuse, dependence, intoxication, and withdrawal (Table 5.1).

Criteria for Diagnosis

The end result of screening, assessing, and/or evaluating the presenting signs and symptoms reported by an individual is the formulation of a diagnosis. Health care professionals, regardless of their discipline and field of expertise, rely on a defined set of elements, or criteria, by which to make a diagnosis (Doweiko, 2006). Professionals in the field of substance use disorders are no different, except for the fact that there is no formal standardization of definitions, terminology, and/or criteria (NIDA, 2005). This is because "a universally accepted comprehensive theory of addiction has yet to be developed" (Doweiko, 2006, p.20).

The medical, or disease, model of addiction states that addiction is a primary medical disorder with the potential for affecting an individual's social, psychologic, spiritual, and economic life (Doweiko, 2006). Chemical or substance addiction is often progressive, may be fatal, and is marked by preoccupation with use regardless of the consequences (Doweiko). The terminology of substance use, abuse, and dependence are frequently used interchangeably; however, these are separate terms and apply to separate patterns of behavior on a drug-use continuum (Table 5.1 on page 140).

Figure 5.1 shows the progression from use to dependence along a continuum. Levels 0 and 1 are reflective of use; level 2 equates to abuse; and at levels 3 and 4, the individual is clearly at a stage of dependence.

Besides understanding the continuum of chemical use, the PCP needs to recognize that there is also a more exact classification system of criteria-based definitions, or diagnostic criteria, for identifying the levels within the state of dependency (Box 5.1 on page 141).

Determining Treatment Level

Once the signs and symptoms displayed by the patient have been evaluated and a diagnosis of dependency has been reached, the next step is to determine the

Text continues on page 140.

Table 5.2 • Process Addictions

Type	Description	Street Name	Signs and Symptoms	Related Information
Pathologic gambling	When gambling interferes with the ability to assume other responsibilities in life resulting in harmful consequences.	Hustle Hustler	• Loss of savings • Loss of property • Direct negative effect on family relationships • Negative effect on personal welfare	• Among activities are lottery, bingo, poker, card games, off-track betting, race track betting, pool, billiards, casino activity, Internet gambling, and others. • Because some of these activities generate revenue for government and municipalities where they are located, access is easy and opportunities to gamble are abundant. • The ability to gamble on the Internet has contributed to this addiction.
Work	When an individual works high-intensity jobs or a position of excitement and danger resulting in lifestyle pattern of isolation from other activities.	Workaholic	• Long hours • Lack of enjoyment with being home or with family • Motivation is excitement and not money • Inflated sense of personal value and responsibility	• Americans work more hours and take less time off than most other nationalities. • May be interpreted as a positive individual trait disregarding the consequence of isolation and lack of interaction with family and others. • The individual truly has an inflated sense of importance related to the job.

Exercise	When fitness becomes a primary goal in the day. Activities often are repetitious and exceed the advice of personal and fitness trainers.	Exercise bulimia Adrenaline junkie	• To feel good about themselves, individuals must work out daily and at times more than once daily; frequently continue to exercise despite physical risks, such as shin splints; or exercise too soon following an injury. • Preoccupation with body image.	• Individuals connect personal worth with numbers on a scale and muscle mass. • Women feel the pressure from society to be thin and shapely at all costs. • Whenever possible, exercise will occur immediately after eating a meal or rich, high-calorie food. • In the workplace, individuals may be seen walking the stairs several times a day to fulfill the craving for exercise and fitness. • Individuals who participate in activities and sports that associate weight to performance are particularly vulnerable, such as wrestlers going to any length to qualify for a weight class.
Internet	When with a click of the mouse one can enter a different world where the problems of the real world are not present. Internet contact replaces face-to-face interactions with others and fosters isolation.	Cyber sex junkie Geek Nerd	• Loses track of time. • Lies about the amount of time spent on the Internet and sites accessed. • Sacrifices sleep to be on the Internet. • Becomes angry when Internet time is interrupted to tend to other responsibilities. • Misses appointments or fails to complete tasks or activities of daily living (ADLs) to be on the Internet.	• Activities, such as surfing the Internet, playing games, and entering chat rooms, consume more than time spent during normal recreation. • The impulse and craving for Internet activity spills over into other ADLs to include Internet use during scheduled work time, often resulting in serious performance issues up to and including job termination. • Maintaining hardware and software to support the addiction can present serious financial burden.

(*Continued*)

Table 5.2 • (Continued)

Type	Description	Street Name	Signs and Symptoms	Related Information
Love	When relationships, good or bad, are needed at all times and at all costs.	Clingy Needy	• When one relationship ends, goal is to immediately establish another. • Pattern resembles that of a chain smoker. • Underlying low self-esteem that is often fed by the immediate excitement and gratification of a love interest. • Self-worth is defined by a relationship. • Numerous phone calls. • General preoccupation with relationships.	• Identified pattern of repeated, dysfunctional relationships. • Little consideration given to the impact of this behavior on the other party. • Presenting problems may be associated with spiritual, physical, and emotional abuse. • Often, willingness to engage in multiple relationships at the same time due to the fear of being alone. • Perceived as stalking when the other party does not want to be involved.
Compulsive spending	Preoccupied with shopping. The impulse to spend is irresistible despite limited resources.	Shopaholic	• Credit card debt • Personal bankruptcy • Frequent borrowing without paying back • Purchasing the same item in various styles, colors	• “Retail therapy” may be recreational for some but out of control for others. • Buyer will go to any length to get the funds to make the purchase including bartering, trading items that are not theirs, stealing from others, and engaging in retail theft or other illegal activities such as prostitution.
Sex	Involves practices to include masturbation, relationships, voyeurism, exhibitionism, and pornography.	Peeping Toms Perverts Sex addict Nympho Flashers	• Constant preoccupation with thoughts of engaging in sexual activities. • Constant effort to engage in sexual activities as often as possible and with as many single or multiple partners. • Excitement is associated with anticipating and carrying out the act.	• Immediate gratification at all costs. • May involve serious, life-threatening, and furtive acts without regard for consequences of discovery and loss of family and/or professional status.

Table 5.3 • Substance Addictions

Name	Description	Street Name(s)	Signs & Symptoms	Related Information
Alcohol	• Can't stop drinking after the first drink. • One drink is never enough. • Associates drinking with the purpose of getting drunk. • Drinking may be in isolation or groups.	Booze Hooch Brew Cocktails Fire water	• Behavior change often accompanies alcoholism. • Blackouts • Motor vehicle accidents and arrests for driving under the influence (DUI) of a substance • Tremors • Loss of appetite • Impaired judgment • Slurred speech	• Binge drinking. • Contributory factors of portrayal in alcohol advertisements and promotion through media. • Financial gain associated with items carrying alcohol labels such as T-shirts, mugs, signs, etc. • Establishing employee assistance programs (EAPs) and substance abuse professionals (SAPs) to identify the presenting behavior or problem behavior that may or may not be associated with drinking.
Street Drugs	Illicit drugs to include but not limited to: Marijuana Cocaine Heroin	 Weed, Dope, Blunts, Mary Jane (too numerous to list) Crack, Blow, Soft, Girl, Smack Horse, Diesel, Hard, H, Boy	• Weight loss • Bruises • Tracks • Insomnia or excessive sleep • Dilated or constricted pupils • Irritability • Memory loss • Skin changes, acne • Picking and itching • Hallucinations • Decline in ADLs • Ataxic gait • Appetite suppression	• Youth experimentation has been reported to occur at an earlier age (primary grades rather than teens). • School dropouts have been directly related to illicit substance use. • Increase in teen pregnancy, hepatitis C, and HIV/AIDS strongly associated with individuals using these substances. • Stricter DUI laws and consequences for all ages. • The effects of these drugs are unpredictable and vary from person to person as well as the circumstances in which they are used. • Psychologic effects can be temporary or more severe with distortions and suicidal behaviors. • Short-term use results in effects to include memory and learning problems, distorted perception, and difficulty with thought processes and problem solving.

(Continued)

Table 5.3 • (Continued)

Name	Description	Street Name(s)	Signs & Symptoms	Related Information
	Ecstasy LSD Quaaludes PCP Ketamine Crystal Methamphetamine Rohypnol	E, X Acid Ludes, Soapers Angel Dust Special K Meth, Ice, Chalk Date rape drug Ruffies		• Physical deterioration is often recognized with malnutrition and lack of attention to personal hygiene. • Many of these substances have been studied as Gen X drugs and club drugs. They may be slipped into drinks and given to unsuspecting individuals to alter judgment associated with ability to fend off undesired sexual advances.
Prescription drugs	When any prescribed medication is used for a purpose other than the original intention or in an amount greater than prescribed by the individual or another.	Pain killer Oxys Uppers Downers Bennies Yellow jackets Roids	• Memory loss • Weight loss • Glassy eyes • Rage or agitation • Excessive sweating • Impaired judgment • Slurred speech • Eye–hand coordination	• Individuals engage in physician shopping and symptom exaggeration. • Frequent emergency room visits. • Prescription drugs are bought, sold, and bartered. • Many different types of prescription drugs have been identified at adolescent "raid parties" when the purpose is to take whatever is available in the family medicine cabinet. • Coordinated efforts among health care providers to include PCPs, pharmacists, case managers, and managed care representatives have identified prescribing practices that decrease duplicate prescriptions and reduce potential to exceed the recommended dosage. • Focus on female body building has increased along with the risk related to steroid use.

Over-the-counter (OTC) drugs	Many OTCs carry the potential for abuse; the most common are caffeine pills, diet preparations, cough preparations, mouthwash, and laxatives.	Black Beauties Robo-Trippin Triple Cs	• Shakiness • Weight loss • Memory loss • Impaired judgment • Irritability • Mood swings • Periods of either excessive sleep or sleeplessness	• Seriousness of use is often minimized. • Occupational hazards have been associated with these substances, as they are not readily identified as a problem or seen as violation of any drug-free policy. • Most school drug policies list all OTC drugs as prohibited substances. • The increase in beverages with "boosts" of caffeine. • See Chapter 6 for more information about laxative abuse.
Inhalants/ Solvents	• Adhesives: glue and cements • Aerosols: paint, hair sprays, fabric sprays such as butane • Anesthetics: gases such as nitrous oxide and local anesthetics, such as ethyl chloride • Cleaning agents including spot removers, dry cleaning fluids, and degreasers. • Gasoline	Huffing Balloons Whippets Poppers Snappers	• User seeks a lightheaded feeling from a substance that has another identified purpose. • Resembles alcohol intoxication but the effects last only for 15 to 45 minutes. • Weakness • Inattentiveness • Depressed mood • Weight loss	• Convenience store items such as whipped cream dispensers and correction fluid are commonly used. • A sensation of warmth and a "rush" can occur and may stimulate sexual pleasure. • Although use of any type of inhaled substance is difficult to identify during assessment, serious neurologic damage is known to occur from use. • Purchasing large amounts of these substances may be an indicator of abuse.

(Continued)

Table 5.3 • (Continued)

Name	Description	Street Name(s)	Signs & Symptoms	Related Information
Nicotine	Includes snuff, cigarettes, chewing tobacco, and cigars.	Smokes Squares Chew Dip Rub Stogies	• Scent of tobacco • Raspy cough • Yellow teeth • Brown fingertips • Ulcers in mouth • Stale breath • Premature aging	• Cigarette smoking kills an estimated 178,000 women in the United States annually. • One of the three leading smoking-related causes of death in women is lung cancer (45,000). • Ninety percent of all lung cancer deaths in women smokers are attributed to smoking. • Since 1950, lung cancer deaths among women have increased by more than 600%. • By 1987, lung cancer had surpassed breast cancer as the leading cause of cancer-related deaths. • Women who smoke have an increased risk for other cancers, including cancers of the oral cavity, pharynx, larynx (voice box), esophagus, pancreas, kidney, bladder, and uterine cervix. • Women who smoke double their risk for developing coronary heart disease and increase by more than 10-fold their likelihood of dying from chronic obstructive pulmonary disease. • Cigarette smoking increases the risk for infertility, preterm delivery, stillbirth, low birth weight, and sudden infant death syndrome (SIDS). • Postmenopausal women who smoke have lower bone density than women who never smoked. • Women who smoke have an increased risk for hip fracture than never smokers (*www.cdc.gov/tobacco/basic_information/index.htm*). • Legislation to ban smoking in public places has stirred much controversy.

				• Secondhand smoke issues are often debated and associated with health consequences. • Increased efforts to control underage use include requiring age identification for purchase of tobacco products. • Employers are taking a more aggressive stand in posting smoking areas and restrictions.
Caffeine	Refers to the liquid stimulant that stirs cravings and exaggerates some sensory and motor processes found in coffee and carbonated beverages.	Java Joe Boost	• Ingested to enhance excitement, mood, and periods of awareness. • Rapid speech • Irritability	• Continued use of caffeinated beverages in spite of identified health risks, such as palpitations, restlessness, and difficulty falling asleep. • Added social value to coffee consumption has increased with establishing coffee houses and flavored hot and cold coffee drinks. The addition of caffeine to carbonated beverages other than the colas (Mountain Dew).

treatment level needed to address the severity of the problem. The classification system used to do this is referred to as patient placement criteria (PPC) or, in some cases, client placement criteria. The most universally known of these is the criteria of the American Society of Addiction Medicine (ASAM). Using the ASAM criteria and a comprehensive biopsychosocial clinical interview, it is possible to determine the most appropriate treatment level (SAMHSA TIP 13, 2002).

Level 4: Clearly addicted represents the individual who demonstrates all the symptoms of the classic addiction syndrome.

Level 3: Heavy problem/early addiction refers to the status of those individuals who are beginning to experience medical complications as a result of their use. They may already have become dependent. Even if dependency is not present, they will likely be experiencing tolerance and withdrawal.

Level 2: Heavy social /early problem use identifies those individuals whose use is clearly above the norm for society and who have begun to experience some consequences as a result of their pattern of use. Many individuals at this level begin to recognize that their use is problematic and are able to change their behavior to prevent the development of dependence.

Level 1: Rare/social use is for individuals who use legal substances socially or experiment with the use of other substances. There might be rare instances of recreational use, but there would not be loss of control over use or any of the consequences that have been identified with that type of use.

Level 0: Total abstinence includes individuals who do not use substances and are at no risk for substance use problems.

Figure 5.1. The progression from use to dependence. (From Doweiko, H. E. [2006]. *Concepts of chemical dependency.* Belmont, CA Thomson Brooks/Cole.)

Box 5.1 • *DSM-IV-TR* Criteria for Substance Dependency

The *DSM-IV-TR* lists the following criteria as possible signs of a drug or alcohol addiction. Any combination of three or more of these criteria is considered diagnostic of dependency:

- A great deal of time is spent obtaining, using, and recovering from the chemical effects.
- Using more of the chemical than had been anticipated
- The development of tolerance to the chemical in question
- A characteristic withdrawal syndrome when the person stops using the chemical
- Repeated efforts to cut back or stop the drug use
- A reduction in social, occupational, or recreational activities in favor of further substance use
- Continuation of chemical use despite having suffered social, emotional, or physical problems related to drug use

Placement Criteria

The clinical interview measures symptoms according to six patient problem areas known as dimensions. These dimensions include the following:

Dimension 1: Acute intoxication and/or withdrawal potential

Dimension 2: Biomedical conditions and complications

Dimension 3: Emotional/behavioral conditions and complications

Dimension 4: Readiness to change

Dimension 5: Relapse, continued use, or continued problem potential

Dimension 6: Recovery/living environment

Within each of these dimensions are criteria that correspond to a level of treatment. Once severity is determined, the patient can be matched either to one of the five levels of detoxification or to one of four levels of treatment: (a) outpatient, (b) intensive outpatient/partial, (c) medically monitored intensive inpatient, or (d) medically managed intensive inpatient.

In addition to the ASAM criteria, each state's substance abuse treatment agency and each managed care company have adopted some type of placement criteria. They may have chosen from existing models or developed their own model. Each PCP should be familiar with the guidelines and standards relative to the medical-necessity criteria defined in the individual's behavioral health care plan and eligibility requirements to include assessment and ongoing treatment benefits. Verification of eligibility should be determined during the assessment phase and prior to every service provision thereafter to ensure authorization and effective resource management. To address issues surrounding this lack of conformity, the CSAT, a part of SAMHSA, formed a consensus panel. The result of the study was the *Treatment Improvement Protocol* (TIP), known as *Patient Placement Criteria* TIP 13. The first consensus panel completed a review of all placement criteria in use since the early 1980s and published the original TIP 13 in 1995. An updated version from 2002 is available online (see Treatment Improvement Exchange in the Websites for Providers and Patients section).

It is unreasonable to expect that PCPs will be skilled in using PPC. However, familiarity with the various dimensions and criteria is necessary to facilitate the appropriate referral for patients screened in the primary care setting. As a complement to the staff in the primary care setting, many providers elect to employ certified addiction professionals as full staff members, contract with addiction professionals as consultants, or establish referral agreements with a variety of community agencies to provide services and/or consultation as indicated. The credentials of certified addiction professionals should be verified directly with the certifying entity to ensure the authenticity of these qualifications. Proactively, the PCP should have this action plan defined so that implementation may be timely when issues related to addiction are identified.

ASSESSMENT

The first step in the assessment process takes place within the normal physical assessment process of the PCP. There are recognizable physical findings that can raise the suspicion of addiction even if the individual denies substance use.

Physical Examination

During the physical examination, the PCP should pay special attention to the following:

- Changes from previous physical exams
- Odors on the breath and clothing
- Poor nutritional status

- Poor personal hygiene
- Intoxicated behavior during the visit, especially slurred speech and staggering gait
- Signs of physical abuse, bruises, lacerations, scratches, burns, needle marks, sores, or abscesses
- Skin rashes or discoloration, hair loss, or excessive sweating
- Head, eyes, ears, nose, and throat status (inflammation, irritation, blanching of any of the mucosa, gum disease, sinus tenderness or sinusitis, rhinitis, or perforated nasal septum)

Disorders of the gastrointestinal tract or the immune, cardiovascular, and pulmonary systems are often complications of addictive behavior. Most frequent are disorders of the liver; hypertension and tachycardia; lymphadenopathy; and coughing with wheezing, rales, and rhonchi. There may be neurologic impairment that presents as cognitive deficits or sensory, motor, or memory impairment. Women may have reproductive disorders (SAMHSA TIP 40, 2004).

Laboratory Values as Indicators of Use

Individuals with addictions are frequently exposed to a number of diseases. Laboratory testing can be conducted for baseline values; blood alcohol levels; and infectious diseases such as HIV/AIDS, hepatitis B and C, and tuberculosis. Other biologic screens may have value in some settings, but there is no current indication for their use in a primary care setting. If it is possible to obtain these results, they may provide some help in offering feedback, encouraging honesty about use, or providing follow-up care (Box 5.2).

Determining Level of Use

Once the PCP suspects that there may be an addictive process occurring, it becomes important to determine the level of the risk and the significance. Quantifying the amount consumed of the substance of choice and the degree of engaging in the addictive behavior is a challenge to all health care providers, because patients may be unclear regarding use and importance. For example, in reporting substance use one time, the patient may overlook an explanation that one-time use includes drinking until passing out or that weekend-only drinking actually means drinking from the end of school or work on Friday until returning to school or work Monday morning. PCPs are encouraged to ask specific questions to obtain a clear pattern of substance abuse. The following may be a

Box 5.2 • Biologic Screening Tools

MCV—Mean Corpuscular Volume
Normal range: 87–103 cubic microns

Measures red blood cell volume and distribution. Elevated levels cause by many other disorders.

GGT—Gamma-glutamyl Transferase
Normal range: Women 7–25 IU/L, men 11–38 IU/L

Measures damage to liver cells; a rise in GGT levels has been correlated with an increase in alcohol intake.

CDT—Carbohydrate-deficient Transferrin, AST—Aspartate Aminotransferase
Normal range CDT: Women 26 IU/L, men 20 IU/L

Normal range AST: 10–34 IU/L

Relatively new tests, the CDT and AST appear to have some value in identifying heavy alcohol consumption. Until large-scale studies begin to confirm their effectiveness for screening and assessment, these tests will be used primarily by researchers.

BAL—Blood Alcohol Level and Breathalyzer
BAL: 20–80 mg/dL indicates alterations in mood, coordination. Helpful only to show recent use.

Breathalyzer: Most states consider that 0.08 on the breathalyzer indicates intoxication.

Urine Toxicology Screens
Urine toxicology screen results are positive or negative. May be useful when screening adolescents who are demonstrating concurrent problems (e.g., legal, school, family problems).

helpful guideline to consistently measure alcohol consumption by defining one drink as:

- A single small glass (8 ounces/half-pint) of beer
- A single glass (5 ounces) of wine
- A single shot/measure (1.5 ounces) of 80-proof distilled spirits

Risky and hazardous drinking is determined by the amount consumed in one session of drinking and varies by population (Table 5.4).

Table 5.4 • Dangerous Amounts of Alcohol When Consumed on Specific Occasions

Population	Daily or On Occasion	Weekly
Men	4 drinks	14 drinks
Women	3 drinks	7 drinks
Pregnant	Any amount	Any amount
Adolescent	Any amount	Any amount
Elderly	3 drinks	7 drinks

The strength of illicit substances can also be questionable, as they may be laced or cut with other identified substances. The purity of heroin and the "reliability" of the marijuana supplier are just a few challenges to the ability to predict the effect that using a substance will have on the individual.

Screening

As chemical dependency is a progressive disease, an essential part of the assessment and screening process for the PCP is developing a relationship with the individual being assessed. In fact, the World Health Organization reported that many patients were pleased to find that their PCPs were interested in their use of chemicals and the problems that may be associated with use (SAMHSA TIP 24, 1999). In the event that addiction-specific services are needed, it is critical for the PCP and addiction provider to communicate, collaborate, and coordinate care. Failing to do so risks contributing to physical and behavioral health consequences and the progression of disease.

The SBIRT Project is an excellent resource to assist PCPs in developing the skills for addiction screening and referring patients to an addiction professional. Manuals are available free of charge through the original state grant recipients and the Addiction Technology Transfer Center. Contact information is included in the Resources for Providers section at the end of this chapter.

PCPs are identified as crucial players in identifying addiction problems early. The patient's personal history may be the simplest means of detecting factors that warrant further assessment. Incorporating questions about substance use and compulsive behaviors into every intake process is advised. PCPs may also utilize more formal screening tools such as self-administered questionnaires or brief face-to-face surveys to evaluate whether a patient may be involved in addiction or whether the presenting symptoms are associated with an addiction. The PCP determines whether the individual would benefit from a more comprehensive assessment by an addiction professional and facilitates the referral. In all instances, there is the opportunity to provide education about addictive behavior and substance abuse as well as the benefit of seeking support to reduce or eliminate the risk of addiction.

While the PCP is challenged to find the time to address these risks during every office visit, many professionals agree that doing so on a routine basis actually saves time in other ways, not to mention delays in treatment or further assessment of abnormal test values or presenting symptoms. Table 5.5 includes many of the commonly used screening instruments. Most of these tools may be obtained by contacting the organization or individual who developed them. Many will provide guides for administration and interpretation. Some are substance specific, while others look at addiction in general.

SPECIFIC CHARACTERISTICS OF WOMEN IN ADDICTIONS

Identifying and recognizing characteristics of women in addiction is a significant component of establishing a comprehensive understanding of all the issues that may impact the behaviors, patterns of addiction, response to treatment, and available resources and supports. Obtaining a thorough history and including queries specific to these variables are essential to the process. Being cognizant of these factors may eliminate delays in treatment response and barriers that may arise as a result of overlooking the need to address them. What follows are a few of the many other factors that may be associated with the woman in addiction.

Families and Children

During the later half of the 20th century, mental health and substance abuse professionals began to alter their developmental theories about individuals and families. Instead of a focus on the inner processes of the individual, the focus became the relationships among the individuals who made up the family. The family systems theory, as it is known, provides a basis for identifying the ongoing interaction and transformation of the members of the system. The child responds to the family, and the family responds to the child; there is no beginning or end but a feedback process that is ongoing, circular, and continuous in nature (SAMHSA TIP 6, 1999).

Text continues on page 157.

Table 5.5 • Screening Tools

Tool	Description	Administration
CONTACT INFO: Can be downloaded from Project Cork website: *www.project-cork.org/clinical_tools/index.html*. There is no fee for use. CAGE-AID	Have you ever felt that you should **C**ut down on your drinking/prescription drug use/illicit drug use? Have people **A**nnoyed you by criticizing your drinking/prescription drug use/illicit drug use? Have you ever felt bad or **G**uilty about your drinking/ prescription drug use/illicit drug use? Have you ever had a drink or used your drug the first thing in the morning to steady your nerves or get rid of a hangover (**E**ye opener) +Instrument Adapted to Include Drugs	• Can be completed by PCP during an office visit. • Information collected provides prescreening data to determine the need for continued assessment whereby responses will be further explored to establish need for treatment with an addiction professional.
TWEAK CONTACT INFO: Can be downloaded from Project Cork website: *www.project-cork.org/clinical_tools/index.html*. There is no fee for use.	How many drinks can you hold? (**T**olerance) Have close friends or relatives worried? (**W**) Do you drink when you first get up? (**E**ye opener) Has a friend told "x" you could not remember? (**A**mnesia) Do you feel the need to cut down on your drinking? (**K**ut) Information collected provides prescreening data to determine the need for continued assessment whereby responses will be further explored to establish criteria for treatment with an addiction professional.	• Can be completed by PCP during an office visit. • Recommended for use with pregnant women. • If respondent reports Tolerance of more than five drinks without falling asleep or passing out, 2 points are awarded. • A positive response to Worry scores 2 points. • A positive response to EAK questions is given 1 point each. • A total score of 2 or more indicates that the woman is a risk drinker and further education/assessment is recommended.

(*Continued*)

Table 5.5 • (Continued)

Tool	Description	Administration
AUDIT—Alcohol Use Disorders Identification Test CONTACT INFO: Can be downloaded from Project Cork website: *www.project-cork.org/clinical_tools/index.html*. There is no fee for use.	• Part I is the core consisting of 10 questions to determine diagnosis and need for treatment for alcohol abuse, dependence, and/or addiction and assesses symptoms and other problems associated with use. How often do you have a drink containing alcohol? How many drinks containing alcohol do you have on a typical day when you are drinking? How often do you have one or more drinks on one occasion? How often during the last year did you find that you were not able to stop drinking once you started? How often during the last year did you fail to do what was normally expected from you because of drinking? How often during the last year did you need a first drink in the morning to get yourself going after a heavy drinking session? How often during the last year did you have a feeling of guilt or remorse after drinking? How often during the last year were you unable to remember what happened the night before because you had been drinking? Have you or someone else been injured as a result of your drinking?	• Administered during office visit. Responder answers each item related to behavior during the past year and must select the statement that most applies to the responder. • A drink is defined by one of the following: • A single small glass of beer (8 oz.; half-pint). • A single shot/measure of liquor/spirits • A single glass of wine • The interviewer reassures the patient that the information is confidential. The questions are easy to understand. PCPs may choose to administer as a self-report questionnaire, instructing the participant prior to beginning and discussing the responses after completion. • The AUDIT includes clear scoring guidelines to assist the clinician with interpretation of the instrument to assist determining the type of follow-up needed.

Table 5.5 • (Continued)

Tool	Description	Administration
	Has a relative or friend or doctor or other health worker been concerned about your drinking or suggested you cut down? • Part II is the clinical assessment consisting of a brief physical exam, several questions about trauma history, and liver function testing. Professional review of this instrument indicates that answers are applicable across cultures, age, and gender.	
MIDAS—Mentally Ill Drug & Alcohol Screening CONTACT INFO: Developed by Kenneth Minkoff, M.D. through the Ohio SAMI CCOE.	Consists of 17 YES/NO questions.	Administered during office visit and easily scored with a score of 1 to 12 indicating probable abuse and a score of 13 to 17 indicating probable dependence.
MAST: Michigan Alcoholism Screening Test CONTACT INFO: Can be downloaded from Project Cork website: *www.project-cork.org/clinical_tools/index.html*. There is no fee for use.	Total of 24 YES or NO questions associated with the effects of drinking too much alcohol such as: Have you ever been in a hospital because of drinking? Have you ever been arrested for drunk driving or driving after drinking? Have you ever neglected your obligations, your family, or your work for 2 or more days in a row because you were drinking?	• Can be completed by PCP during an office visit. • Information collected provides prescreening data to determine the need for continued assessment whereby responses will be further explored to establish criteria for treatment with an addiction professional. • Each question is assigned a point value associated with alcoholism, suggested alcoholism, or no alcoholism.

(*Continued*)

Table 5.5 • (Continued)

Tool	Description	Administration
	Has your wife, husband (or other family member) ever gone to anyone for help about your drinking? Have you ever lost a job because of drinking? Do you drink before noon fairly often? Have you gotten into physical fights when drinking? Have you ever attended a meeting of Alcoholics Anonymous (AA)?	
SMAST: Short MAST	Total of 13 questions taken from the full MAST.	Same as MAST.
MAST G: MAST Geriatric Version	These 24 questions are different from both the MAST and SMAST. All responses are YES or NO and associate drinking with changes in ADLs and previous patterns of drinking to include some of the following examples: After drinking have you ever noticed an increase in your heart rate or beating in your chest? Does having a drink help you sleep? Do you hide your alcohol bottles from family members? Are you drinking more now than in the past? Have you ever made rules to manage your drinking?	Recommended use to screen individuals over the age of 60 years.

Table 5.5 • (Continued)

Tool	Description	Administration
GAIN SS: Global Assessment of Individual Needs - Short Screener CONTACT INFO: Download possible from the Lighthouse Institute website.	Twenty questions covering psychologic, behavioral, and personal effects of use as well as recent drug/alcohol use within the last month, 2 to 12 months, or more than 1 year, divided into 5 items for substance disorders; 5 for internalizing disorders, such as depression, suicide and anxiety; 5 for externalizing disorders, such as behavioral disorders; and 5 for crimes and violence.	• Can be completed by PCP during an office visit. • Information collected provides prescreening data to determine the need for continued assessment whereby responses will be explored to establish criteria for treatment with an addiction professional.
SAAST: Self-Administered Alcohol Screening Test CONTACT INFO: This scale is not copyrighted for use and may be obtained by contacting the Mayo Foundation for Medical Education and Research.	• Consists of 37 items. Responses are YES or NO. Each question is assigned a + or −, with + sign indicating alcoholic responses. • Questions include patterns of use, such as "Do you ever drink in the morning?"; physical/cognitive effects of use, such as "Have you ever had severe shaking, heard voices, or seen things that weren't there after heavy drinking?"; and can you identify relatives with or history of alcohol problems.	Test can be administered during an office interview or self-administered via paper or reproduced on a computer.

(Continued)

Table 5.5 • (Continued)

Tool	Description	Administration
CIWA-Ar: Addiction Research Foundation Clinical Institute Withdrawal Assessment for Alcohol CONTACT INFO: SAMHSA Tip 24	Tool asks patient to rate the following 9 areas using a scale from 0 to 7: Nausea and vomiting Tactile disturbances Tremor Auditory disturbances Paroxysmal sweats Visual disturbances Anxiety Headache, fullness in head Agitation The 10th area is Orientation and Clouding of Sensorium and is scored between 0 and 4.	• Takes 2 to 5 minutes to administer. • Three areas are scored by the PCP's observation (tremor, paroxysmal sweats, and agitation). • One area, anxiety, is scored combining the response and observation. • The maximum possible score is 67 points with a score of 10 or more indicating clinical concern.
CRAFFT CONTACT INFO: Can be downloaded from Project Cork website: *www.project-cork.org/clinical_tools/index.html*. There is no fee for use.	Have you ever ridden in a **C**ar driven by someone (including yourself) who was "high" or who had been using alcohol or drugs? Do you ever use alcohol or drugs to **R**elax, feel better about yourself, or fit in? Do you ever use alcohol/drugs while you are by yourself? (***A***) Do your family or **F**riends ever tell you that you should cut down on your drinking or drug use? Do you ever **F**orget things you did while using alcohol or drugs? Have you gotten into **T**rouble while you were using alcohol or drugs?	• Can be completed by PCP during an office visit. • Information collected provides prescreening data to determine the need for continued assessment whereby responses will be further explored to establish criteria for treatment with an addictions professional.

Table 5.5 • (Continued)

Tool	Description	Administration
POSIT: Problem Oriented Screening Instrument for Teenagers CONTACT INFO: This noncopyrighted document as well as the scoring template may be obtained at no cost from the National Clearinghouse for Alcohol and Drug Information, DHHS publication no. ADM 91-1735.	Consists of 139 YES or NO questions. Including personality traits and high-risk behaviors that may or may not be associated with addiction. Several examples include the following: Do you have so much energy you don't know what to do with it? Do you get into trouble because you use drugs or alcohol at school? Do your friends get bored at parties when there is no alcohol served? Are most of your friends older than you? Do you threaten to hurt people? Have the whites of your eyes ever turned yellow? Do you forget things you did while drinking or using drugs? Do you miss school or arrive late for school because of your alcohol or drug use? Do you worry a lot? Are you restless and can't sit still? Have you ever had sexual intercourse without using a condom?	• Estimated to take 25 minutes to administer. • Can be self-administered in writing, adapted to computerized administration, or completed during a structured interview. • Participants are instructed to answer each question even if a question does not fit exactly. Participants may ask for explanations if they do not understand a word or question.

(Continued)

Table 5.5 • (Continued)

Tool	Description	Administration
ASI - Addiction Severity Index CONTACT INFO : Thomas McLellan, PhD, Department of Psychiatry and the University of Pennsylvania.	This 161-item instrument is multidimensional.	• Administered as part of an interview and takes approximately 45 minutes to complete and score. • This form and administration manual are available at no charge by contacting the developer. • Recommended use during the ongoing maintenance/ reassessment process (Grupp, 2006).
CSSA – Cocaine Selective Severity Assessment CONTACT INFO: Kampman, K. M., Volppicelli, J. R., McGinnis, D. E., et al. (1998). Reliability and validity of the CSSA. *Addictive Behaviors,* 23(4), 449–461.	Consists of 18 items.	• Takes 10 minutes to administer. The higher the score, the greater the clinical concern.
SOWS – Subjective Opiate Withdrawal Scale CONTACT INFO: Handelsman, L., Cochrane, K. J., Aronson, M. J., et al. (1987). Two new rating scales for opiate withdrawal. *American Journal of Alcohol Abuse,* 13, 293–308.	A 16-item questionnaire seeking responses to the extent the individual is currently experiencing each of the characteristics described.	Each item is scored between 0 and 4. The higher the score, the greater the severity of the associated withdrawal.

Table 5.5 • (Continued)

Tool	Description	Administration
OOWS—Objective Opiate Withdrawal Scale CONTACT INFO: Handelsman, L., Cochrane, K. J., Aronson, M. J., et al. (1987). Two new rating scales for opiate withdrawal. *American Journal of Alcohol Abuse, 13*, 293–308.	Thirteen manifestations of withdrawal are identified. Staff completing this assessment must be familiar with the signs and symptoms of opiate withdrawal. The clinician completes this by direct observation of the individual.	• Observation takes approximately 10 minutes. The rater scores each item on a scale of 0 to 13. The more pronounced the presenting symptom, the higher the score. The higher score indicates the risk of more severe withdrawal.
FTND—Fagerstrom Test for Nicotine Dependence CONTACT INFO: Personality Research website: *www.personalityresearch.org.*	This test is a modification of the FTQ—Fagerstrom Tolerance Questionnaire known to be the standard instrument used to measure physical dependence on nicotine. Contains 6 questions.	May be self-administered or during brief interview. Each question has more than one response to choose and each is assigned a point value from 0 to 3. Total scores greater than 7 are considered nicotine dependence.
GN-SBQ—The Glover-Nilsson Smoking Behavioral Questionnaire CONTACT INFO: Personality Research website: *www.personalityresearch.org.*	Eleven questions; identifies behaviors associated with smoking and evaluates the impact of these behaviors and patterns that develop as result.	This test is self-administered. The information will help both the treating clinician and individual to better understand the factors that influence physical and behavioral dependence.
T-ACE— Tolerance Annoyed Cut Eye-opener	Four simple questions: How many drinks does it take for you to feel high? (T) Have people annoyed you by criticizing your drinking? (A)	Easily incorporated into every office visit questionnaire. Has been tested and found to be appropriate for pregnant women.

(Continued)

Table 5.5 • (Continued)

Tool	Description	Administration
CONTACT INFO: Sokol, R. J., Martier, S. S., Ager, J. W. (1989). The T-ACE questions: Practical prenatal detection of risk-drinking. *American Journal of Obstetrics and Gynecology, 160*(4), 863–868.	Have you ever felt you should to cut down on your drinking? (C) Have you ever had a drink first thing in the morning to steady your nerves or get rid of a hangover? (E)	Any woman who answers more than two drinks on the tolerance question is scored 2 points. Each yes to the ACE questions is given a score of 1. A total score of 2 or more is considered a positive screen, and further assessment is recommended.
4 Ps CONTACT INFO: Developed by the Born Free Project in Martinex , California	Four simple questions with responses of YES or NO: Have you ever used drugs or alcohol during this ***P***regnancy? Have you had a problem with drugs or alcohol in the ***P***ast? Does your ***P***artner have a problem with drugs or alcohol? Do you consider one of your ***P***arents to be an addict or alcoholic?	• Although most often used for screening pregnant females, these questions may be added to any intake process. • Any woman who answers yes to one or more question should be given educational material to include where to turn for additional support or assessment.
SASSI—Substance Abuse Subtle Screening Inventory CONTACT INFO: SASSI Institute website: *www.sassi.com.*	One-page questionnaire rates probability of a substance use disorder. There is an adult version, the Adult SASSI-3, and an adolescent version, the SASSI-2. There is also a Spanish version. A web-based option has been developed for the adult screening with progress toward the adolescent version.	• Brief, easily administered during scheduled office visit. • Takes 15 minutes to complete and 5 minutes to score. • There is a fee for these tests. • Administration guides and test administrator training information are also available on the website.

Families have identifiable and predictable patterns of behavior among their members as they strive to preserve the status quo. All families have rules, roles, verbal and nonverbal communication, closeness or distance, boundaries, and hierarchy. Healthy families have clear but flexible rules and roles: Parents make the decisions and provide support and a positive example. Nonverbal communication is the same as what is communicated verbally, family members feel interrelated but are able to be together or separate without discomfort, and change takes place at a pace that is comfortable for all members (SAMHSA TIP 6, 1999).

Dysfunctional families show very different patterns of interaction. Rules and roles may be so rigid that families are unable to adapt as needed or are so flexible that only chaos is possible; unspoken rules may be more important than spoken rules. The pattern of communication may become so distorted that it is difficult to determine who is in charge, family members may begin to have difficulty determining what is real and what is not, and boundaries may blur and anxiety may increase (SAMHSA TIP 6, 1999).

Substance use disorders do not appear in isolation. Interaction with the family of origin and the current family provide the patterns and dynamics for addictive behaviors (SAMHSA TIP 34, 1999). Parents with substance use disorders may model drug use. Parental drug use or other disturbances in family function may make parents ineffective or inattentive in their child-rearing behaviors. Children reared in families with long-standing family issues may find themselves at risk physically and emotionally. They have no example for developing healthy boundaries or communication skills. Their transition into young adulthood may be difficult due to a lack of skill in negotiating change as well as a lack of parental intercession to mediate the influence of peer practice and other social forces (SAMHSA TIP 6, 1999).

Adolescent Females

The 2005 survey conducted by SAMHSA found that 56.2% of females age 18 and younger accounted for the reported first use of illicit drugs. Every opportunity to identify factors associated with substance use or addictive behavior should be taken. Inquiring about recent or past substance use as well as sexual contact and relationships and the date of the last menstrual period (LMP) may prompt further discussion about high-risk behaviors. Refer to Chapter 6 to understand how significant the LMP may be in identifying the presence of an eating disorder.

Little information is available that separates adolescent male and female substance abuse. Unless specified, most reports about adolescent substance use refers across the genders. Often, adolescent female use is minimized, and male use is assumed to account for the majority. PCPs need to take into account that their female adolescent patients are equally as likely to be using or abusing substances and engaging in related addictive behavior. Overall, adolescent substance use and addictive disorders have caused a 39% increase in professional intervention. This includes treatment for substance dependency (SAMHSA, NSDUH, 2005). Alarmingly, more than half of the referrals for professional intervention and treatment were initiated through the criminal justice system. Adolescent substance use is rarely in isolation and often includes binge episodes. More times than not, school performance and family relationships suffer negative consequences as substance use and associated addictive behaviors become more prominent in an adolescent's life. One in seven adolescents admits to drinking and driving at least once a year (Fornili, 2004). This behavior has continued even though most states strongly enforce the drinking age. The consequences of underage drinking or drinking and driving can include suspension of driving privileges or delays in obtaining a license.

As discussed later in this chapter, clinicians must be aware of the Health Information Portability Accountability Act (HIPAA) of 1996 and its regulations regarding disclosure of personal health information to parents of a minor. This is equally important for the adolescent and the parents to understand. It is the responsibility of the PCP to communicate within the boundaries of these regulations and know what instances may be identified as exceptions to obtaining consent or authorization from the minor.

Again, the role of the PCP is multifaceted and presents many challenges to find the time to communicate with all involved in the care of the adolescent. For the guardian or parent of the adolescent, the PCP may be recognized as a reliable support for immediate assessment and intervention. For the adolescent, the staff in the primary care setting may provide an opportunity to establish a relationship with a caring, concerned adult.

Elderly Women

Symptoms of substance abuse and addiction are often overlooked or unjustly associated with dementia, depression, adverse drug reactions, or other conditions common to older adults. Because of this, little attention has been paid to associate findings or even study gender-specific patterns of substance use or abuse and related addictive behavior in the elderly population. In fact, researchers are just beginning to identify the concern of addiction in the elderly. Psychosocial and physiologic changes that accompany aging may alter the effects of substances on the individual and increase risks for injury and illness as well as emotional and socioeconomic decline (Fornili, 2004). A simple assessment of the ability to complete ADLs or notable changes in them may prompt further investigation.

While older adults are more likely to hide their substance use and addiction, the families of older adults are often embarrassed when treatment or intervention is needed (SAMHSA TIP 26C, 2006). Although attempts are made to maintain the autonomy of the elderly, family members or friends may need to be contacted to obtain information, especially if it appears that the older adult may not be coherent or capable of giving reliable information. If it is necessary to contact other individuals on behalf of the older adult, the PCP is reminded that confidentiality regulations require obtaining signed releases of information.

Adults 65 years of age and older consume more prescribed and over-the-counter medications than any other age group in the United States. Prescription drug misuse and abuse is prevalent among older adults not only because more drugs are prescribed to them but also because, as with alcohol, aging makes the body more vulnerable to drug effects. Any use of drugs in combination with alcohol carries risk; abuse of these substances raises that risk, and multiple drug abuse raises it even further (SAMHSA TIP 26C, 1998).

Women of Childbearing Age

From menarche through late adulthood, the date of the LMP should be identified during each office visit. In addition, inquiring whether the individual believes that she could be pregnant may prompt further discussion about sexual activity, safe sex practices, and education opportunities. This dialogue offers the PCP the opportunity to specifically inquire about the degree of substance use and assist in determining the need for a pregnancy test or other tests related to sexually transmitted diseases in the event that the information indicates symptoms.

PCPs are encouraged to have pamphlets and other resources available in the waiting area for the individual to take without threat of discovery until she is more comfortable with disclosure. Although alcohol consumption during pregnancy was prohibited in the past, some PCPs believe that alcohol may be used in moderation. Being prepared to answer the question about drinking during pregnancy is essential to include what "one" drink means and the period of time in which the allowable amount may be consumed.

Women in the Workforce

Substance use and its associated issues can affect a woman's ability to work and/or the quality of her work, which can have a far-reaching effect on the individual, families, and society. Public safety can be threatened when these individuals are members of health care or other professions that deal with the public. Often, women have children and families for whom they are caring. Research has identified this as a factor that impacts their ability to seek help (Grupp, 2006). Obtaining information related to resources and supports can remove this barrier to obtaining counseling and other treatment services.

Employers recognize that employees may display job-performance problems at some point in their work life. For example, coming to work late may be just an isolated incident or a symptom of a much larger problem. Supervisors are in a position to evaluate behavior and determine if there is a pattern of decline that may need to be addressed with corrective action or a referral for assessment counseling or treatment. Boxes 5.3 and 5.4 may be used as checklists to determine whether substance-related job-performance problems exist. When performance declines as a result of substance use, employers and professional credentialing and licensing boards are usually involved.

Corrective and/or disciplinary action are usually taken when there are issues regarding job performance. In an effort to promote public safety and retain competent professionals, various professional organizations have begun to look at the problem and develop peer assistance or alternatives-to-discipline programs. PCPs should become familiar with these work-related characteristics of addiction. In the event that concerns are identified, PCPs need to be knowledgeable about employee assistance programs that are available to families in addition to the employee, which will help to establish a partnership between the PCP and peer assistance/alternatives-to-discipline programs that will best meet the woman's needs.

Pregnant Addicts

Between 5% and 10% of all women have substance abuse problems during pregnancy. This finding is consistent among women of all ethnic, geographic, and socioeconomic groups. In 2001, the rates of current illicit drug use were similar for white (4.0%), black (3.7%), and Hispanic (3.3%) pregnant women (SAMHSA TIP 45, 2006).

Substance abuse contributes to both obstetric and pediatric complications, including fetal alcohol syndrome, prematurity, and placental abruption. The opportunity to intervene and treat addiction during pregnancy has been significantly more effective than efforts that occur at other times in a woman's life (Health Resources and Services Administration, 2001). Because the PCP may be the first person to identify the pregnancy and presenting symptoms, providing

Box 5.3 • Warning Signs at Work

Decline in Job Efficiency

- Decrease in overall work quality
- Inconsistent work quality
- Errors in judgment
- Periods of confusion
- Lack of concentration
- Unrealistic excuses for lowered work quality
- Missed deadlines
- Increased carelessness/mistakes
- Excessive time completing tasks
- Difficulty handling complex tasks
- Loss of memory

Impaired Interpersonal Relationships

- Frequent arguments with coworkers
- Excessive blaming of others
- Unwilling to cooperate or compromise with coworkers
- Overreactions to coworkers
- Wide swings in mood from isolation to angry outbursts
- Avoidance of contact with supervisor
- Complaints of irritability, physical roughness, verbal abuse

Absenteeism

- Repeated absenteeism (above average)
- Pattern of absenteeism around scheduled days off
- Excessive tardiness (Monday and Friday) or after days off
- Leaving work early
- Repeated absenteeism due to vaguely defined illnesses
- Improbable reasons for absenteeism
- Unauthorized leave
- Last-minute request for leave
- Excessive use of sick leave

(Continued)

Box 5.3 • (Continued)

On-the-job Absenteeism
- Extended lunch breaks
- Physical illnesses developed on the job
- Unexplained disappearances on the job
- Excessive breaks, trips to bathroom
- Vacant look

Attitude/Mood
- Dramatic mood shifts
- Tendency to isolate
- Irritability
- Secretive and or suspicious
- Teary/crying
- Inflexible

Physical/Emotional Problems
- Change in physical/emotional condition during workday
- Marked nervousness on the job
- Excessive sweating
- Tremors of hands
- Lack of attention to personal cleanliness or grooming
- Reports to duty despite not being fit

Inconsistent Work Patterns
- Alternate periods of high and low efficiency
- Becoming or currently less dependable
- Substandard work compared with that of peers
- Frequent requests for help with assignments

Other Areas
- Excessive time spent making personal telephone calls
- Physically threatening to others
- Excessive talkativeness

Retrieved January 23, 2007, from *www.peerassist.org*; 2007 assessment forms are available for download on the website.

Box 5.4 • Warning Signs of Addictive Behaviors in Nurses and Pharmacists

- Difficulty concentrating
- Assignments take more time despite skill/experience
- Difficulty prioritizing
- Medication errors
- Omitted, illogical, incomplete, or illegible charting
- Deteriorating handwriting or performance during shift
- Errors in transcribing orders or taking verbal orders
- Overlooking signs of a patient's deteriorating condition

Retrieved January 23, 2007, from *www.peerassist.org*; 2007 assessment forms are available for download on the website.

support and promptly accessing resources to include referral are critical. Coordinating care between the PCPs and obstetric services will be essential to effective management of existing medical or psychiatric conditions warranting medications that have the risk of abuse by the mother and harm to the fetus.

Incarcerated Women

The growing female prison population has been recognized throughout the United States, with the northeastern regions reporting the lowest incidence. In contrast to the 1977 statistic of 11,212 incarcerated women, a total of 96,125 women were incarcerated in 2004 (Join Together, 2006). In 2005, a total of 2.3 million persons age 12 and older received substance use treatment, with 229,000 of those being treated in prison or jail (SAMHSA TIP 45, 2006). Approximately 19.1% of the 1,357,841 state and local arrests for drug abuse violations in the United States have involved females (Office of National Drug Control Policy, 2006). The Bureau of Justice Statistics reported that 60.2% of state and 42.8% of federal female prisoners surveyed in 2004 met criteria to be diagnosed with an addiction. A report released by the Institute on Women and Criminal Justice in May 2006 cited drugs as significantly contributing to this increase (Frost, Greene, and Pranis, 2006). Methamphetamine use has been identified as the primary drug of choice associated with offenses warranting involvement with the criminal justice system.

Because the PCP's goal may be to access alternatives to incarceration, he or she may be involved with drug testing or treating the physical conditions associated with high-risk behaviors. The predominant risk for women of all ages is engaging in sexually promiscuous behaviors that may result in contracting sexually transmitted diseases, hepatitis C, and/or HIV/AIDS. Disease-state management protocols are available to include patient education about personal health management, risks of continued behavior(s), and chronic disease management to include HIV/AIDS. PCPs may not be given this information during the intake of the patient for requested services; however, in the event that the patient is involved in the criminal justice system and mandated for treatment to include care provided by the PCP, a clear definition of expectations related to reporting compliance needs to be established.

Culture, Race, Ethnicity, and Sexual Orientation

Minimizing barriers is key to developing a relationship between the PCP and patient. Most initial patient histories include race, although the primary care setting is challenged to identify methods to obtain information related to other personal characteristics. Simple modifications to how questions are worded may invite more discussion informing the PCP of beliefs and values that may impact treatment response, including the following:

- Family organization and relational roles (both traditional and nontraditional)
- Effects of ethnically related stress factors, such as poverty and discrimination
- Beliefs and practices related to physical and mental health
- Spirituality
- Sexual orientation
- History of past treatment and help-seeking efforts
- Changes in the individual and family related to immigration, assimilation, or acculturation (SAMHSA National Mental Health Information Center, 2006)
- Language barriers

The PCP must ensure that both formal and informal assessment processes are reliable and valid for use with all consumers. This also requires awareness of how important it is for forms and conversations to be clearly understood to avoid misinterpretation. In addition, the PCP must be cognizant of a client's linguistic differences, which may affect symptom expression (SAMHSA National Mental Health Information Center, 2006).

Managed care standards require providers to demonstrate cultural competence to address individual characteristics of persons seeking treatment. The standards stress the importance of providing a safe and nonjudgmental treatment environment. Providers are encouraged to obtain information during the credentialing and contracting process to ensure compliance with standards set forth by all regulatory entities, because compliance impacts the ability to deliver services and receive reimbursement.

SAMHSA's 2005 national survey provides details about the trends specific to geographic location as well as substance use preferences. Awareness of the patterns specific to a group and practice location as well as nationally identified trends may provide significant insight to the PCP. Establishing resources in the clinical practice to address trends identified both nationally and with the population served will strengthen the effectiveness of health assessment and treatment outcomes.

CO-OCCURRING DISORDERS IN WOMEN

SAMHSA found that 54% of women who were dependent on or abused illicit drugs or alcohol experienced serious psychologic distress (SAMHSA TIP 42, 2005). Recognizing and appropriately treating comorbid substance use and mental disorders in women are especially important. Drugs are more readily available and females now are represented in almost equal numbers with their male counterparts, but they continue to be assessed and treated with male-derived protocols. The presence of substance use disorders in women is accompanied with a higher incidence of mental disorders—by slightly more than half (Evans and Sullivan, 2001), stigma, and social problems associated with child rearing and relationships. The assessment process may be complicated by the difference in presenting symptomatology and accompanying coping mechanisms (Fornili, 2004; SAMHSA TIP 42).

SAMHSA TIP 42 (2005) offers the estimate that between 55% and 99% of women receiving treatment for substance abuse have experienced some type of trauma. Because 33% to 59% (SAMHSA TIP 42) of these women currently meet the diagnostic criteria for posttraumatic stress disorder, it is recommended that treatment programs screen for abuse histories as a part of the assessment process and provide treatment and/or education as indicated. As mixed-gender programs continue to be the rule, treatment programs need to begin to offer women-only groups that address the sensitive issues of trauma, parenting, and self-esteem.

Coexisting medical problems have often presented a challenge for the PCP, especially when treating an individual with a substance addiction. Often, pain can be a symptom of the medical disorder or the result of some aspect of the treatment process for that disorder. The goal is to manage pain without exacerbating abuse and promoting relapse. One of the difficulties is helping the individual to distinguish between the need for medication to relieve pain and the cravings that are occurring. Personal control of analgesia is not recommended, and a fixed administration schedule is recommended rather than prescribing as-needed medications (Ziegler, 2007).

In patients identified with a very high risk for relapse, a "medication administrator" may be identified. This person actually holds the medication and administers it according to schedule (Ziegler, 2007). In all cases, a concerted effort by the prescribing physician and pharmacist administering the prescription refills is critical. Many prescription plans have defined and strict regulations associated with the time frame when a prescription may be refilled. For the patient who reports that she is engaged in agonist treatment for opioid dependence including methadone or buprenorphine, the PCP should obtain a release for information so that the prescribing physician may be involved in the pain management plan.

TREATMENT OPTIONS

Patient outcomes have been successful by utilizing approaches that include the harm reduction model and behavioral health counseling in conjunction with 12-step programs. Harm reduction refers to gradually reducing the amount and frequency of substance use and related behaviors as opposed to total abstinence. Behavioral health counselors develop comprehensive treatment plans that include community and support group involvement as well as family education and family therapy. This allows significant others the opportunity to openly discuss the impact that addiction has had on their lives, address the feelings associated with the negative consequences and the relationship with the individual, and learn to "let go" and heal as they begin a new relationship with the individual working a lifelong recovery program.

In each treatment modality, monitoring all substance use or activity identified with the addictive behavior as well as periods of abstinence is critical. Further insight into the patterns of addiction comes from understanding the relationship of addictive behaviors and the feelings experienced during abstinence and any periods of use, whether use involves one episode, binge episodes, or repeated use. Giving greater strength to the ability to recover results from recognizing near misses and discussing the urge to pick up, use, or engage in the addictive behavior. The value of having resources available and ensuring that individuals use them during these trying times keeps them focused on recovery and allows them to recognize the tools that keep them healthy and addictionfree.

This education becomes even more valuable when the concerned significant others involved in the patients' lives are involved. Support groups, including 12-step programs, for families and friends are strongly encouraged. Providing brochures with hotline numbers and support group information in the PCP lobbies can be a first step.

Complementary and Alternative Therapies

Due to the high percentage of relapse, noncompliance, and early termination of treatment in the substance-abusing population, treatment professionals have looked to complementary and alternative medicine (CAM) for additional therapeutic approaches. The National Center for Complementary and Alternative Medicine at the National Institutes of Health (NIH, 2007) defines CAM as a grouping of medical and health care systems, practices, and products that are considered different from, and not a part of, conventional medicine. CAM therapies are considered to be complementary when they are combined with conventional medicine and alternative medicine and replace conventional medicine. As research studies determine the safety and efficacy of CAM therapy for a certain medical problem, these methods may be combined with mainstream approaches and considered integrative medicine. (See Chapter 16.)

Auricular Acupuncture

The major form of alternative medicine being used to treat substance disorders is auricular acupuncture, which is the insertion of flexible, fine stainless steel needles bilaterally in specific locations in the outer ear. Proponents believe that this approach is effective for all forms of substance dependence. More than 300 treatment facilities are using protocols based on the Chinese theory of detoxification to treat acute opiate withdrawal and cocaine addiction. It is believed that acupuncture can be used to reduce cravings for all substances, calm disruptive individuals, and increase retention rates in treatment programs. Most of the supporting data, 25 years of it, is anecdotal or program-outcomes based.

Researchers cite the difficulties of setting up a true clinical trial but encourage continued study of the efficacy of acupuncture-based protocols for treating substance disorders (Janssen, Demorest, and Whynot, 2005; Kim, Schiff, Waalen, et al., 2005; Margolin, 2003; Otto, 2003).

Eye Movement Desensitization and Reprocessing

Another frequently used alternative treatment for substance disorders is eye movement desensitization and reprocessing (EMDR). Not considered to be part of CAM, EMDR is a set protocol that incorporates alternating eye movements or alternating auditory or kinesthetic stimuli with a cognitive process. Through neurobiologic study, it has been determined that EMDR is effective because of the apparent stimulation of the corpus callosum. Currently, EMDR is a methodology that uses multiple psychotherapeutic approaches in a focused protocol for the treatment of a number of disorders. Manfield (1998) reports that a number of controlled clinical trials have been conducted that uphold the safety and efficacy of this treatment approach when used alongside or with other treatment methods. A number of EMDR-certified clinicians are using the traditional EMDR treatment approach and incorporating it into other treatment approaches to develop extended protocols. The addiction protocol is one of these extended protocols. Although not as rigorously tested as the traditional approach, initial results support continued use and research (Manfield).

Pharmacotherapy

For many years, the treatment of addiction has focused on psychologic and behavioral approaches. As knowledge grows of the underlying neurologic and physiologic basis for the addictive process, medication-assisted addiction treatment is becoming more acceptable. However, a great deal of research, education, and clinical trials must be completed.

As PCPs become more aware of the cost of addiction for individuals, families, and the community, the interest in understanding how to use pharmacologic approaches to treat individuals with substance misuse disorders has increased. In particular, the National Institute on Alcohol Abuse and Addiction (NIAAA) and the NIDA are interested in increasing opportunities for neurologic and neurochemical research (Thayer, 2006). The NIAAA has formed an integrated medication development program to develop new medications (Thayer). Table 5.6 provides an overview of medications currently in use and/or development.

Table 5.6 • Medications Used in Treating Addictions

Brand Name (Generic Name)	Drug Classification	Indication	Use
Antabuse (disulfiram)	Alcohol sensitivity	Alcohol dependence	Maintenance
Atretol, Tegretol (carbamazepine)	Anticonvulsant	Alcohol dependence	Withdrawal
Campral (acamprosate calcium)	Benzodiazepine	Alcohol dependence	Relapse-prevention agent
Catapres (clonidine)	Antihypertensive	Presence of hypertension	Withdrawal
Chantix (varenicline)	Nicotine receptor partial agonist	Nicotine addiction	Reduce craving and withdrawal
LAAM (levo-alpha-acetyl methadol)	Opioid agonist	Opiate addiction	Longer half-life compared to methadone use during withdrawal and maintenance
Librium (chlordiazepoxide)	Benzodiazepine	Alcohol	Increase seizure threshold; reduce withdrawal agitation
Luvox (luvoxamine)	Partial opioid agonist/ selective serotonin reuptake inhibitor (SSRI)	Obsessive D/O	Detoxification and maintenance
Methadone (methadone hydrochloride)	Narcotic analgesic	Narcotics	Detoxification and maintenance
Paxil (paroxetine hydrochloride)	SSRI	Co-occurring disorders	Depressive disorder or obsessive thinking
Phenobarbital (phenobarbital)	Barbiturate	Alcohol	Withdrawal
Quetiapine fumarate (dibenzothiazepine derivative)	Psychotropic	—	Detoxification with reduced craving

(*Continued*)

Table 5.6 • (Continued)

Brand Name (Generic Name)	Drug Classification	Indication	Use
Subutex, oral Buprenex, injectable (buprenorphine)	Partial opioid agonist	Opiate addiction	Detoxification and maintenance
Suboxone (buprenorphine and naloxone)	Partial opioid agonist	Opiate addiction	Detoxification and maintenance
Trexan (naltrexone hydrochloride)	Opioid antagonist	Heroin	Detoxification and maintenance
		Opiates	Detoxification and maintenance
		Pathologic gambling	Reduce impulsive and compulsive behaviors
Valium (diazepam)	Benzodiazepines	Alcohol	Withdrawal
Sabril (vigabatrin)			
Vigabatrin	GABA derivative	Cocaine	*Clinical trial
TA-CD	Cocaine vaccine	—	*Clinical trial
Selegiline (l-deprenyl)	Antispasmodic	—	*Clinical trial
InterveXin-PCP	Monoclonal antibody	PCP	*Clinical trial
InterveXin-METH	Monoclonal antibody	Methamphetamine	*Clinical trial
DAS-431	Dopamine receptor agonist	Cocaine/ methamphetamine	*Clinical trial
Vivitrol, injectable, Revia, Depade, oral (naltrexone)	Opioid receptor antagonist	Alcohol	Withdrawal; relapse prevention
Zimulti (rimonabant)	Endocannabinoid	Nicotine and obesity	Maintenance of body weight
Zyban (bupropion) Includes patches, gums, lozenges, nasal sprays, and inhalers	Norepinephrine and dopamine reuptake inhibitor	Nicotine	Withdrawal from smoking

Maintenance

Since addiction is pervasive across the entire life span, recovery is a lifelong process as well. Recognizing the individuality of each person whose life is touched by addiction, maintaining a clean, sober, and healthy lifestyle must also be individualized. Former beliefs discouraging the use of medications in recovery have been modified so that, in some instances, working a 12-step recovery program may not be enough to minimize relapse and maintain abstinence from substance use and addictive behaviors. Theories to include recognizing comorbidity and harm reduction have proved effective when efforts associated with counseling and the supports in the recovery community are concerted. Some researchers recommend maintaining a period of 3 months of pharmacotherapy (National Institutes of Health/National Institutes of Alcohol Abuse and Addiction (2005)).

The "aftercare plan" or "sober living plan" will need to address all of the characteristics that have been mentioned in this chapter—and more. For individuals dealing with significant health-related consequences of addiction such as cirrhosis, gastrointestinal disorders, and sexually transmitted diseases, the PCP will not only monitor the related laboratory tests and severity of physical symptoms but will need to ask at each office visit about the status of the contributing substance use, new substance use, and compliance with the established treatment plan. The risk for relapse, especially for alcohol abuse, is greatest within the first 3 months of recovery. In fact, 60% of women who receive treatment will relapse and require more treatment to achieve long-term sobriety (Grupp, 2006). Further, the first 12 months after initiating abstinence is strongly associated with testing high-risk behaviors to include the people, places, and things that were previously identified with substance use and addiction and may continue to expose the individual to the opportunity to relapse. When individuals stop using substances but continue to associate with former people, places, and things related to the substance abuse, they put themselves at risk for relapse. Involvement in self-help support groups such as Alcoholics Anonymous is recommended. In the 2005 National Survey on Drug Use and Health, SAMHSA reported that more than half (1.4 million) of the 2.3 million persons 12 years of age and older who received substance use treatment also received support through a self-help group (SAMHSA, NSDUH, 2005).

Coordinating service delivery and monitoring progress is essential in conjunction with a managed care provider's case manager and other professionals from the legal system or employee/student assistance network. Information regarding the status of the individual must be updated regularly to ensure that those involved in the process have the most current information on which to base recommendations and actions.

CONCLUSION

PCPs have varying levels of knowledge relative to understanding addiction and assessment processes. More often than not, the patient/family has a long-standing relationship with the PCP, which increases the comfort level in discussing substance use or addictive behavior and related physical, legal, or emotional consequences. Establishing a nonthreatening environment in which individuals feel comfortable discussing such matters is critical for all patients receiving services. The display of posters and printed educational materials in the waiting area is a first step in showing individuals that the PCP will be empathetic and supportive during discussions such as these and is willing to provide direction as needed. Further enhancing these resources to include some of the self-administered questionnaires referred to in the Screening section of this chapter as well as recovery/support group pamphlets listed in the Resources for Providers are often of no cost or available at a minimal fee to the PCP.

Frequently, situations may present as emergencies associated with the severity of the symptoms. The management of emergencies associated with substance use disorders and other consequences of addiction warrant the establishment of collaborative agreements and partnerships with other professionals in the community. All staff in the practice location or branch offices on all shifts need to be fully aware of the disease-state management protocol for such emergencies. If the primary practice has an addiction professional on site, assessment of the severity of symptoms should begin immediately as arrangements for referral and/or transport are being confirmed.

It is also important to remember that PCPs are responsible for ensuring the qualifications of the addiction provider they select. This may include verifying licensure and certification as well as confirming that the provider is in good standing without sanctions against license to include suspension and disbarment. Box 5.5 provides detail related to the skill level and competency of individuals working in addictions.

The PCP must be cognizant of the federal and state regulations associated with HIPAA and alcohol and other drug confidentiality during all verbal or written interaction with professionals or agencies outside of the practice. Although releases of information are often obtained with the consent for treatment, it is advised to confirm authorization to release specific information as well as to whom the information is being released prior to each episode. In the case of an

Box 5.5 • Skill Levels and Competencies for Substance Use Professionals

Transdisciplinary Foundations

The following knowledge and attitudes are *prerequisite* to the development of competency in the professional treatment of substance use disorders. Such knowledge and attitudes form the basis of understanding on which discipline-specific proficiencies are built.

A. Understanding Addiction

1. Understand a variety of models and theories of addiction and other problems related to substance use.
2. Recognize the social, political, economic, and cultural context within which addiction and substance abuse exist, including risk and resiliency factors that characterize individuals and groups and their living environments.
3. Describe the behavioral, psychologic, physical health, and social effects of psychoactive substances on the user and significant others.
4. Recognize the potential for substance use disorders to mimic a variety of medical and psychologic disorders and the potential for medical and psychologic disorders to coexist with addiction and substance abuse.

B. Treatment Knowledge

1. Describe the philosophies, practices, policies, and outcomes of the most generally accepted and scientifically supported models of treatment, recovery, relapse prevention, and continuing care for addiction and other substance-related problems.
2. Recognize the importance of family, social networks, and community systems in the treatment and recovery process.
3. Understand the importance of research and outcome data and their application in clinical practice.
4. Understand the value of an interdisciplinary approach to addiction treatment.

C. Application to Practice

1. Understand the established diagnostic criteria for substance use disorders, and describe treatment modalities and placement criteria within the continuum of care.
2. Describe a variety of helping strategies for reducing the negative effects of substance use, abuse, and dependence.

(*Continued*)

Box 5.5 • (Continued)

3. Tailor helping strategies and treatment modalities to the client's stage of dependence, change, or recovery.
4. Provide treatment services appropriate to the personal and cultural identity and language of the client.
5. Adapt practice to the range of treatment settings and modalities.
6. Be familiar with medical and pharmacologic resources in the treatment of substance use disorders.
7. Understand the variety of insurance and health maintenance options available and the importance of helping clients access those benefits.
8. Recognize that crisis may indicate an underlying substance use disorder and may be a window of opportunity for change.
9. Understand the need for and the use of methods for measuring treatment outcome.

D. Professional Readiness

1. Understand diverse cultures and incorporate the relevant needs of culturally diverse groups, as well as people with disabilities, into clinical practice.
2. Understand the importance of self-awareness in one's personal, professional, and cultural life.
3. Understand the addiction professional's obligations to adhere to ethical and behavioral standards of conduct in the helping relationship.
4. Understand the importance of ongoing supervision and continuing education in the delivery of client services.
5. Understand the obligation of the addiction professional to participate in prevention as well as treatment.
6. Understand and apply setting-specific policies and procedures for handling crisis or dangerous situations, including safety measures for clients and staff.

From SAMHSA TIP 21. (2004.) *Addiction counseling competencies: the knowledge, skills and attributes of professional practice. Technical Assistance Publication* (TAP) Series 21. Washington, DC: U.S. Department of Health and Human Services.

emergent situation in which the individual is unable to give authorization, the PCP should obtain information related to the client from an individual who has written authority to act on behalf of the client.

Confidentiality regulations and the rights of adolescents may differ per state. PCPs are encouraged to become familiar with the behavioral health regulations established by the state in which they practice before proceeding with referral or treatment.

Resources for Providers

American Psychiatric Association. (2000). *Diagnostic and statistical manual of mental disorders* (Revised 4th ed.). Washington, DC: Author.

Barbor, T. F., de la Fuente, J. R., Saunders, J., et al. (1992). *AUDIT: The alcohol use disorders identification test: Guidelines for use in primary health care*. Geneva: World Health Organization.

Carnes, P. (2001). *Out of the shadows: Understanding sexual addiction.* Center City, MN: Hazelden.

Health Resources and Services Administration (HRSA). (2001). *Screening for substance abuse during pregnancy: Improving care, improving health*. Maternal and Child Health Bureau. National Center for Education in Maternal and Child Health. Arlington, VA: Author.

Helping patients who drink too much: A clinician's guide. (2005). NIH Publication No. 07-3769. Retrieved January 16, 2007, from *www.niaaa.nih.gov/guide*.

International Nurses Society on Addictions, *Journal of Addictions Nursing: A Journal for the Prevention and Management of Addictions.*

Mayo Foundation for Medical Education and Research, 200 First Street, S.W., Rochester, MN, 55905

Minkoff, K., M.D. Mentally ill drug and alcohol screening (MIDAS).

Morse, B., Gehshan, S., Hutchins, E. (1997). *Screening for substance abuse during pregnancy: Improving care, improving health.* Arlington, VA: National Center for Education in Maternal and Child Health.

National Clearinghouse for Alcohol and Drug Information, P.O. Box 2345, Rockville, MD, 20847-2345

National Drug and Alcohol Treatment Referral Routing Service, (800) 662-HELP.

NIAAA Publications Distribution Center, P.O. Box 10686, Rockville, MD, 20849-0656, (301) 443-3860.

SAMHSA TIP 13: *Patient placement criteria*. (2002).Substance Abuse and Mental Health Services Administration (SAMHSA).

SAMHSA TIP 24: *A guide to substance abuse services for primary care clinicians*. (1998) SAMHSA/SCATR Treatment Improvement Protocols.

SAMHSA TIP 26C: *Substance abuse among older adults*. (1998). SAMHSA/SCATR Treatment Improvement Protocols.

SAMHSA TIP 34: *Brief interventions and brief therapies for substance abuse*. (1999) SAMHSA.

SAMHSA TIP 39: *Substance abuse and family therapy*. (2004). SAMHSA.

SAMHSA TIP 42: *Substance abuse treatment for persons with co-occurring disorders*. (2005). SAMHSA/SCATR Treatment Improvement Protocols.

SAMHSA TIP 45: *Detoxification and substance abuse treatment*. (2006). SAMHSA Treatment Improvement Protocols.

Schmidt, S. N. (2006). A simple approach to pathological gambling? Don't bet on it. *Journal of Addictions Nursing, 16*, 4, 237–238.

Screening for substance abuse during pregnancy: Improving care, improving health. (2001). Health Resources and Services Administration (HRSA), Maternal and Child Health Bureau. National Center for Education in Maternal and Child Health, Arlington, VA: U.S. Department of Health.

Substance Abuse and Mental Health Services Administration, Clearinghouse for Alcohol and Drug Information. (2001). *Cultural competence standards in managed care mental health services: Four underserved/underrepresented racial/ethnic groups*. Retrieved January 23, 2007, from *www.ncadi.samhsa.gov/govpubs/M5500/*.

Swenson, W. M., & Morse, R. M. (1975). The use of a Self-Administered Alcoholism Screening Test (SAAST) in a medical center. *Mayo Clinic Proceedings, 50*, 204–208.

U.S. Department of Health and Human Services and SAMHSA's National Clearinghouse for Alcohol and Drug Information. *Quick facts: Pregnant women*. Retrieved January 23, 2007, from *http://noadistore.samhsa.gov/catalog/facts.aspx?topic=11*

Websites for Providers and Patients

Addiction Technology Transfer Center, *www.nattc.org*

Alcoholics Anonymous, *www.aa.org*

American Nurses Association (ANA), *www.nursingworld.org*

American Society of Addiction Medicine (ASAM), *www.asam.org*

Centers for Disease Control and Prevention (CDC), *www.cdc.gov/tobacco/basic_information/index.htm*

Centers for Disease Control and Prevention, Department of Health and Human Services. (n.d.) *Fact sheet: Women and tobacco*. Retrieved December 14, 2007, from *www.cdc.gov/tobacco/basic_information/index.htm*.

Chemical and Engineering News, *www.CEN-ONLINE.org*

Institute for Research, Education, and Training in Addictions (IRETA), *www.ireta.org/sbirt*

International Nurses Society on Addictions, *www.intnsa.org*

Join Together, *www.jointogether.org*

National Center for Education in Maternal and Child Health, Maternal and Child Health Bureau, Health Resources and Services Administration, *www.mchb.hrsa.gov*

National Center on Addiction and Substance Abuse (CASA), *www.casacolumbia.org*

National Clearinghouse for Alcohol and Drug Information, *www.health.org*

National Institute on Alcohol Abuse and Alcoholism (NIAAA), *www.niaaa.nih.gov/guide*

National Institute on Alcohol Abuse and Alcoholism (NIAAA), *http://pubs.niaaa.nih.gov/publications/Practitioner/CliniciansGuide2005/clinicians_guide.htm*

National Institute on Drug Abuse (NIDA), *www.drugabuse.gov*

National Organization of Alternative Programs (NOAP), *www.alternativeprograms.org*

National Survey on Drug Use and Health (NSDUH) *http://nsduhweb.rti.org*

Office of National Drug Control Policy, Drug Facts, *www.whitehousedrugpolicy.gov*

Pathologic Gambling, *www.robertperkinson.com*

Peer Assistance Services, *www.peerassist.org*

Project MAINSTREAM, *www.projectmainstream.net*

Psychiatric Times, *www.psychiatrictimes.com*

Sex Addicts Anonymous, *www.sexaa.org/addict.htm*

Sexual Addiction Recovery Resources, *www.sarr.org*

Substance Abuse Facility Treatment Locator, *http://findtreatment.samhsa.gov*

Substance Abuse Subtle Screening Inventory, *www.sassi.com*

Treatment Improvement Exchange, *www.treatment.org*

U.S. Department of Health and Human Services, Substance Abuse and Mental Health Services Administration Center for Substance Abuse Treatment, *www.ncadi.samhsa.gov*

Virginia Department of Mental Health, Mental Retardation, and Substance Abuse Services, *www.dmhmrsas.virginia.gov*

World Health Organization (WHO), *www.who.int/substance/publications/alcohol/en/index.html*

References

American Psychiatric Association. (2000). *Diagnostic and statistical manual of mental disorders* (4th ed., text revision). Washington, DC: Author.

Antai-Otong, D. (2006). Women and alcoholism: Gender-related medical complications: Treatment considerations. *Journal of Addictions Nursing, 17*(1), 33.

Back, S. E., Contini, R., & Brady, K. T. (2007). *Substance abuse in women: Does gender matter?* Retrieved January 27, 2007, from *www.psychiatrictimes.com/display/article/10168/46496.*

Bouchez, C. (2006). Cycles of addiction. *Psychiatric Times*. Retrieved December 10, 2006, from *www.twilightbridge.com.*

Doweiko, H. E. (2006). *Concepts of chemical dependency.* Belmont, CA Thomson Brooks/Cole.

Evans, K., & Sullivan, J. M. (2001). *Dual diagnosis: Counseling the mentally ill* (2nd ed.). New York: Guilford Press.

Fornili, K. (Ed.). (2004). *Substance abuse tool box.* Richmond, VA: Virginia Office of Substance Abuse Services.

Freimuth, M. (2005). *Hidden addictions.* New York: Jason Aronson.

Frost, N., Greene, J., & Pranis, K. (2006). The punitiveness report: Hard hit. *Institute on Women and Criminal Justice.* Retrieved May 23, 2006, from www.wpaonline.org/institute/hardhit/index.htm.

Grupp, K. (2006). Women one year following gender-specific treatment for alcohol and/or other drug dependency. *Journal of Addictions Nursing, 17*, 1, 5–11.

Health Resources and Services Administration (HRSA). (2001). *Screening for substance abuse during pregnancy: Improving care, improving health.* Maternal and Child Health Bureau. National Center for Education in Maternal and Child Health. Arlington, VA: Author.

Janssen, P. A., Demorest, L. C., & Whynot, E. M. (2005). Acupuncture for substance abuse treatment in the Downtown Eastside of Vancouver. *Journal of Urban Health, 82*(2), 285–295.

Join Together. (2006). Addiction, mental illness common in U.S. *Archives of General Psychiatry.* Retrieved July 15, 2005, from *www.jointogether.org/sa/news/summaries/print/0,1856,577244,00.html.*

Kim, Y. J., Schiff, E., Waalen, J., et al. (2005). Efficacy of acupuncture for treating cocaine addiction: A review paper. *Journal of Addictive Diseases, 24*(4), 115–132.

Manfield, P. (Ed.). (1998). *Extending EMDR: A casebook of innovative applications.* New York: W. W. Norton & Company.

Margolin, A. (2003). Acupuncture for substance abuse. *Current Psychiatry Reports, 5*(5), 333–339.

National Center for Complementary and Alternative Medicine, National Institutes of Health (NIH), *What is CAM?* Retrieved January 18, 2007, from *www.nccam.nih.gov/health/whatiscam/_*

Otto, K. C. (2003). Acupuncture and substance abuse: A synopsis, with indications for further research. *American Journal on Addictions, 12*(1), 43–51.

Power, C. (2005). Food and sex addiction: Helping the clinician recognize and treat the interaction. *Sexual Addiction and Compulsivity, 12*, 219–234.

Snow, D., & Delaney, K. R. (2006). Substance use and recovery: Charting a course toward optimism. *Archives of Psychiatric Nursing, 20*(6), 288–290.

Substance Abuse and Mental Health Services Administration (SAMHSA). Mental Health Information Center. http://mentalhealth.samhsa.gov/ U.S. Department of Health and Human Services.

Substance Abuse and Mental Health Services Administration, National Survey on Drug Use and Health (SAMHSA, NSDUH). (2005). *Results from the 2005 national survey on drug use and health: National findings.* Washington, DC: U.S. Department of Health and Human Services.

SAMHSA TIP 6. (1999). *Empowering families, helping adolescents* (Treatment Improvement Protocol [TIP] Series 6). Washington, DC: U.S. Department of Health and Human Services.

SAMHSA TIP 13. (2002). *Patient placement criteria.* Retrieved January 2, 2007, from *www.ncbi.nlm.nih.gov/books.*

SAMHSA TIP 24. (1999). *A guide to substance abuse services for primary care clinicians.* Retrieved January 2, 2007, from *www.ncbi.nlm.nih.gov/books.*

SAMHSA TIP 26C. (1998). *Substance abuse among older adults.* Retrieved January 17, 2007, from *http://tie.samhsa.gov/Externals/tips.html.*

SAMHSA TIP 34 (1998) *Brief interventions and brief therapies for substance abuse* (Treatment Improvement Protocol [TIP] Series 34). Washington DC: U.S. Department of Health and Human Services.

SAMHSA TIP 39. (2004). *Substance abuse and family therapy.* Retrieved January 17, 2007, from *http://tie.samhsa.gov/Externals/tips.html.*

SAMHSA TIP 40. (2004). *Clinical guidelines for the use of buprenorphine in the treatment of opioid addiction* (Treatment Improvement Protocol [TIP] Series 40). Washington, DC: U.S. Department of Health and Human Services.

SAMHSA TIP 42. (2005). *Substance abuse treatment for persons with co-occurring disorders* (Treatment Improvement Protocol [TIP] Series 42). Washington, DC: U.S. Department of Health and Human Services.

SAMHSA TIP 43. *Medication assisted treatment.* Retrieved January 23, 2007, from *www.samhsa.gov.*

SAMHSA TIP 45. (2005). *Detoxification and substance abuse treatment* (Treatment Improvement Protocol [TIP] Series 45). Washington, DC: U.S. Department of Health and Human Services.

Thayer, A. M. (2006). Drugs to fight addictions. *Chemical and Engineering News, 84*(39), 21–44.

Wieland, D. (2005). Computer addiction: Implications for nursing psychotherapy practice. *Perspectives in Psychiatric Care, 41*(4), 153–161.

Women and Drugs. Office of National Drug Policy. Retrieved January 18, 2007 from *http://www.whitehousedrugpolicy.gov/drugfact/women/index.html.*

Ziegler, P. (2007). Safe treatment of pain in the patient with a substance use disorder. *Psychiatric Times, 24,* 1. Retrieved January 27, 2007, from *www.psychiatrictimes.com.*

Judy Sargent
Karen Stein
David Rosen

chapter 6

Eating Disorders

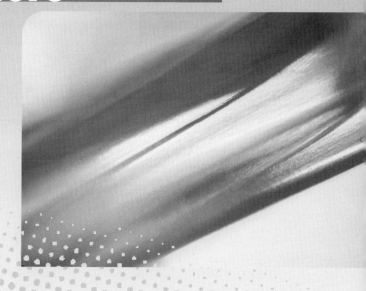

Eating problems are among the most common major mental disorders that affect young women, and these problems carry a high burden of morbidity and mortality (Kreipe and Birndorf, 2000). An estimated 0.9 percent of females will suffer from anorexia nervosa in their lifetime, while an estimated 1.5 percent will suffer from bulimia nervosa, 2.4 percent will suffer from an eating disorder not otherwise specified (EDNOS), and 3.5 percent will experience a binge eating disorder (Hudson, 2007; Kessler, Berglung, Chiu, et al., 2004; Kessler, Chiu, Dernier, et al., 2005). Eating disorders carry the highest rate of mortality of any of the major mental disorders (Millar, Wardell, Vyvyan, et al., 2005). The mortality rate for individuals with anorexia nervosa has been estimated at 5 to 10 percent, a rate which is about 12 times higher than the annual death rate due to all causes of death among females ages 15 to 24 years in the general population (Steinhausen, 2002). Unfortunately, the diagnosis of eating disorders can be elusive, and some studies suggest that more than half of all cases go undetected (Becker, Grinspoon, Klibanski, et al., 1999). Another large percentage of individuals with eating disordered symptoms suffer from clinically significant effects, yet fail to meet *Diagnostic and Statistical Manual of Mental Disorders (DSM-IV-TR)* criteria for a specific eating disorder (Wonderlich, Joiner, Keel, et al., 2007). The primary care provider (PCP) is in an ideal setting to identify eating disorders and initiate early treatment. Earlier identification of eating disorders with intervention and earlier age at diagnosis are associated with improved outcomes (Herzog, Nussbaum, and Marmor, 1996). This chapter provides an overview of the diagnostic criteria, differential diagnoses, assessment, and treatment guidelines for PCPs for the *DSM-IV-TR*-recognized eating disorders (anorexia nervosa, bulimia nervosa, EDNOS, and binge eating).

EATING DISORDERS

Eating disorders were once thought to affect primarily white, adolescent, or young-adult women from higher socioeconomic groups in Western cultures (Cooper, 2005). However, no relationship has been shown between socioeconomic status and eating disorders (Favaro, Ferrara, and Santonastaso, 2003). Studies have shown that eating disorders are also prevalent among diverse cultures, males, and females across the life span (Boroughs and Thompson, 2002; Chatoor and Surles, 2004; Hraborsky and Grilo, 2007; Mangweth-Matzek, Raup, Hausman, et al., 2006). Often, eating disorders go unrecognized and undiagnosed in these nontraditional populations assumed to be low risk for eating disorders.

Eating disorders often begin during high school or college, when patients are in their teens and 20s, although earlier and later onsets also occur. Children with early onset anorexia nervosa may experience delayed growth, and they may be especially prone to osteopenia and osteoporosis (Katzman, 2005). Later onsets of eating disorders have been associated with the physical changes of aging (Lewis and Cachelin, 2001) as well as significant stressors including the death of a spouse, divorce, or other major loss (Forman and Davis, 2005).

Although eating disorders are more common in women, they also occur in men. Lifetime prevalence rates of *DSM-IV-TR* anorexia nervosa, bulimia nervosa, and binge eating disorder are estimated to be 0.3, 0.5, and 2.0 percent, respectively among men (Hudson, Hiripi, Pope, et al., 2007). Many cases of anorexia nervosa and bulimia may go unrecognized and undiagnosed in men because of the association of eating disorders as primarily affecting women (Striegel-Moore and Bulik, 2007).

Etiology

The etiology of eating disorders is complicated and likely multidetermined (Garner & Magana, 2006). A critical combination of biologic, genetic, psychological, social, cultural, and environmental factors are believed to play a role in the development and maintenance of eating disorders (Garner and Magana; Striegel-Moore and Bulick, 2007). Societal ideals and values concerning weight and body shape vary among different cultures. Eating disorders appear to be more prevalent in industrialized societies where there is an abundance of food and where beauty and attractiveness are linked to a thin ideal (Striegel-Moore and Bulick). Unrealistic cultural ideals portrayed in various forms of Western media may encourage individuals to strive for beauty and acceptance according to the stereotypes they perceive in the media, contributing to disordered eating attitudes and behaviors (Striegel-Moore and Bulick).

Feminist theorists have suggested a few mechanisms that may explain the higher prevalence of eating disorders in women (Striegel-Moore and Bulick, 2007). Two elements of femininity, as defined by Western culture, are thought to contribute to women's enhanced risk for eating disorders. First, feminine identity tends to be relationally defined. Women are often raised in an environment that places great value on interpersonal relationships, and they tend to define themselves in terms of their relationships with others. The relational orientation renders women more vulnerable to the opinions of others, especially during adolescence. Often, self-worth becomes linked to one's ability to engage in empathetic and mutually empowering relationships. An extensive body of social psychological research has shown that physical attractiveness is a powerful determinant of interpersonal success. Failed attempts to achieve mutuality and understanding in relationships may be experienced as a fundamental insult on individual identity and evoke feelings of self-doubt and low self-esteem. Second, in Western culture, femininity and beauty are inextricably linked (Moradi, Dirks, and Matteson, 2005). It makes sense that women may place a high priority on achieving the culturally defined beauty ideal because they are highly motivated to find social approval and achieve meaningful interpersonal relationships and realize the importance of beauty for interpersonal attraction (Striegel-Moore, 1995).

Studies have shown a higher incidence of diagnosed eating disorders in first-degree relatives of individuals diagnosed with anorexia and bulimia nervosa, suggesting a genetic or inherited component (Fairburn, Cowen, and Harrison, 1999; Klump, Miller, Keel, et al., 2001; Kortegaard, Hoerder, Jorgensen, et al., 2001; Strober, Freeman, Lampert, et al., 2000; Wade, Bulik, Neale, et al., 2000). Personality characteristics including perfectionism and obsessive-compulsive traits may also contribute to eating disorder vulnerability for some individuals (Forsberg and Lock, 2006).

From a cognitive psychological standpoint, identity impairments have long been thought to contribute to the development of anorexia and bulimia nervosa (Bruch, 1973; Chernin, 1994; Stein, 1996; Tan, Hope, and Stewart, 2006). Impaired identity formation, lacking a clear and consistent sense of self, may make some women more vulnerable to cultural pressures for achieving the unrealistic stereotypic cultural ideal body image (Garner and Magana, 2006). Since positive self-schemas function to motivate and direct one's patterns of daily behavior, the absence of positive identities lead to self-confusion, dissatisfaction, and a high reliance on body weight as a source of self-definition and esteem. In turn, the taking on of body weight as a key source of self-definition is predictive of eating disordered behaviors in clinical and community samples (Stein and Corte, 2007).

Critical periods with associated life stressors (Garner and Magana, 2006) have also been linked to the onset of the development of eating disorders (i.e., transitioning from high school to college, parental divorce, loss of a spouse, moving away from home for the first time, etc.). Furthermore, certain sports like ballet, gymnastics, figure skating, and competitive running, where there is an undue emphasis on body weight and physical appearance, tend to see higher rates of eating disorders (Forsberg and Lock, 2006). Parents and coaches in disciplines such as gymnastics, ballet, and figure skating often encourage individuals in these sports to maintain sometimes unrealistic weight goals to enhance performance in the discipline.

Diagnosis

Eating problems are patterns of thinking, feeling, and behaving that develop over time. Box 6.1 lists common signs and symptoms of eating disorders. The *Diagnostic and Statistical Manual of Mental Disorders (DSM-IV-TR;* American Psychiatric Association [APA], 2000) has established criteria for the diagnosis of anorexia nervosa, bulimia nervosa, and EDNOS. The diagnostic criteria set forth in the *DSM-IV-TR* are the product of a synthetic process reflecting published research and clinical knowledge. Rather than naturally defined categories, the eating disorder diagnoses reflect that state of knowledge at a specific point in time. Consistent with that view, contemporary models are suggesting that the eating disorders of anorexia, bulimia, and binge eating disorder may not be discrete syndromes. Rather, eating disorder theorists have suggested that eating disorder symptoms could be profitably conceptualized as falling on a continuum (Wonderlich et al., 2007), with points on the continuum ranging from normal thoughts and feelings about one's body weight and normal eating behavior to anorexia, bulimia, and binge eating disorder. For example, up to 50 percent of patients with anorexia nervosa develop bulimic symptoms, and some patients who are initially bulimic develop anorexic symptoms (Bulik, Sullivan, Fear, et al., 1997). Furthermore, many patients who initially present with subclinical levels of eating disordered symptoms and a diagnosis of EDNOS will eventually be diagnosed with the full-blown syndrome of anorexia or bulimia nervosa.

Box 6.1 • Signs and Symptoms Common to Eating Disorders

- Unreasonable fear of being fat or overweight
- Self-evaluation excessively influenced by shape and weight
- Extensive effort to control/reduce weight (dieting, purging, exercise)
- Denial that weight or eating habits are a problem (anorexia nervosa)
- Obsessive symptoms
- Relationship difficulties
- Increasing withdrawal
- School and work problems

From the World Health Organization (2004).

Many more individuals experience clinically significant levels of disordered eating symptoms yet never meet the full *DSM-IV-TR* diagnostic criteria for an eating disorder (Wonderlich et al., 2007). In recent years, researchers have described a variety of atypical eating disordered symptom patterns including purging disorder (characterized by recurrent purging in the absence of objective binge eating episodes among normal-weight individuals; Keel, Haedt, and Edler, 2005), anorexia athletica (characterized by loss of weight and caloric restriction along with high levels of physical activity in an effort to improve competitive athletic performance, often without body-image distortion; Sudi, Ottl, Payerl, et al., 2004), and night eating syndrome (characterized by morning anorexia, evening hyperphagia, and insomnia with awakening followed by nocturnal food intake; O'Reardon, Peshek, and Allison, 2005). Some clinical researchers have suggested that the current *DSM-IV-TR* eating disorder classification system is inadequate in categorizing the diversity of eating disorders seen in current clinical practice, while suggesting there may be as many as six different distinct clinical syndromes, including (1) bulimia nervosa, (2) binge eating disorder, (3) restricting anorexia nervosa, (4) anorexia nervosa, binge-purge type, (5) purging disorder, and (6) subjective binge eating disorder (Wonderlich et al., 2007). All of these "atypical" eating disordered patterns emphasize the need for an improved classification system that adequately addresses the diversity of clinically significant eating disorders commonly seen in clinical practice.

Obesity is included in the International Classification of Diseases as a general medical condition but does not appear in the *DSM-IV-TR* because it has not been established that it is consistently associated with a psychological or behavioral syndrome. However, when there is evidence that psychological factors are of importance in the etiology or course of a particular case of obesity, this may be indicated using the *DSM-IV-TR* (APA, 2000) diagnosis "316 Psychological Factors Affecting Medical Condition" (p. 731). Some research suggests that 3.5 percent of the general population and 8 percent of the obese population engage in recurrent binge eating episodes without compensatory purging behaviors (Grilo, 2002; Hudson et al., 2007). These individuals may meet the diagnostic criteria for EDNOS or binge eating disorder.

ANOREXIA NERVOSA

The *DSM-IV-TR* has established criteria for the diagnosis of anorexia nervosa (Box 6.2). Common signs and symptoms of anorexia nervosa are listed in Box 6.3. The essential characteristics of this disorder are that an individual refuses to

Box 6.2 • *DSM-IV-TR* Criteria for Anorexia Nervosa

DSM

A. Refusal to maintain body weight at or above a minimally normal weight for age and height (e.g., weight loss leading to body weight less than 85 percent of that expected or failure to make expected weight gain during period of growth, leading to body weight less than 85 percent of that expected)
B. Intense fear of gaining weight or becoming overweight, even though patient is underweight
C. Disturbance in the way in which one's body weight or shape is experienced, undue influence of body weight or shape on self-evaluation, or denial of the seriousness of the current low body weight
D. Amenorrhea in postmenarchal females (i.e., the absence of at least three consecutive menstrual cycles; a woman is considered to have amenorrhea if her periods occur only following hormone administration)

Specify Type:

Restricting type: During the current episode, the patient has not regularly engaged in binge eating or purging (i.e., self-induced vomiting or the misuse of laxatives, diuretics, or enemas)

Binge eating/purging type: During the current episode, the patient has regularly engaged in binge eating or purging

From the American Psychiatric Association (APA) (2000).

Box 6.3 • Common Signs and Symptoms of Anorexia Nervosa

- Severe dietary restriction despite very low body weight (BMI <17.5 kg/m^2)
- Morbid fear of fatness
- Distorted body image (unreasonable belief that one is overweight)
- Amenorrhea
- Compulsive exercise
- May binge and purge

From the World Health Organization (2004).

maintain a minimally normal body weight, is intensely afraid of gaining weight, and displays a significant disturbance in body image. Furthermore, postmenarcheal females with the disorder are amenorrheic (APA, 2000). Although individuals with anorexia nervosa may engage in patterns of binge eating and purging that are consistent with bulimia nervosa, the diagnosis of anorexia nervosa prevails when the physical criteria are met (Box 6.2).

Differential Diagnosis

Other possible causes of significant weight loss should be considered in the differential diagnosis of anorexia nervosa. In general medical conditions (e.g., malignancies, gastrointestinal disorders, AIDS), serious weight loss may occur, but individuals with these disorders do not usually have body weight concerns and desire for further weight loss. In major depression and schizophrenia, serious weight loss may occur, but individuals with these disorders do not usually show an excessive fear of gaining weight or a further desire for excessive weight loss is absent (APA, 2000). For individuals with anorexia nervosa, their extreme weight loss is seldom viewed as a problem, whereas weight loss stemming from depression or other causes may be recognized by the individual as problematic.

Course

The percentage of individuals with anorexia nervosa who fully recover is modest. Although many patients improve symptomatically over time, a substantial proportion of individuals continue to have distorted body image, psychiatric problems, and disordered eating (APA, 2006). Aggregate results from long-term follow-up studies show that nearly 50 percent of patients will eventually make a full recovery, 20 to 30 percent show residual symptoms, 10 to 20 percent remain severely ill, and 5 to 10 percent will die of related causes (Steinhausen, 2002).

CASE A

Melissa, a 14-year-old girl, was referred to her PCP for evaluation on the request of her parents and school officials. Melissa is 5 feet, 3 inches tall. Nine months ago, she weighed 112 pounds. At the time of her office visit, her weight is just 68 pounds. Melissa denies any physical complaints, while her physical exam is remarkable for wasting, cachexia, malnutrition, poor perfusion, bradycardia, and low blood pressure. Melissa reports that her menses became irregular and then stopped several months earlier. A social history reveals that Melissa is the eldest of three children, her parents are both working professionals, and she is a straight-A student. Melissa's parents complain that she has been increasingly socially withdrawn and obsessed with compulsive running (she is on the competitive cross-country team at school). Her family tells you that she finds any excuse she can to avoid family mealtimes. Melissa tells her PCP that she doesn't know what her parents are concerned about and says, "Please don't make me gain weight and get fat."

Case A illustrates a fairly classic presentation of anorexia nervosa. Melissa is young, her disorder was identified quite early, and therefore she is a good candidate for aggressive treatment. Melissa's symptoms are ego-syntonic, that is, the symptoms are not recognized as problematic or leading to feelings of distress. Consequently, enlisting Melissa's support and cooperation in the treatment process may prove challenging. It will be important for the PCP to work with Melissa to earn her trust, which will be essential for cooperation and participation in the treatment plan.

BULIMIA NERVOSA

The *DSM-IV-TR* has established criteria for the diagnosis of bulimia nervosa (Box 6.4). Common signs and symptoms of bulimia nervosa are listed in Box 6.5. The essential characteristics of bulimia nervosa are behavioral and attitudinal, including both binge eating and inappropriate compensatory methods (i.e., purging, excessive exercise) to prevent weight gain. Attitudinal symptoms include self-evaluation of individuals with bulimia nervosa excessively influenced by weight and shape. To qualify for the diagnosis, the binge eating and inappropriate compensatory behaviors must occur, on average, at least twice a week for 3 months (APA, 2000) (Box 6.4).

Differential Diagnosis

In certain general medical conditions, there is disturbed eating behavior (e.g., Kleine-Levin syndrome), but the characteristic psychological features of bulimia

Box 6.4 • *DSM-IV-TR* Criteria for Bulimia Nervosa

DSM

A. Recurrent episodes of binge eating. An episode of binge eating is characterized by both of the following:
   1. In a discrete period of time (e.g., within any 2-hour period), eating an amount of food that is larger than what most people would eat during a similar period of time and under similar circumstances
   2. A sense of lack of control over eating during the episode

B. Recurrent inappropriate compensatory behavior in order to prevent weight gain, such as self-induced vomiting; misuse of laxatives, diuretics, enemas, or other medications; fasting; or exercising excessively

C. The binge eating and inappropriate compensatory behaviors both occur, on average, at least twice a week for 3 months

D. Self-evaluation is unduly influenced by body shape and weight

E. The disturbance does not occur exclusively during episodes of anorexia nervosa

Specify Type:

Purging type: During the current episode, the patient has regularly engaged in self-induced vomiting or the misuse of laxatives, diuretics, or enemas

Nonpurging type: During the current episode, the patient has used inappropriate compensatory behaviors such as fasting or exercising excessively but has not regularly engaged in self-induced vomiting or the use of laxatives, diuretics, or enemas

From the American Psychiatric Association (APA) (2000).

Box 6.5 • Common Signs and Symptoms of Bulimia Nervosa

- Binge eating (discrete episodes of uncontrolled overeating)
- Purging (attempts to eliminate food by self-induced vomiting, laxative use, and/or diuretic use)
- Strict dieting and other compensatory measures such as excessive exercise
- Self-evaluation unduly influenced by shape and body weight

From the World Health Organization (2004).

nervosa (i.e., overconcern with body shape and weight) and inappropriate compensatory behaviors (i.e., self-induced vomiting and other forms of purging) are absent.

Individuals whose binge eating behavior occurs only during anorexia nervosa are given the diagnosis of anorexia nervosa, binge eating/purging type and should not be given the additional diagnosis of bulimia nervosa. For an individual who binges and purges but no longer meets the full diagnostic criteria for anorexia nervosa, binge eating/purging type (e.g., when the weight is normal or menses have returned), it is a matter of clinical judgment whether the most appropriate current diagnosis is anorexia nervosa, binge eating/purging type; in partial remission; or bulimia nervosa (APA, 2000).

Course

The prognosis for individuals with bulimia nervosa is modest. Estimates of remission over time range from 37 to 74 percent (Ben-Tovim, Walker, Gilchrist, et al., 2001; Grilo, Sanislow, Shea, et al., 2003; Milos, Spindler, Schnyder, et al., 2005). However, remission is often fleeting and relapse has been estimated at 47 percent (Grilo, Pagano, Skodol, et al., 2007).

Factors that predict improved outcomes in patients with eating disorders include an earlier age at the time of diagnosis, a brief interval from onset to initiation of treatment, a good parent–child relationship, and a history of having other healthy relationships with family and friends (APA, 2006; Herzog et al., 1996).

CASE B

Kathy is a 19-year-old college student who presented to the primary care university health clinic requesting treatment for chronic constipation. Kathy is 5 feet, 4 inches tall and weighs 146 pounds. The physical exam finds erosion of the dental enamel. Lab tests reveal hypokalemia, hypochloremia, and metabolic alkalosis with elevated blood urea nitrogen (BUN). Further questioning shows that Kathy has been on intermittent diets since she was 12 years old. She tells you that she learned how to "vomit" from several friends and the behavior has gotten "out of control." Although she started vomiting to control her weight, Kathy's weight has remained steady, even increased during this time, which forced her to "try using laxatives." Kathy says that every time she tries stopping the laxatives she becomes constipated, which initiates the vicious cycle all over again. Kathy says that she is ashamed to admit that she spends a good part of her day bingeing and purging and wishes she could stop. When asked about what factors she thinks may have contributed to the eating problems, Kathy identifies a stressful childhood and positive history of childhood sexual abuse.

Case B illustrates one way in which bulimia nervosa may appear in primary care. Unlike the case of Melissa (Case A) with anorexia nervosa, Kathy's symptoms are ego-dystonic and distressing to her. This should help provide motivation for change and facilitate her engagement in the treatment and recovery process.

EATING DISORDER NOT OTHERWISE SPECIFIED

The diagnosis of EDNOS is used for individuals with significant levels of disordered eating that do not meet the diagnostic criteria for any specific eating disorder. The diagnosis of EDNOS is often given when the physical and behavioral symptoms are of shorter duration (e.g., less than 3 months) or less severe intensity (e.g., binge-purge cycles that occur on average once rather than twice weekly) than those set for anorexia and bulimia nervosa (Box 6.6).

Examples of cases that might fall into this diagnostic classification include (1) individuals who have all of the signs and symptoms of anorexia nervosa yet still menstruate regularly, (2) individuals who have all of the signs and symptoms of bulimia nervosa yet have not had the symptoms for a long enough time period or of significant intensity (i.e., binge and purge, on average, less than twice a week), and (3) individuals with symptoms of night-eating syndrome, anorexia athletica, or purging disorder.

BINGE EATING DISORDER

The essential characteristics of binge eating disorder are both behavioral and attitudinal, including recurrent binge eating episodes followed by feelings of emotional distress. Box 6.7 lists the common signs and symptoms of binge eating disorder.

Compulsive overeating (binge eating disorder) is a common eating problem that has not yet been fully recognized in the *DSM-IV-TR* as a legitimate and distinct eating disorder. However, research criteria have been established for further evaluation of a new diagnostic category: binge eating disorder (Box 6.8).

Box 6.6 • *DSM-IV-TR* Criteria for Eating Disorder Not Otherwise Specified

DSM

A. For females, all of the criteria for anorexia nervosa are met except that the individual has regular menses.

B. All of the criteria for anorexia nervosa are met except that despite significant weight loss, the individual's weight is in the normal range.

C. All of the criteria for bulimia nervosa are met except that the binge eating and inappropriate compensatory mechanisms occur at a frequency of less than twice a week or for a duration of less than 3 months.

D. The regular use of inappropriate compensatory behavior by an individual of normal body weight after eating small amounts of food (e.g., self-induced vomiting after the consumption of two cookies).

E. Repeatedly chewing and spitting out, but not swallowing, large amounts of food.

F. Binge eating disorder: Recurrent episodes of binge eating in the absence of the regular use of compensatory behaviors characteristic of bulimia nervosa.

Specify Type:

Purging type: During the current episode, the patient has regularly engaged in self-induced vomiting or the misuse of laxatives, diuretics, or enemas

Nonpurging type: During the current episode, the patient has used inappropriate compensatory behaviors such as fasting or exercising excessively but has not regularly engaged in self-induced vomiting or the use of laxatives, diuretics, or enemas

From the American Psychiatric Association (APA) (2000).

Box 6.7 • Common Signs and Symptoms of Binge Eating Disorder

- Binge eating (discrete episodes of uncontrolled overeating)
- Feeling "out-of-control" during binge eating episodes
- Feeling guilty or depressed after binge eating episodes
- Binge eating is associated with emotional distress.

From Grilo, C. M. (2002).

Box 6.8 • *DSM-IV-TR* Research Criteria for Binge Eating Disorder

A. Recurrent episodes of binge eating. An episode of binge eating is characterized by both of the following:
   (1) In a discrete period of time (e.g., within any 2-hour period), eating an amount of food that is larger than what most people would eat during a similar period of time and under similar circumstances
   (2) A sense of lack of control over eating during the episode

B. The binge eating episodes are associated with three (of more) of the following:
   (1) Eating much more rapidly than normal
   (2) Eating until feeling uncomfortably full
   (3) Eating large amounts of food when not feeling physically hungry
   (4) Eating alone because of being embarrassed by how much one is eating
   (5) Feeling disgusted with oneself, depressed, or very guilty after overeating

C. Marked distress regarding the binge eating is present.

D. The binge eating occurs, on average, at least 2 days a week for 6 months.

E. The binge eating is not associated with the regular use of inappropriate compensatory behaviors (e.g., purging, fasting, excessive exercise) and does not occur exclusively during the course of anorexia nervosa or bulimia nervosa.

From the American Psychiatric Association (APA) (2000).

Individuals meeting the DSM-IV-TR research diagnostic criteria for binge eating disorder would be a smaller subset of individuals currently diagnosed with EDNOS.

Differential Diagnosis

The differential diagnosis for binge eating disorder must rule out general medical or other psychiatric conditions that may be responsible for the eating behavioral symptoms. Some medical conditions (e.g., Prader-Willi syndrome) are characterized by marked hyperphagia and inability to regulate oral intake. Clinical depression is sometimes accompanied by significant changes in appetite (hyperphagia in some cases, anorexia in others). These conditions must be ruled out before coming to the diagnosis of binge eating disorder.

Course

High rates of remission (binge abstinence) have been reported, even in the absence of treatment, for individuals with binge eating disorder. As well, there appears to be no tendency for binge eating disorder to evolve into any other eating disorder (Fairburn and Walsh, 2002).

ASSESSMENT OF EATING DISORDERS

Early diagnosis with treatment and earlier age of diagnosis are correlated with improved outcomes in eating disorder patients (Herzog et al., 1996). PCPs have an important role in early identification of these disorders.

Instruments for the Assessment of Eating Disorders

Several paper-and-pencil questionnaires exist for the purpose of aiding in the assessment or identification of individuals with high levels of eating disordered cognitions, attitudes, and behaviors. These instruments may be a useful adjunct in the assessment process but do not replace a careful diagnostic interview. A few common instruments for the assessment of eating disordered signs and symptoms are listed in Table 6.1.

Although these instruments can be useful tools to aid in case identification, their practical utility in a primary care setting may be limited due to time constraints with their administration and interpretation. For this reason, a brief five-item screening tool, the SCOFF, was developed for use with primary care patients (Morgan, Reid, and Lacey, 1999). The SCOFF has a reported sensitivity of 53.3 percent and specificity of 93.2 percent among a sample of college women (Parker, Lyons, and Bonner, 2005). This test has a 12.5 percent false-positive rate, and thus it is best used as a screening tool (Pritts et al., 2007). With this measure, a score of 2 or greater yields a high degree of suspicion for an eating disorder and indicates the need for further evaluation, referral, and/or treatment. This brief screening tool has been effectively integrated into primary care practice (Pritts et al., 2007) and could easily be incorporated into a standard PCP's general screening questionnaire (Box 6.9).

Table 6.1 • Common Instruments for the Assessment of Eating Disorders

Eating Attitudes Test (EAT)	Brief, 26-item, standardized, self-report screening assessment of the symptoms, attitudes, and behaviors characteristic of eating disorders. Completion time = approx. 5–10 minutes (Garner, Olmstead, Bohr, et al., 1982).
Eating Disorders Examination (EDE)	Semistructured interview. Assesses the presence and severity of eating disorder symptoms. Uses operational *DSM-IV* diagnostic features (Fairburn & Cooper, 1993).
Eating Disorders Inventory (EDI)	Standardized measure of psychological traits and clusters of symptoms common to eating disorders. Eleven subscales: three subscales assess attitudes and behaviors concerning eating, weight, and shape; eight subscales assess more general psychological characteristics. Completion time = approx. 20 minutes (Garner, Olmstead, & Polivy, 1983).

Eating Disorder History

Patients with eating disorders may present with a wide range of symptoms or mild nonspecific symptoms (fatigue, dizziness, lack of energy), or they might deny any symptoms at all while their family members, friends, or school officials

Box 6.9 • SCOFF Questions

1. Do you make yourself **S**ick (induce vomiting or purge) because you feel uncomfortably full or like you've eaten too much?
2. Do you worry that you have lost **C**ontrol over how much you eat?
3. Have you recently lost more than **O**ne stone (6.4 kg/14 pounds) in a 3-month period of time?
4. Do you think you are too **F**at, even though others say you are too thin?
5. Would you say that **F**ood dominates your life?

Note: Give 1 point for every "yes" answer. A score of ≥2 indicates a likely case of anorexia or bulimia nervosa (sensitivity: 100%; specificity: 87.5%).

From Morgan, J. F., Reid, F., & Lacey, J. H. (1999).

express concern. Individuals with anorexia nervosa often present with no expressed concern about significant weight loss (Pritts and Susman, 2003). Menstrual disorders are among the most common reasons that women seek medical consultation (Mehler, 2001).

PCPs can do a quick assessment of a patient to determine the possibility of an eating disorder by using SCOFF, a brief 5-item screening tool that was developed by a group of primary care providers (Morgan, Reid, and Lacey, 1999). A score of 2 or greater yields a high degree of suspicion for an eating disorder, and indicates the need for further evaluation, referral, and/or treatment. This brief screening tool could easily be incorporated into a standard PCP's general screening questionnaire (Box 6.9). A few additional instruments for the assessment of eating disordered signs and symptoms are listed in Table 6.1.

A careful interview assessment is the most reliable approach to case finding in primary practice (Johnson, Fornai, Cabrini, et al., 2007; Pritts et al., 2003). During the interview, the individual's current weight, height, and weight history should be noted. Weight during childhood and early adolescence should also be explored. Questions about desired and ideal weight may provide valuable information regarding eating and weight control problems. Assessment of current and past eating disordered attitudes and behaviors should be included in the interview in an effort to gain a better understanding of the eating problem and to determine the eating disorder differential diagnosis (Crowther and Sherwood, 1997). This part of the interview may include questions about when the eating disordered symptoms first started, the type of symptoms (dieting, fasting, exercise for the purpose of weight control, vomiting, laxative, diuretic, diet pill, emetic usage, etc.), the duration and intensity of symptoms, and the course of these symptoms over time. Questions related to frequency and pattern of binge eating and compensatory behavior cycles are also important.

Box 6.10 shows some sample questions for use in assessing eating disordered behaviors. These questions could be used to assess the current level of eating disordered symptoms and behaviors and provide a baseline assessment for future reference.

The establishment of a therapeutic alliance is central to successful case identification, ongoing management, and treatment referral (Leichsenring, 2005). Throughout the process, an attitude of genuine interest and concern for the individual, along with a nonjudgmental interest and support, is critical to effective communication and intervention. The clinician may gently ask questions to determine the client's understanding of how and why the eating disorder

Box 6.10 • Eating Disorder Assessment Questions

1) **WEIGHT HISTORY**

Current weight? ________ pounds

Current height? ________ feet, __________ inches

2) **MENSTRUAL HISTORY**

In the last 3 months, have you had your menstrual period?

If no, for how long have you missed your period?

If yes, have you noticed any changes in your period?

1) Changes in length (flow days)? Describe changes (longer or shorter).
2) Changes in flow? Describe changes.
3) Changes in cycle length? Describe changes.
4) Date changes occurred (month/year, if known)?
5) Duration of changes in your period (# months, if known)?

Describe typical menses.

1) # days of flow
2) Strength of flow
3) Cycle length

Are you currently taking birth control pills?

1) **If yes,** when did you start using the pill (month/year)?
   a. Why did you start using the pill (regulate menses, contraception, PMS Symptoms)?
   b. Name of your birth control pill?
2) **If no,** have you ever taken birth control pills?
   a. If yes, why did you start taking the pill?
   b. If yes, the name of the birth control pill you took?

3) **RESTRICTING**

During the last month, have you restricted calories due to concern about body size or weight?

Estimated calories/day

(Continued)

Box 6.10 • *Continued*

During the last month, have you restricted fat due to concern about body size or weight?

Estimated fat grams/day

4) **BINGEING**

During the last month, have you eaten an amount of food that others would consider unusually large in a brief (less than 2-hour) period of time?

If yes, describe the typical type and amount of food.

If yes, how often have you typically binged in the last month?

5) **FASTING**

In the last month, have you used fasting to control your weight?

If yes, have you fasted until noon?

If yes, have you fasted until dinner time?

If yes, have you fasted all day?

In the last month, how many days did you fast?

6) **VOMITING**

During the last month, have you induced vomiting in order to get rid of food eaten?

If yes, how often have you typically induced vomiting in the last month?

7) **LAXATIVE USE**

During the last month, have you used laxatives to control your weight or "get rid of food"?

If yes, during the last month, how often have you taken laxatives for weight control?

What kind of laxatives do you take?

How many laxatives do you usually take each time?

8) **DIET PILLS**

During the last month, have you taken diet pills?

If yes, during the last month, how often have you typically taken diet pills?

What kind of diet pills do you take?

How many diet pills do you take each time?

(*Continued*)

Box 6.10 • *Continued*

9) **DIURETICS**

During the last month, have you taken diuretics (water pills) to control your weight?

If yes, during the last month, how often have you typically taken diuretics?

What kind of diuretics do you take?

How many diuretics do you take each time?

10) **EXERCISE**

During the last month, how many times did you exercise per week?

What type of exercise do you do?

How long do you exercise each time?

What percentage of your exercise is aimed at controlling your weight?

11) **GENERAL QUESTIONS**

Are you afraid of becoming fat?

Are parts of your body too fat?

developed and also the factors that may be maintaining the behaviors in the present state. Physical complications, when they develop, may be used as opportunities for teaching about the consequences of eating disordered behavior.

General Psychiatric History: Current and Past

A general psychiatric history should be completed during the same interview. Comorbid major mental disorders are extremely common in eating disordered patients (Woodside and Staab, 2006). Eating disordered patients may also struggle with substance abuse issues (Conason and Sher, 2006) or have unresolved issues of past sexual abuse (Wonderlich et al., 2007). It is not uncommon for individuals with eating disorders to experience an Axis I psychiatric disorder in the form of clinical depression or a comorbid anxiety disorder (Blinder, Cumella, and Sanathara, 2006). Comorbid anxiety and substance disorders have been associated with greater severity of eating disordered symptoms (Spindler and Milos, 2007). Axis II personality disorders are also present in some patients with eating disorders. Borderline and histrionic personality disorders have been associated with recurrent bingeing and purging eating disordered behaviors, while antisocial and schizotypal personality disorders have been associated with recurrent bingeing and binge eating disorder (Johnson, Cohen, Kasen, et al., 2006). Thus, it is important to obtain a general psychiatric history from the client, so comorbid major mental health problems may be identified and addressed in the client's individualized treatment plan.

The PCP should consider the following: Has the individual ever sought psychiatric or psychological help before? If so, for what type of symptoms? What was the diagnosis (depression, anxiety disorder, etc.)? What was the treatment? Is the individual currently experiencing any of these symptoms? Is the patient currently receiving any type of treatment for these symptoms?

Medical Considerations

The medical history is an essential tool for diagnosing eating disorders (Pritts and Susman, 2003). All patients should be screened during routine office visits.

Physical examination and laboratory findings may be normal, especially during the early course of these disorders. A full physical exam should be performed by the PCP. Particular attention should be paid to vital signs, physical growth and development (including height and weight), the cardiovascular system, evidence of dehydration, acrocyanosis, lanugo, salivary gland enlargement, and scarring on the dorsum of the hands (Russell's sign) from self-induced vomiting (APA, 2006). A dental exam should also be performed (looking for erosion of enamel on the teeth).

The need for laboratory analyses should be determined on an individual basis, depending on the patient's condition. The following laboratory tests should be considered for all patients with eating disorders: blood chemistries including serum magnesium and serum phosphorus, complete blood count, serum electrolyte levels, BUN, serum creatinine level, thyroid function studies, urinalysis, and electrocardiogram (ECG) (APA, 2006). Medical complications are common and often serious in patients with eating disorders (Mitchell and Crow, 2006). Table 6.2 shows common laboratory abnormalities and medical complications associated with anorexia and bulimia nervosa. Because medical complications in patients with eating disorders are not uncommon, the PCP will need to provide careful medical evaluation and ongoing medical management in the care of these patients.

Fluids and Electrolytes

- Electrolyte abnormalities are quite common in patients with eating disorders, especially among patients who frequently purge by vomiting

Table 6.2 • Laboratory Abnormalities and Medical Complications of Anorexia Nervosa and Bulimia Nervosa

Metabolic	Hypercarotenemia Hypoglycemia Hypercholesterolemia Abnormal liver function Abnormal glucose tolerance
Gastrointestinal	Gastric dilatation Salivary gland swelling (due to vomiting) Amylase elevation Delayed gastric emptying Constipation Superior mesenteric artery syndrome Pancreatitis Esophagitis Esophageal tears or rupture Gastric rupture
Cardiovascular	ECG abnormalities Bradycardia Arrhythmias Syncope Pericardial effusion Edema Congestive heart failure (refeeding syndrome) Cardiomyopathy (ipecac abuse)
Fluid & Electrolytes	Hypokalemia Hypochloremia Hyponatremia Hypocalcemia Hypophosphatemia (anorexia nervosa) Hyperphosphatemia (bulimia nervosa) Hypomagnesemia Metabolic acidosis (due to laxative abuse) Metabolic alkalosis (due to self-induced vomiting)

(*Continued*)

Table 6.2 • (Continued)

	Dehydration Weakness Tetany
Hematologic	Pancytopenia Leukopenia Neutropenia Relative lymphocytosis Bone marrow hypocellularity Thrombocytopenia Bleeding diathesis Anemia
Dental	Decalcification Enamel erosion Caries
Endocrine	Low luteinizing hormone Low follicle-stimulating hormone Low urinary gonadotropins Low urinary estrogen Low triiodothyronine Blunted TSR response to TRH Glucose elevation Prolactin elevation Elevated growth hormone Elevated cortisol Amenorrhea Lack of sexual interest Impotence Dexamethasone suppression test nonsuppression
Renal	Elevated BUN Decreased GFR Urinary concentrating defect Kaliopenic nephropathy Dehydration Hypokalemic nephropathy

(Continued)

Table 6.2 • (Continued)

Neurologic	EEG abnormalities Seizures Reversible brain atrophy
General Complications	Weakness Hypothermia Lanugo Hypercarotenemia Alopecia Dry skin Russell's sign (calluses on knuckles from self-induced vomiting)
Laxative Abuse Complications	Hyperuremia Hypocalcemia Tetany Osteomalacia Clubbing Hypomagnesemia Fluid retention Malabsorption syndromes Protein-losing enteropathy Cathartic colon

From Mehler, P. S. (2001); Mehler, P. S., & Anderson, A. D. (1999); Mehler, P. S., Crews, C., & Weiner, K. (2004); Pomeroy, C., & Mitchell, J. E. (2002).

or taking laxatives or diuretics (Pomeroy and Mitchell, 2002). Some of the deaths attributable to anorexia and bulimia nervosa have been linked to hypokalemia, which may result from both dehydration and increased potassium loss because of volume contraction, vomiting, laxative abuse, and/or diuretic use. Hypokalemia will reverse with cessation of the provoking behaviors. Sometimes, a potassium replacement supplement is required. Because potassium is predominantly intracellular, normal serum potassium is maintained even in the face of significant total body potassium deficiency. Thus, in the absence of concurrent acid-base derangements, any hypokalemia represents a significant total body potassium deficit and should be replaced. The effect of serum bicarbonate level on extracellular potassium should also be considered. In the case of long-standing dehydration and hypovolemic metabolic alkalosis (the most common acid-base disturbance seen in eating disordered patients), it is likely that total body potassium stores are depleted because of renal losses as the kidney preferentially reabsorbs sodium in order to retain water. In this case, adequate potassium replacement cannot be achieved until the contraction alkalosis has been corrected by reduction or cessation of self-induced vomiting. If serum potassium levels remain low after correction of acid-base disturbance, additional replacement is indicated. A drop of 1 mEq/L represents a total body deficit of approximately 350 mEq/L. Assuming normal kidney function, an oral potassium replacement is usually started at 40 to 80 mEq per day. Serum potassium and bicarbonate levels should be assessed frequently (Mehler, Crews, and Weiner, 2004).

- Other electrolyte abnormalities include hypomagnesemia (which may be associated with hypocalcemia or hypokalemia, both of which will only resolve with correction of the magnesium deficiency) and hypophosphatemia. Refeeding early in the course of treatment for anorexia nervosa often leads to a further drop in serum phosphorus levels, which can lead to rhabdomyolysis, severe myocardial dysfunction, acute renal failure, seizures, or death. Refeeding syndrome can be prevented by starting refeeding slowly. In order to avoid phosphate depletion, supplemental phosphorus (e.g., Nutra-phos 500 mg) orally twice daily for the 5 days of refeeding may help to compensate for the increased tissue phosphate requirements (Rome and Ammerman, 2003). It is important for the PCP to carefully monitor serum magnesium, calcium, potassium, and phosphorus levels in this group of patients, especially during early refeeding (Katzman, 2005).

Cardiovascular

- Ipecac abuse in bulimic patients has been associated with cardiomyopathy (Mehler et al., 2004).
- ECG abnormalities, including prolongation of the QT interval, may predispose some patients to the development of life-threatening arrhythmias (Katzman, 2005). Drugs that prolong the QT interval

should be avoided with these patients. Other ECG changes, including decreased QRS amplitude, nonspecific ST segment, and T-wave changes, are more benign and have been associated with the decrease in left ventricular wall thickness and cardiac chamber size with loss of muscle mass (Katzman).

- Cardiac arrhythmias are a potentially fatal complication that may develop secondary to electrolyte abnormalities (e.g., hypokalemia). Hypokalemia is associated with decreased amplitude or inversion of the T wave on the ECG assessment, QT prolongation, and increased risk for ventricular arrhythmias (Facchini, Sala, Malfatto, et al., 2006).

Gastrointestinal

- Delayed gastric emptying may be associated with complaints of stomach bloating and abdominal pain in some patients with eating disorders. Although these symptoms will improve with nutritional therapy and weight gain, there may be a limited role for prokinetic agents during the early stages of refeeding (Rome and Ammerman, 2003).
- Starvation and laxative abuse both contribute to constipation. The chronic use of stimulant laxatives containing phenolphthalein may lead to irreversible damage to colonic innervation. However, in most cases, withdrawal of the laxatives combined with a high-fiber diet and a bulking agent (e.g., Metamucil) are effective (Mehler et al., 2004).
- Vomiting and malnutrition can result in gastrointestinal bleeding, secondary to esophagitis and erosion. Esophageal rupture or Boerhaave syndrome is a rare but emergent and potentially life-threatening complication in patients who engage in self-induced vomiting (Mehler et al., 2004).

Bone Mineral Density

Hypoestrogenemia and amenorrhea have been associated with osteopenia and osteoporosis in eating disordered patients (Katzman, 2005; Miller, Grinspoon, Ciampa, et al., 2005; Misra, Aggarwal, Miller, et al., 2004). Calcium replacement may be considered in low-weight anorexics with documented osteoporosis, although dietary calcium has been found to be superior to oral calcium supplementation for its effects on enhancing bone mineral density (Napoli,

Thompson, Civitelli, et al., 2007), and restoration of a healthy weight is the preferred treatment (APA, 2006; Katzman, 2005; Misra and Klibanski, 2006). The use of alendronate 10 mg daily has been shown to increase bone mineral density in anorexic individuals with osteopenia (Golden, Iglesias, Jacobson, et al., 2005).

TREATMENT OF EATING DISORDERS

The treatment of eating disorders requires a multidisciplinary team approach. The PCP should be an integral part of that team and coordinate the team of professionals (e.g., psychiatrist, psychologist, dietician) needed for the care of individuals with eating disorders. Referral of patients to a registered dietician is often helpful (American Dietetic Association [ADA], 2006). The dietician should work with the patient to set up a healthy eating plan and educate her about healthy nutrition and the effects of nutrition on one's body. Furthermore, referral of patients to psychological counseling services is essential. Although eating disorders often present with physical manifestations (extreme loss of weight, cachexia) and disturbing behaviors (binge episodes and self-induced vomiting), the root cause of these eating disorders is believed to lie in underlying psychological conflicts (Bruch, 1973; Chernin, 1994; Stein, 1996). The empirically supported eating disorder practice guidelines recommend engaging a psychological counselor to treat and address these critical underlying issues (APA, 2006; National Institute for Clinical Excellence [NICE], 2004; Wilson, Grilo, and Vitousek, 2007).

The treatment setting and intensity of treatment should be determined by the severity of illness. Patients presenting with mild forms of eating disorders can often be managed on an outpatient basis. Individuals who are medically or psychiatrically unstable will require more intensive and sometimes inpatient treatment. Aggressive early treatment of young adults, before the behaviors and attitudes have had a chance to get firmly rooted and entrenched, may help improve long-term outcome. Guidelines have been established for the determination of level of care required for patients with eating disorders (Table 6.3). Treatment goals generally include (1) reducing eating disordered attitudes and behaviors, (2) attainment and maintenance of a healthy weight, (3) management of physical complications, and (4) prevention of relapse.

For a small subgroup of very chronic and treatment refractory patients, treatment goals may be revised to include stabilization of current weight, achievement of a minimally safe weight compatible with life, and achievement of medical and psychiatric stability (Strober, 1997).

Treatment Guidelines for Patients with Anorexia Nervosa

Nutritional Intervention

For patients with anorexia nervosa who are severely underweight, a program of nutritional rehabilitation should be established (ADA, 2006; APA, 2006; NICE 2004). Inpatient hospital-based programs should be considered for seriously nutritionally compromised patients (i.e., those whose weight is less than 75 percent of the recommended weight for their height or for children and adolescents whose weight loss may not be as severe but who are losing at a rapid rate). The nutritional rehabilitation program should aim to establish a healthy target weight and have expected rates of controlled weight gain (i.e., 2 to 5 pounds per week in inpatient settings, and 0.5 to 1.0 pound a week for outpatient programs). Caloric intake levels should usually start at 30 to 40 kcal/kg per day (approximately 1,000 to 1,600 kcal per day) and should be advanced progressively. During the weight-gaining phase, caloric intake may be increased to as high as 70 to 100 kcal/kg per day for some patients. During the weight maintenance (and for ongoing growth and development in children and adolescents), caloric intake should be around 40 to 60 kcal per day. Patients who require higher caloric intakes may be discarding food, vomiting, or exercising or may have higher metabolic rates. In addition to caloric intake, patients may benefit from vitamin and mineral supplements (in particular, phosphorus). Medical monitoring during refeeding is essential and should include assessment of food and fluid intake and output, monitoring of vital signs and electrolytes (including phosphorus), observation for edema (rapid weight gain in severely underweight patients may be associated with fluid overload and congestive heart failure), and observation for gastrointestinal symptoms (particularly constipation and bloating). Physical activity during the refeeding phase should be adapted to the food intake and energy expenditure of the client along with the current medical condition (APA, 2006; NICE, 2004).

Other treatment options for nutritional intervention include temporary supplementation or replacement of regular food with liquid supplements. On occasion, nasogastric feedings may be required. In life-threatening or very unusual circumstances, parenteral feedings for brief periods of time may be considered; however, infection is a serious risk with parenteral feedings in emaciated and possibly immune-compromised individuals with anorexia nervosa. These types of extreme interventions should be considered only when patients are unwilling to cooperate with oral feedings; when the patient's health, physical safety, and recovery are threatened; and after legal and ethical considerations have been taken into account (APA, 2006; NICE, 2004).

Table 6.3 • Level-of-Care Criteria for Patients with Eating Disorders

Characteristic	Level 1: Outpatient	Level 2: Intensive Outpatient	Level 3: Full-Day Outpatient	Level 4: Residential Treatment Center	Level 5: Inpatient Hospitalization
Medical complications	Medically stable to the extent that more extensive monitoring, as defined in Levels 4 and 5, is not required			Medically stable (not requiring NG feeds, IV fluids, or multiple daily laboratories)	Adults: HR <40 beats per minute; BP <90/60 mm Hg; glucose <60 mg per dL (3.3 mmol per L); K^+ <3 mg per dL (0.8 mmol per L); temperature <36.1°C (97°F); dehydration; renal, hepatic, or cardiovascular compromise Children and adolescents: HR <50 beats per minute; orthostatic BP; BP <80/50 mm Hg; hypokalemia; hypophosphatemia
Suicidality	No intent or plan			Possible plan but no intent	Intent and plan
Weight, as percent of healthy body weight	>85%	>80%	>70%	<85%	Adults: <75% Children and adolescents: acute weight decline with food refusal

Motivation to recover (cooperativeness, insight, ability to control obsessive thoughts)	Good to fair	Fair	Partial; preoccupied with ego-syntonic thoughts more than 3 hours per day; cooperative	Fair to poor; preoccupied with ego-syntonic thoughts 4 to 6 hours per day; cooperative with highly structured treatment	Poor to very poor; preoccupied with ego-syntonic thoughts; uncooperative with treatment or cooperative only with highly structured environment
Comorbid disorders (substance abuse, depression, anxiety)	Presence of comorbid condition may influence choice of level of care				Any existing psychiatric disorder that would require hospitalization
Structure needed for eating/gaining weight	Self-sufficient		Needs some structure to gain weight	Needs supervision at all meals or will restrict eating	Needs supervision during and after all meals, or NG/special feeding
Impairment and ability to care for self; ability to control exercise	Able to exercise for fitness; able to control obsessive exercise		Structure required to prevent excessive exercise	Complete role impairment, cannot eat and gain weight by self; structure required to prevent patient from compulsive exercising	
Purging behavior (laxatives and diuretics)	Can greatly reduce purging in nonstructured settings; no significant medical complications, such as ECG abnormalities or others suggesting the need for hospitalization			Can ask for and use support or skills if desires to purge	Needs supervision during and after all meals and in bathrooms
Environmental stress	Others able to provide adequate emotional and practical support and structure		Others able to provide at least limited support and structure	Severe family conflict, problems, or absence so as unable to provide structured treatment in home or lives alone without adequate support system	
Treatment availability/living situation	Lives near treatment setting			Too distant to live at home	

NG, nasogastric; IV, intravenous; HR, heart rate; BP, blood pressure; K^+, potassium level; ECG, electrocardiogram.
Adapted from the American Psychiatric Association Work Group on Eating Disorders (2000).

Nutritional intervention programs should also include ongoing education, emotional support, and efforts to help the patients deal with their concern about gaining weight and the associated body image changes (APA, 2006).

Psychosocial Intervention

Individual Therapy Identity impairments and other psychological conflicts are believed to contribute to the onset and maintenance of anorexia nervosa (Bruch, 1973; Stein, 1996). As a result, successful outcomes usually require the affected individual to work through these issues. Consequently, all individuals with anorexia nervosa should be referred for psychological counseling. Ideally, the referral should be to a professional who is familiar and experienced with treating clients who have eating disorders.

Psychosocial interventions aim to help patients understand and cooperate with nutritional and physical rehabilitation, to understand and change dysfunctional attitudes and behaviors associated with the eating disorder, to improve interpersonal and social functioning, and to address comorbid psychiatric issues that are reinforcing and maintaining the eating disorder (APA, 2006; NICE 2004). Various forms of psychotherapeutic techniques have been used in patients with anorexia nervosa, including psychodynamic therapy (Herzog, 1995) and cognitive behavioral therapy (CBT; Wilson et al., 2007), although no one form of therapy stands out as being clearly superior (McIntosh, Jordan, Carter, et al., 2005). Psychosocial interventions are best when individually tailored to a particular patient's needs. In severely malnourished patients with anorexia nervosa, there is general agreement that the effectiveness of psychotherapy is limited until the effects of malnutrition can be corrected and a minimally healthy weight is restored (Strober, 1997).

Family Therapy Family psychotherapy may be useful for addressing family relational problems that may be contributing to and maintaining the eating disorder (APA, 2006; NICE, 2004; Wilson et al., 2007). Some research has shown that patients with anorexia nervosa, with an onset before the age of 18 years and a duration of fewer than 3 years, treated with family therapy demonstrated greater improvement 1 year after hospital discharge than patients receiving individual psychotherapy alone (Russell, Szmukler, Dare, et al., 1987). The 5-year follow-up study also showed continuing effects of the family therapy, further supporting the efficacy of family therapy for this group of patients (Eisler, Dare, Russell, et al., 1997). Family therapy can be especially helpful for younger patients who still live at home with their parents.

Medications

Psychotropic medications should not be used as the primary or sole treatment for anorexia nervosa (APA, 2006; NICE, 2004). Empirical support for the use of medication and its efficacy in the treatment of anorexia nervosa has been disappointing (Pederson, Roerig, and Mitchell, 2003; Steffan, Roerig, Mitchell, et al., 2006; Walsh, Kapplan, Attia, et al., 2006). Medication therapy should not be used routinely during the weight-restoration period (APA, 2006; NICE 2004). The need for antidepressants is often best assessed following weight gain, when the psychological effects of malnutrition are resolved. However, antidepressant medication may be considered to prevent relapse among weight-restored patients or for the treatment of concurrent, associated disorders including depression and obsessive-compulsive disorder (APA, 2006). When prescribing antidepressant and other psychotropic medication for those with eating disorders, careful attention must be paid to prescribing black-box warnings. Antipsychotic medication, particularly second-generation antipsychotics, may be useful during the weight-restoration stage of treatment and also for treating associated symptoms including severe anxiety, obsessionality, and psychoticlike thinking (APA, 2006; NICE, 2004). Occasionally, anxiolytics (such as lorazepam) may be briefly useful to help with anxiety associated with early refeeding (Garner and Garfinkel, 1997).

Treatment Guidelines for Patients with Bulimia Nervosa

Nutritional Intervention

The primary focus of nutritional rehabilitation for most individuals with bulimia nervosa concerns monitoring patterns of binge eating and purging. Most patients with bulimia nervosa are of normal weight, so nutritional restoration is not usually a central focus of the treatment. However, nutritional counseling may be useful for reducing behaviors related to the eating disorder, minimizing food restriction, increasing the variety of foods eaten, and encouraging healthy eating patterns (ADA, 2006; APA, 2006).

Psychosocial Intervention

Individual Therapy Psychological intervention using a cognitive behavioral approach is regarded as the leading form of psychotherapeutic treatment for bulimia nervosa (NICE, 2004; Wilson et al., 2007). CBT is based on the view that certain cognitive processes are responsible for initiating and maintaining the eating disordered behaviors. Cognitions that are thought to contribute to the eating disorder include the tendency to judge self-worth according to body shape and weight, the presence of low self-esteem, perfectionism, and the tendency for dichotomous ("black-and-white") patterns of thinking. Treatment generally is conducted on a one-to-one basis and usually involves about 20 sessions over the course of 4 to 5 months. CBT involves a series of efforts to address and correct both the cognitive and behavioral aspects of the eating disorder. Numerous studies have found CBT to be superior to other forms of psychotherapy and also have shown on average at least a 70-percent reduction in the frequency of binge eating and purging, while nearly one third to one half of patients cease binge eating altogether (Wilson et al., 2007). Follow-up studies have found that the progress made following CBT tends to be fairly well maintained (Fairburn, Jones, Peveler, et al., 1993).

Group Therapy Cognitive behavioral group psychotherapy is sometimes used for individuals with bulimia nervosa and has been shown to be effective in reducing symptoms (Wilson et al., 2007). There is some evidence that programs that include dietary counseling and management as part of the group treatment (Laessle, Zoettle, and Pirke, 1987) and more frequent group sessions (Mitchell, Pyle, Pomeroy, et al., 1993) result in improved outcomes. Often, individuals are treated with a combination of group and individual therapy.

Family Therapy Family therapy may be helpful in the treatment of bulimia nervosa (APA, 2006; NICE, 2004). It may be particularly useful for adolescents who still live with their parents.

Medications

Antidepressants may be effective as one component of an initial treatment program for many patients with bulimia nervosa (APA, 2006; NICE 2004). Fluoxetine is currently the only FDA drug approved for use in the treatment of bulimia nervosa, although antidepressant medications from a variety of classes can help to reduce symptoms of binge eating and purging and may prevent relapse among patients in remission. Careful attention must be paid to black-box warnings when prescribing these medications for individuals with eating disorders. The selective serotonin reuptake inhibitors (SSRIs) may be especially helpful for patients with significant symptoms of depression, anxiety, obsessive-compulsive behavior, or certain impulsive disorder symptoms and for patients who have failed or had suboptimal response to previous attempts at strictly psychosocial intervention.

Fluoxetine at high doses (60 mg per day) has been studied and is shown to be superior to lower doses of the drug for reducing bulimic symptoms (Fluoxetine Bulimia Nervosa Collaborative Study Group, 1992). Fluoxetine is generally well tolerated by this group of patients, and some have suggested starting bulimic patients on doses of 60 mg per day and titrating downward if necessary due to side effects (Goldstein, Wilson, Thompson, et al., 1995; NICE 2004). Studies have shown that the combination of medication with CBT is superior to either one therapy alone (Bacaltchuk, Hay, and Trefiglio, 2002).

Practitioners should try to avoid prescribing tricyclic antidepressants for patients who may be suicidal and monoamine oxidase inhibitors (MAOIs) for individuals with chaotic binge eating and purging (APA, 2006). Bupropion should be avoided in patients with eating disorders (or in those individuals with a history of an eating disorder) due to its propensity to lower the seizure threshold and induce seizures in these individuals. In general, lithium should be avoided in eating disordered patients with fluid and electrolyte disturbances (APA, 2006).

Treatment Guidelines for Patients with Eating Disorder Not Otherwise Specified

In the absence of evidence to guide the management of atypical eating disorders included under the broad classification of EDNOS, except for binge eating disorder, practice guidelines recommend that the guideline for the eating problem that most closely resembles the patient's eating disorder symptoms should be followed (NICE, 2004).

Treatment Guidelines for Patients with Binge Eating Disorder

Nutritional Intervention

All psychological treatments for binge eating disorder have only a limited effect on body weight. Evidence-based practice guidelines recommend providing concurrent or consecutive intervention focusing on the management of comorbid obesity (ADA, 2006; NICE, 2004). Many individuals who experience binge eating disorder also struggle with overweight or obesity. Both biology and environment have been found to play a significant role in obesity (Silventoinen, Pietilainen, Tynelius, et al., 2007). Since it is impossible to alter genetics and biology, environmental modifications may be undertaken including altering energy expenditure by increasing exercise and decreasing energy intake by modifying diet. Behavioral weight control programs including very-low- or low-calorie diets may help overweight or obese individuals with binge eating disorder lose weight and usually reduce symptoms of binge eating, although some degree of weight gain often follows the weight loss, and weight gain after weight loss may be accompanied by a return of binge eating behavior (APA, 2006). Guidelines have been established for safe weight-loss practices (Box 6.11). Healthy weight-loss programs often include a combination of nutritional counseling, exercise, and psychological counseling (Powell, Calvin, and Calvin, 2007).

Psychosocial Intervention

Individual Therapy Individuals with binge eating problems may benefit from a modified version of the treatment program that is used for the treatment of bulimia nervosa, along with psychotherapy (interpersonal psychotherapy, modified dialectical behavioral therapy, and/or CBT), nutritional counseling, and pharmacotherapy (NICE, 2004). Studies have shown that individuals who received some form of psychological intervention (most often CBT) demonstrated greater overall improvements in binge frequency and binge abstinence at follow-up compared with individuals treated with SSRI medication alone (Devlin, Goldfein, Petkova, et al., 2007; Grilo, Masheb, and Wilson, 2005; Molinari, Baruffi, Croci, et al., 2005). Studies have found that individual interpersonal psychotherapy and individual CBT for the treatment of binge eating disorder result in a similar improvement in binge abstinence (59 percent for CBT and 61 percent for interpersonal therapy) at 1-year follow-up (Wilfley, 2002; Wilfley and Cohen, 1997). However, improvements in binge frequency and binge abstinence were poorly correlated with changes in individual weight.

Medications

SSRI antidepressants may be an effective component of the initial treatment program for patients with binge eating disorder (NICE, 2004). The SSRIs may be especially helpful for patients with significant symptoms of depression, anxiety, obsessive-compulsive behavior, or certain impulsive behaviors and for patients who have failed or had suboptimal response to previous attempts at strictly psychosocial intervention.

EATING DISORDERS IN SPECIAL POPULATIONS

Eating Disorders in Patients with Diabetes Mellitus

Eating disorders are quite common among young women with type 1 diabetes mellitus. Up to one third of women with this type of diabetes may have some

Box 6.11 • Recommendations for Adult Weight-Loss Programs

Reasonable Weight Goal

The weight goal for the patient should be based on personal and family history and not exclusively on height and weight charts.

Rate of Weight Loss

The rate of weight loss should not exceed 2 pounds per week.

Calories Per Day

The daily caloric intake should not be below 1,000 kcal per day without medical supervision.

Diet Composition

a) **Protein:** Between 0.8 to 1.5 g protein per kg body weight, but not more than 100 g protein per day.
b) **Fat:** 10% to 30% of energy as fat.
c) **Carbohydrate:** At least 100 g per day without medical supervision.
d) **Fluid:** At least 1 quart of water per day.

Nutritional Education

Nutritional education that teaches healthy eating patterns should be incorporated into the weight-loss program.

Exercise

The weight loss program should include an exercise component that is safe for the individual patient.

a) The patient should be screened for medical conditions that would require medical clearance before starting any exercise program.
b) The patient should be instructed on how to recognize and deal with potentially dangerous responses to exercise.
c) The patient should work toward 30 to 60 minutes of continuous exercise 5 to 7 times per week, with gradual increases in intensity and duration.

Psychological Component

Appropriate behavior modification techniques should be incorporated into the individual weight-loss program.

From the Task Force to Establish Weight Loss Guidelines (1990).

form of eating disorder, and these women are at an especially high risk of microvascular and other metabolic complications (Herzog et al., 1996; Peveler, 2000). Diabetics with eating disorders often underdose insulin in order to lose weight. Nutritional counseling and aggressive management of eating disordered symptoms are important to prevent long-term consequences in the form of diabetic complications.

Eating Disorders in Pregnant Patients

Eating disorders sometimes have an onset during pregnancy, but many patients get pregnant even while they are actively symptomatic with an eating disorder. The behaviors associated with eating disorders (poor nutrition, binge eating, purging) can result in both fetal and maternal complications (Micali, Simonoff, and Treasure, 2007). Women with lifetime histories of anorexia nervosa appear to be at a greater risk for birth complications and of giving birth to lower-weight babies (Bulik, Sullivan, Fear, et al., 1999). Therefore, care of the pregnant patient with an eating disorder usually requires the collaboration of a psychiatrist and an obstetrician specializing in high-risk pregnancies (Micali et al., 2007).

CONCLUSION

The role of the PCP in the treatment of eating disorders is usually identification of the problem and coordination of the treatment program. This involves collaboration with other health care providers including psychologists, psychiatrists, and nutritional counselors. Since anorexia nervosa and bulimia nervosa tend to be fairly chronic conditions, the PCP will often have an ongoing role in the coordination of treatment and medical monitoring of these patients. It is important for the PCP to work to establish trust and a good working relationship with the eating disordered patient. Referral to psychological and nutritional counselors who are familiar with treating eating disorders, and ongoing communication with these professionals in the collaborative care of these patients, is essential. The PCP has an invaluable role in helping patients recover from eating disorders by detecting them early, diligently monitoring and assessing the patient's physical condition, and providing emotional support and encouragement to facilitate the recovery process.

Resources for Providers

Books for Professionals

Brownell, K. D., & Foreyt, J. P. (1986). *Handbook of eating disorders: Physiology, psychology, and treatment of obesity, anorexia, and bulimia.* New York: Basic Books.

Bruch, H. (1978). *The golden cage: The enigma of anorexia nervosa.* New York: Random House.

Fairburn, C. G. (1995). *Overcoming binge eating.* New York: Guilford Press.

Fairburn, C. G., & Brownell, K. D. (Eds.). (2005). *Eating disorders and obesity: A comprehensive handbook,* 2nd ed. New York: Guilford Press.

Fairburn, C. G., & Wilson, G. T. (Eds.). (1993). *Binge eating: Nature, assessment, and treatment.* New York: Guilford Press.

Garner, D. M., & Garfinkel, P. E. (Eds.). (1985). *Handbook of psychotherapy for anorexia nervosa and bulimia.* New York: Guilford Press.

Garner, D. M., & Garfinkel, P. E. (Eds.). (1997). *Handbook of treatment for eating disorders.* New York: Guilford Press.

Levenkron, S. (1982). *Treating and overcoming anorexia nervosa.* New York: Scribner Books.

Mehler, P. S., & Anderson, A. D. (1999). *Eating disorders: A guide to medical care and complications.* Baltimore, MD: Johns Hopkins University Press.

Striegel-Moore, R., & Smolak, L. (Eds.). (2001). *Eating disorders: New directions for research and practice.* Washington, DC: American Psychological Association.

Resources for Patients

Organizations

National Association of Anorexia Nervosa and Associated Disorders (ANAD)
P.O. Box 7
Highland Park, IL 60035
(847) 831-3438
Monday–Friday, 9 a.m.–5 p.m., Central Time
E-mail: anad20@aol.com

National Eating Disorder Association (NEDA)
603 Stewart Street, Suite 803
Seattle, WA 98101
(206) 382-3587
Toll-Free Information and Referral Helpline: (800) 931-2237
E-mail: info@nationaleatingdisorders.org

Websites

ANAD, National Association for Anorexia and Associated Eating Disorders: *www.anad.org*

Eating Disorders, Mirror Mirror: *www.mirror-mirror.org/eatdis.htm*

National Eating Disorders Association: *www.nationaleatingdisorders.org*

Something Fishy, Website on Eating Disorders: *www.something-fishy.org*

Books for Families and Friends

Lask, B., & Bryant-Waugh, R. (2004). *Eating disorders: A parent's guide*. London: Routledge.

Lock, J., & LeGrange, D. (2005). *Help your teenager beat an eating disorder*. New York: Guilford Press.

Lock, J., LeGrange, D., Agras, W. S., et al. (2002). *Treatment manual for anorexia nervosa: A family-based approach*. New York: Guilford Press.

Siegel, M., Brisman, J., & Weinshel, M. (1988). *Surviving an eating disorder: Strategies for families and friends*. New York: HarperCollins.

Way, K. (1993). *Anorexia nervosa and recovery: A hunger for meaning*. Binghamton, NY: Haworth Press.

Books for Eating Disorder Sufferers

Hall, L. (Ed.). (1993). *Full lives: Women who have freed themselves from food and weight obsession.* Carlsbad, CA: Gurze Books.

Hall, L., & Cohn, L. (1998). *Bulimia: A guide to recovery*. Carlsbad, CA: Gurze Books.

Hall, L., & Ostroff, M. (1998). *Anorexia nervosa: A guide to recovery*. Carlsbad, CA: Gurze Books.

References

American Dietetic Association (ADA). (2006). Position of the American Dietetic Association: Nutrition intervention in the treatment of anorexia nervosa, bulimia nervosa and other eating disorders. *Journal American Dietetic Association, 106*, 2073–2082.

American Psychiatric Association (APA). (2000). *Diagnostic and statistical manual of mental disorders* (Revised 4th ed.). Washington, DC: Author.

American Psychiatric Association (APA). (2006). *Practice guideline for the treatment of patients with eating disorders* (3rd ed.). Washington, DC: Author.

Bacaltchuk, J., Hay, P., & Trefiglio, R. (2002). Antidepressants versus psychological treatments and their combination for bulimia nervosa, *Evidence Based Mental Health, 5*(3), 74–75.

Becker, A. E., Grinspoon, S. K., Klibanski, A., et al. (1999). Eating disorders. *New England Journal of Medicine, 340*, 1092–1098.

Ben-Tovim, D. I., Walker, K., Gilchrist, P., et al. (2001). Outcome in patients with eating disorders: A 5-year study. *Lancet, 357*, 1254–1257.

Blinder, B. J., Cumella, E. J., & Sanathara, V. A. (2006). Psychiatric comorbidities of female inpatients with eating disorders. *Psychosomatic Medicine, 68*, 454–462.

Boroughs, M., & Thompson, J. K. (2002). Exercise status and sexual orientation as moderators of body image disturbance and eating disorders in males. *International Journal of Eating Disorders, 31*, 307–311.

Bruch, H. (1973). *Eating disorders: Obesity, anorexia nervosa, and the person within*. New York: Basic Books.

Bulik, C., Sullivan, P. F., Fear, J., et al. (1997). Predictors of the development of bulimia nervosa in women with anorexia nervosa. *Journal of Nervous and Mental Disorders, 185*, 704–707.

Bulik, C., Sullivan, P. F., Fear, J., et al. (1999). Fertility and reproduction in women with anorexia nervosa: A controlled study. *Journal of Clinical Psychiatry, 60*, 130–135.

Chatoor, I., & Surles, J. (2004). Eating disorders in mid-childhood. *Primary Psychiatry, 11*(4), 34–39.

Chernin, K. (1994). *The hungry self: Women, eating & identity*. New York: HarperCollins.

Conason, A. H., & Sher, L. (2006). Alcohol use in adolescents with eating disorders. *International Journal of Adolescent Medicine and Health, 18*(1), 31–36.

Cooper, Z. (2005). The development and maintenance of eating disorders. In K. D. Brownell & C. G. Fairburn (Eds.), *Eating disorders and obesity* (pp. 199–211). New York: Guilford Press.

Crowther, J. H., & Sherwood, N. E. (1997). Assessment. In D. M. Garner & P. E. Garfinkel (Eds.), *Handbook of treatment for eating disorders* (pp. 34–49). New York: Guilford Press.

Devlin, M. J., Goldfein, J. A., Petkova, E., et al. (2007). Cognitive behavioral therapy and fluoxetine for binge eating disorder: Two-year follow-up. *Obesity, 15*(7), 1702–1709.

Eisler, I., Dare, C., Russell, G., et al. (1997). Family and individual therapy in anorexia nervosa: A 5-year follow-up. *Archives of General Psychiatry, 54*, 1025–1030.

Facchini, M., Sala, L., Malfatto, G., et al. (2006). Low K+ dependent QT prolongation and risk for ventricular arrhythmia in anorexia nervosa. *International Journal of Cardiology, 106*(2), 170–176.

Fairburn, C. G., Cowen, P. J., & Harrison, P. J. (1999). Twin studies and the etiology of eating disorders. *International Journal of Eating Disorders, 26*, 349–358.

Fairburn, C. G., Jones, R., Peveler, R. C., et al. (1993). Psychotherapy and bulimia nervosa: The longer-term effects of interpersonal psychotherapy, behavior therapy, and cognitive behavioral therapy. *Archives of General Psychiatry, 50*, 419–428.

Fairburn, C. G., & Walsh, B. T. (2002). Atypical eating disorders (eating disorder not otherwise specified). In C. G. Fairburn & K. D. Brownell (Eds.), *Eating disorders and obesity* (pp. 171–177). New York: Guilford Press.

Favaro, A., Ferrara, S., & Santonastaso, P. (2003). The spectrum of eating disorders in young women: A prevalence study in a general population sample. *Psychosomatic Medicine, 65*, 701–708.

Fluoxetine Bulimia Nervosa Collaborative Study Group. (1992). Fluoxetine in the treatment of bulimia nervosa. *Archives of General Psychiatry, 49*, 139–147.

Forman, M., & Davis, W. N. (2005). Characteristics of middle-aged women in inpatient treatment for eating disorders. *Eating Disorders: The Journal of Treatment and Prevention, 13*(3), 231–243.

Forsberg, S., & Lock, J. (2006). The relationship between perfectionism, eating disorders and athletes: A review. *Minerva Pediatrica, 58*(6), 525–536.

Garner, D. M., & Garfinkel, P. E. (Eds.). (1997). *Handbook of treatment for eating disorders.* New York: Guilford Press.

Garner, D. M., & Magana, C. (2006). Cognitive vulnerability to anorexia nervosa. In L. B. Alloy & J. H. Riskind (Eds.), *Cognitive vulnerability to emotional disorders* (pp. 365–403). Mahwah, NJ: Lawrence Erlbaum Press.

Garner, D. M., Olmstead, M. J., & Polivy, J. (1983). Development and validation of a multidimensional eating disorder inventory for anorexia nervosa and bulimia. *International Journal of Eating Disorders, 2*, 15–34.

Garner, D. M., Olmstead, M. P., Bohr, Y., et al. (1982). The Eating Attitudes Test: Psychometric features and clinical correlates. *Psychological Medicine, 12*, 871–878.

Golden, N. H., Iglesias, E. A., Jacobson, M. S., et al. (2005). Alendronate for the treatment of osteopenia in anorexia nervosa: A randomized, double-blind, placebo-controlled trial. *Journal of Clinical Endocrinology and Metabolism, 90*(6), 3179–3185.

Goldstein, D. J., Wilson, M. G., Thompson, V. L., et al. (1995). Long-term fluoxetine treatment of bulimia nervosa. *British Journal of Psychiatry, 166*, 660–666.

Grilo, C. M. (2002). Binge eating disorder. In C. G. Fairburn & K. D. Brownell (Eds.), *Eating disorders and obesity* (pp. 178–187). New York: Guilford Press.

Grilo, C. M., Masheb, R. M., & Wilson, G. T. (2005). Efficacy of cognitive behavioral therapy and fluoxetine for the treatment of binge eating disorder: A randomized double-blind placebo-controlled comparison. *Biological Psychiatry, 57*(3), 301–309.

Grilo, C. M., Sanislow, C. A., Shea, M. T., Skodol, A. E., Stout, R. L., Pagano, M. E. et al. (2003). The natural course of bulimia nervosa and eating disorder not otherwise specified is not influenced by personality disorders. *International Journal of Eating Disorders, 34*, 319–330.

Grilo, C., Pagano, M., Skodol, A., et al. (2007). Natural course of bulimia nervosa and of eating disorder not otherwise specified: 5-year prospective study of remissions, relapses, and the effects of personality disorder psychopathology. *Journal of Clinical Psychiatry, 68*(5), 738–746.

Herzog, D. B. (1995). Psychodynamic psychotherapy for anorexia nervosa. In K. D. Brownell & C. G. Fairburn (Eds.), *Eating disorders and obesity* (pp. 330–335). New York: Guilford Press.

Herzog, D. B., Nussbaum, K. M., & Marmor, A. K. (1996). Comorbidity and outcome in eating disorders. *Psychiatric Clinics of North America, 19*, 843–859.

Hrabosky, J. I., & Grilo, C. M. (2007). Body image and eating disordered behavior in a community sample of black and Hispanic women. *Eating Behaviors, 8*(1), 106–114.

Hudson, J. I., Hiripi, E., Pope, H. G., et al. (2007). The prevalence and correlates of eating disorders in the National Comorbidity Survey Replication. *Biological Psychiatry, 61*(3), 348–358.

Johnson, J. G., Cohen, P., Kasen, S., et al. (2006). Personality disorder traits evident by early adulthood and risk for eating and weight problems during middle adulthood. *International Journal of Eating Disorders, 39*, 184–192.

Johnson, O., Fornai, G., Cabrini, S., et al. (2007). Feasibility and acceptability of screening for eating disorders in primary care. *Family Practice, 24*(5), 511–517.

Katzman, D. K. (2005). Medical complications in adolescents with anorexia nervosa: A review of the literature. *International Journal of Eating Disorders, 37*, 552–559.

Keel, P. K., Haedt, A., & Edler, C. (2005). Purging disorder: An ominous variant of bulimia nervosa? *Journal of Eating Disorders, 38*, 191–199.

Kessler, R. C., Berglund, P., Chiu, W. T., et al. (2004). The US National Comorbidity Survey Replication (NCS-R): Design and field procedures. *International Journal of Methods in Psychiatric Research, 13*(2), 69–92.

Kessler, R. C., Chiu, W. T., Dernier, O., et al. (2005). Prevalence, severity, and comorbidity of 12-month DSM-IV disorders in the National Comorbidity Survey Replication. *Archives of General Psychiatry, 62*, 617–627.

Klump, K. L., Miller, K. B., Keel, P. K., et al. (2001). Genetic and environmental influences on anorexia nervosa syndromes in a population-based twin sample. *Psychological Medicine, 31*, 737–740.

Kortegaard, L. S., Hoerder, K., Joergensen, J., et al. (2001). A preliminary population-based twin study of self-reported eating disorder. *Psychological Medicine, 31*, 361–365.

Kreipe, R. E., & Birndorf, S. A. (2000). Eating disorders in adolescents and young adults. *Medical Clinics of North America, 84*, 1027–1049.

Laessle, R. G., Zoettle, C., & Pirke, K. M. (1987). Meta-analysis of treatment studies for bulimia. *International Journal of Eating Disorders, 6*, 647–654.

Leichsenring, F. (2005). Are psychodynamic and psychoanalytic therapies effective?: A review of empirical data. *International Journal of Psychanalysis, 86*(3), 841–868.

Lewis, D. M., & Cachelin, F. M. (2001). Body image, body dissatisfaction, and eating attitudes in midlife and elderly women. *Eating Disorders: The Journal of Treatment and Prevention, 9*(1), 29–39.

Mangweth-Matzek, B., Rupp, C., Hausman, A., et al. (2006). Never too old for eating disorders or body dissatisfaction: A community study of elderly women. *International Journal of Eating Disorders, 39*(7), 583–586.

McIntosh, V., Jordan, J., Carter, F. A., et al. (2005). Three psychotherapies for anorexia nervosa: A randomized, controlled trial. *American Journal of Psychiatry, 162*(4), 741–747.

Mehler, P. S. (2001). Diagnosis and care of patients with anorexia nervosa in primary care settings. *Annals of Internal Medicine, 134*, 1048–1059.

Mehler, P. S., & Anderson, A. D. (1999). *Eating disorders: A guide to medical care and complications.* Baltimore, MD: Johns Hopkins University Press.

Mehler, P. S., Crews, C., & Weiner, K. (2004). Bulimia: Medical complications. *Journal of Women's Health, 13*(6), 668–675.

Micali, N., Simonoff, E., & Treasure, J. (2007). Risk of major adverse perinatal outcomes in women with eating disorders. *British Journal of Psychiatry, 190*(3), 255–259.

Millar, H. R., Wardell, F., Vyvyan, J. P., et al. (2005). Anorexia nervosa mortality in Northeast Scotland 1965-1999. *American Journal of Psychiatry, 162*, 753–757.

Miller, K. K., Grinspoon, S. K., Ciampa, J., et al. (2005). Medical findings in outpatients with anorexia nervosa. *Archives of Internal Medicine, 165*, 561–566.

Milos, G., Spindler, A., Schnyder, U., et al. (2005). Instability of eating disorder diagnoses: Prospective study. *British Journal of Psychiatry, 187*, 573–578.

Misra, M., Aggarwal, A., Miller, K. M., et al. (2004). Effects of anorexia nervosa on clinical, hematologic, biochemical, and bone density parameters in community-dwelling adolescent girls. *Pediatrics, 114*, 1574–1583.

Misra, M., & Klibanski, A. (2006). Anorexia nervosa and osteoporosis. *Review of Endocrinology and Metabolic Disorders, 7*, 91–99.

Mitchell, J. E., & Crow, S. (2006). Medical complications of anorexia nervosa and bulimia nervosa. *Current Opinion in Psychiatry, 19*(4), 438–443.

Mitchell, J. E., Pyle, R. L., Pomeroy, C., et al. (1993). Cognitive-behavioral group psychotherapy of bulimia nervosa: Importance of logistical variables. *International Journal of Eating Disorders, 14*(3), 277–287.

Molinari, E., Baruffi, M., Croci, M., et al. (2005). Binge eating disorder in obesity: Comparison of different therapeutic strategies. *Eating and Weight Disorders, 10*(3), 154–161.

Moradi, B., Dirks, D., & Matteson, A. (2005). Roles of sexual objectification experiences and internalization of standards of beauty in eating disorder symptomatology: A test and extension of objectification theory. *Journal of Counseling Psychology, 52*, 420–428.

Morgan, J. F., Reid, F., & Lacey, J. H. (1999). The SCOFF questionnaire: Assessment of a new screening tool for eating disorders. *British Medical Journal, 319*, 1467–1468.

Napoli, N., Thompson, J., Civitelli, R., et al. (2007). Effects of dietary calcium compared to calcium supplements on estrogen metabolism and bone mineral density. *American Journal of Clinical Nutrition, 85*, 1428–1433.

National Institute for Clinical Excellence (NICE). (2004). *Eating disorders—Core interventions in the treatment and management of anorexia nervosa, bulimia nervosa, and related eating disorders.* Clinical Guideline No. 9. London: Author. Retrieved October 15, 2007, from *www.nice.org.uk/guidance/CG9.*

O'Reardon, J. P., Peshek, A., & Allison, K. C. (2005). Night eating syndrome: Diagnosis, epidemiology, and management. *CNS Drugs, 19*(12), 997–1008.

Parker, S. C., Lyons, J., & Bonner, J. (2005). Eating disorders in graduate students: Exploring the SCOFF questionnaire as a simple screening tool. *Journal of American College Health, 54*(2), 103–107.

Pederson, K. J., Roerig, J. L., & Mitchell, J. E. (2003). Towards the pharmacotherapy of eating disorders. *Expert Opinion in Pharmacotherapy, 4*, 1659–1678.

Peveler, R. (2000). Eating disorders and insulin-dependent diabetes. *European Eating Disorders Review, 8*(2), 164–169.

Pomeroy, C., & Mitchell, J. E. (2002). Medical complications of anorexia nervosa and bulimia nervosa. In C. G. Fairburn & K. D. Brownell (Eds.), *Eating disorders and obesity: A comprehensive handbook* (2nd ed., pp. 278–285). New York: Guilford Press.

Powell, L. H., Calvin, J. E. III, & Calvin, J. E., Jr. (2007). Effective obesity treatments. *American Psychologist, 62*(3), 234–246.

Pritts, S. D., & Susman, J. (2003). Diagnosis of eating disorders in primary care. *American Family Physician, 67*(2), 297–304.

Rome, E. S., & Ammerman, S. (2003). Medical complications of eating disorders: An update. *Journal of Adolescent Health, 33*, 418–426.

Russell, G. F., Szmukler, G. I., Dare, C., et al. (1987). An evaluation of family therapy in anorexia nervosa and bulimia nervosa. *Archives of General Psychiatry, 44*, 1047–1056.

Silventoinen, K., Pietilainen, K. H., Tynelius, P., et al. (2007). Genetic and environmental factors in relative weight from birth to age 18: The Swedish young male twins study. *International Journal of Obesity, 31*(4), 615–621.

Spindler, A., & Milos, G. (2007). Links between eating disorder symptoms severity and psychiatric comorbidity. *Eating Behavior, 8*(3), 364–373.

Steffen, K. J., Roerig, J. L., Mitchell, J. E., et al. (2006). Emerging drugs for eating disorder treatment. *Expert Opinion on Emerging Drugs, 11*(2), 315–336.

Stein, K. F. (1996). The self-schema model: A theoretical approach to the self-concept in eating disorders. *Archives of Psychiatric Nursing, 10*(2), 96–109.

Stein, K. F., & Corte, C. (2007). Identity impairment and the eating disorders: Content and organization of the self-concept in women with anorexia nervosa and bulimia nervosa. *European Eating Disorder Review, 15*, 58–69.

Steinhausen, H. C. (2002). The outcome of anorexia nervosa in the 20th century. *American Journal of Psychiatry, 159*, 1284–1293.

Striegel-Moore, R. H. (1995). A feminist perspective on the etiology of eating disorders. In K. D. Brownell & C. G. Fairburn (Eds.), *Eating disorders and obesity: A comprehensive handbook* (pp. 224–229). New York: Guilford Press.

Striegel-Moore, R. H., & Bulik, C. M. (2007). Risk factors for eating disorders. *American Psychologist, 62*(3), 181–193.

Strober, M. (1997). Consultation and therapeutic engagement in severe anorexia nervosa. In D. M. Garner & P. E. Garfinkel (Eds.), *Handbook of treatment for eating disorders* (pp. 229–247). New York: Guilford Press.

Strober, M., Freeman, R., Lampert, C., et al. (2000). Controlled family study of anorexia nervosa and bulimia nervosa: Evidence of shared liability and transmission of partial syndromes. *American Journal of Psychiatry, 157*(3), 393–401.

Sudi, K., Ottl, K., Payerl, D., et al. (2004). Anorexia athletica. *Nutrition, 20*, 657–661.

Tan, J., Hope, T., & Stewart, A. (2006). Anorexia nervosa and personal identity. *International Journal Law Psychiatry, 26*(5), 533–548.

Task Force to Establish Weight Loss Guidelines. (1990). Toward safe weight loss: Recommendations for adult weight loss programs in Michigan. Full text of the Michigan Guidelines published by the Michigan Department of Public Health, Center for Health Promotion. Lansing, MI: Michigan Department of Public Health.

Wade, T. D., Bulik, C. M., Neale, M., et al. (2000). Anorexia nervosa and major depression: Shared genetic and environmental risk factors. *American Journal of Psychiatry, 157*(3), 469–471.

Walsh, B. T., Kaplan, A. S., Attia, E., et al. (2006). Fluoxetine after weight restoration in anorexia nervosa: A randomized controlled trial. *Journal of the American Medical Association, 295*(22), 2659–2660.

Wilfley, D. E. (2002). Psychological treatment of binge eating disorder. In C. G. Fairburn & K. D. Brownell (Eds.), *Eating disorders and obesity* (pp. 350–353). New York: Guilford Press.

Wilfley, D. E., & Cohen, L. R. (1997). Psychological treatment of bulimia nervosa and binge eating disorder. *Psychopharmacology Bulletin, 33*, 437–454.

Wilson, G. T., Grilo, C. M., & Vitousek, K. M. (2007). Psychological treatment of eating disorders. *American Psychologist, 62*(3), 199–216.

Wonderlich, S. A., Joiner, T. E., Keel, P. K., et al. (2007). Eating disorder diagnoses: Empirical approaches to classification. *American Psychologist, 62*(3), 167–180.

Woodside, B. D., & Staab, R. (2006). Management of psychiatric comorbidity in anorexia nervosa and bulimia nervosa. *CNS Drugs, 20*(8), 655–663.

World Health Organization. (2004). *WHO guide to mental and neurological health in primary care: A guide to mental and neurological ill health in adults, adolescents, and children* (2nd ed.). London: Author.

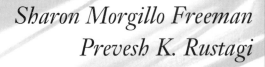

Sharon Morgillo Freeman
Prevesh K. Rustagi

chapter 7

Personality Disorders

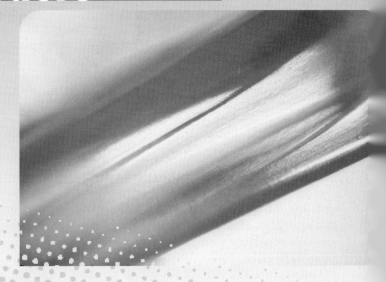

Many mental health disorders have identifiable signs and symptoms such as emotional, behavioral, and physiologic manifestations (some of which are measurable) that may lead to a clear diagnosis of the disorder. However, assessment and diagnosis of personality disorder (PD) in individuals is not as clear cut, and the clinician may be required to combine categories of PDs by cluster, symptom, or other manifestation.

Individuals with PD tend to be less amenable to change and their behaviors tend to be more deeply entrenched and inflexible. Most of the behaviors attributed to individuals with PD include conflict-ridden relationships, including their health care providers who might characterize them as "difficult", "noncompliant", or "attention-seeking." Their unpredictable and maladaptive behaviors leave significant others and treatment providers confused, disappointed, and angry with an end result of compromised health care.

Some of the more severe problems encountered in individuals with PD include behavior that is violent, demanding, aggressive, and rude (Steinmetz and Tabenkin, 2001). Less severe, though just as difficult, problems include acting withdrawn and hard to reach; exhibiting demanding, clingy, attention-seeking, and manipulating behaviors; and being verbally aggressive (Koekkoek, van Meijel, and Hutschemaekers, 2006). This chapter will focus on methods of identification, intervention, and treatment of individuals with PDs in health care settings.

CHARACTERISTICS OF PERSONALITY DISORDERS

By definition, personality is an enduring pattern of perceiving, relating to, and thinking about the environment and oneself (American Psychiatric Association [APA], 2000). PDs include behaviors that are inflexible, pervasive, stable, and enduring and that lead to clinically significant distress or impairment in functioning (APA). Disordered behaviors typically manifest by early adulthood, although beginning symptoms may be seen as early 6 years of age (APA; Freeman and Reineke, 2007). Although they need and demand help, individuals with PD often ultimately reject it when it is provided. A key defining factor that the patient may have a PD is an ongoing series of conversations that include the phrase "Yes, but . . . ." (Freeman, 2005).

According to one study, difficult patients defined as "dependent clingers, entitled demanders, manipulative help rejecters, and self-destructive deniers" made up 15 to 30 percent of the primary care practice population (Hahn, Kroenke, and Spitzer, 1996). Physiologic or functional health outcomes may be worse for this group. They make more frequent medical visits, have lower Short Form Health Survey scores, receive more prescriptions, undergo more laboratory investigations, and receive more referrals than "nondifficult" control subjects (Hahn et al., 1996). Primary care providers (PCPs) suffer significant stress from interactions with these patients (McCue, 1982).

PDs often coexist with affective disorders. This is because individuals with PDs often exhaust, frustrate, or anger most people around them, leaving the individual alone, angry, and/or distrustful. In addition, the individual with a PD often lacks understanding or insight as to the part she may have played in her own misery. It is estimated that approximately 1 to 3 percent of the general population has a diagnosable PD (APA, 2000). In a study of individuals presenting for outpatient therapy, approximately one third were diagnosed with one of the ten official *Diagnostic and Statistical Manual of Mental Disorders* (*DSM-IV*) PDs ($N = 270$, 31.4%) (Zimmerman, Rothschild, and Chelminski, 2005).

Many individuals suffer from subclinical levels of character pathology. No two people typically present with the exact same combination of diagnostic criteria. It was once suggested that borderline personality disorder (BPD) has 247 possible symptom combinations (Arntz, 1994). Individuals with PD do not usually seek help for their PD; however, they may seek help for the aftermath (i.e., divorce, job loss, loneliness, depression, and lack of friends). Stress, especially due to a major life change, will bring about increases in PD symptoms. For example, the prevalence of PD was estimated to be 6.4 percent in a study of women presenting for antenatal care for first pregnancies in Sweden (Borjesson, Ruppert, and Bajedahl-Strindlund, 2005). Having a PD was the single most important factor associated with onset of Axis I psychiatric symptoms during and after pregnancy (Borjesson et al., 2005).

Approximately 30 to 80 percent of individuals with PD are diagnosed with an Axis I major depressive disorder (MDD) during their lifetimes and will have higher rates of relapses, poorer responses to pharmacologic treatments (PTs), and more frequent relapses (Feske, 2004). Of the various PDs, BPD and dependent personality disorder (DPD) are diagnosed more frequently in women (Table 7.1). The *DSM-IV-TR* lists PDs as Axis II disorders and further divides them into diagnostic clusters. Cluster A includes paranoid, schizoid, and schizotypal PDs; Cluster B includes antisocial, borderline, histrionic, and narcissistic PDs; and Cluster C includes avoidant, dependent, and obsessive-compulsive PDs.

Table 7.1 • Incidence of Various Personality Disorders*

Personality Disorder	Prevalence
Paranoid	Between 0.5 and 2.5 percent of the general population of the United States; approaches 2–10 percent of outpatients receiving psychiatric care; between 10 and 30 percent of institutionalized psychiatric patients; more common in men than in women
Schizotypal	3 percent of the general population; more common in males
Antisocial	3 percent of males and 1 percent of females in the general population
Borderline	2 percent of the general population; accounts for 30–60 percent of all PDs; affects women more frequently than men—75 percent of all diagnosed patients are female
Histrionic	2–3 percent of the general population
Narcissistic	2–16 percent of the clinical population; slightly less than 1 percent of the general population of the United States; between 50 and 75 percent of those diagnosed with NPD are males
Avoidant	Between 0.5 and 1.0 percent of the general population
Dependent	Diagnosed more often in females
Obsessive-Compulsive	1 percent of the population; 3–10 percent among psychiatric outpatients In the United States, OCPD occurs almost twice as often in men as in women. (Some researchers attribute this disproportion to gender stereotyping, in that men have greater permission from general Western culture to act in stubborn, withholding, and controlling ways.)

*Estimated rates.
From the American Psychiatric Association (2000). *Diagnostic and statistical manual of mental disorders* (Revised 4th ed.). Washington, DC: Author.

GENDER ISSUES AND PERSONALITY DISORDERS

Societal and stereotypical expectations become exaggerated for the individual with a PD. Traditional gender roles defined as masculine, which include competitiveness, independence, control, ambition, anger, and possibly violence, may become exaggerated in the individual with a narcissistic personality disorder (NPD).

Likewise, characteristics traditionally described as feminine, such as weakness, helplessness, insecurity, intimacy needs, and worry, become exaggerated in the individual with histrionic or dependent PD. It is important that the PCP understand the sociocultural context of a behavior pattern. Roles that are interpreted based on traditional expectations or familial rules may be different from manifestations of PDs. Health care professionals must be adept at assessment to determine the basis of the behavior and not be too quick to diagnose PDs without fully understanding sociocultural context of behavior patterns.

Despite anecdotal reports that bias appears to exist regarding diagnostic criteria, diagnostic criteria do not seem to display sex bias with the exception of the borderline diagnosis (Boggs, Morey, Shea, et al., 2005). Gender may point to diagnosis and, therefore, the treatment of PDs. According to *DSM-IV-TR*, paranoid, schizoid, schizotypal, narcissistic, antisocial, and obsessive-compulsive PDs are more common in males, while histrionic, dependent, and borderline PDs are more commonly diagnosed in females (APA, 2000). This does not mean that these diagnoses are not etiologically more gender specific; they are just more commonly diagnosed in one gender or the other. Empirical evidence evaluating gender differences for most PDs is rare; however, there is evidence that there are differences in gender manifestations in the antisocial PDs. For example, in one study of Swedish general criminal offenders, female diagnosed (antisocial) psychopaths showed significantly more lying, deceitfulness, and lack of control than their male counterparts (Strand and Belfrage, 2005).

There is some evidence that females with PDs benefit more from psychotherapy than males and gain insight into self-concept as well as understand how this impacts their relationships. Men, on the other hand, are more likely to resist help and see it as an intrusion into their self-reliance (Loffler-Stastka, Ponocny-Seliger, Meissel, et al., 2006).

ASSESSMENT AND DIAGNOSIS OF PERSONALITY DISORDERS

Individuals with a primary mood disorder that falls under Axis I are often willing to provide a detailed history and any other information needed in the hope that they will obtain relief from their suffering. An individual with a primary Axis II disorder, on the other hand, may be reluctant to disclose information, provide sketchy details, and otherwise be a more difficult patient to interview. The assessment becomes difficult for both the patient and the interviewer because the individual may not recognize her own problems or may be unwilling to disclose detailed information. Some patients with PD are recognizable from the onset of the first session, while others may take some time to recognize (Sass and Junemann, 2001). If the therapist is adept in conceptualization, he or she will be able to make sense of the patient's past and present behavior and help predict future behavior (Freeman, 2001).

Box 7.1 includes criteria to assist in making the diagnosis of PD.

A variety of instruments have been developed to help identify PDs. One of the gold standards is the Millon Clinical Multiaxial Inventory-III (MCMI-III), which is a widely used comprehensive psychiatric measure of PD (Millon and Davis, 1997). The MCMI was first developed in 1977 and, now, the third edition,

Box 7.1 • *DSM-IV-TR* Criteria for Personality Disorder

DSM

A. Experience and behavior that deviates markedly from the expectations of the individual's culture. This pattern is manifested in two (or more) of the following areas:
   1. Cognition (perception and interpretation of self, others, and events)
   2. Affect (the range, intensity, lability, and appropriateness of emotional response)
   3. Interpersonal functioning and impulse control

B. The enduring pattern is inflexible and pervasive across a broad range of personal and social situations.

C. The enduring pattern leads to clinically significant distress or impairment in social, occupational, or other important areas of functioning.

D. The pattern is stable and of long duration, and its onset can be traced back at least to adolescence or early adulthood.

E. The enduring pattern is not better accounted for as a manifestation or consequence of another mental disorder.

F. The enduring pattern is not due to the direct physiologic effects of a substance or a general medical condition such as head injury.

Individuals must meet the criteria by the age of 18 years. Antisocial PD cannot be diagnosed at all in individuals under 18 years.

Adapted from the American Psychiatric Association (2000). *Diagnostic and statistical manual of mental disorders* (Revised 4th ed.). Washington, DC: Author.

MCMI-III, is specifically designed to produce a profile that corresponds with the *DSM* criteria. Comprehensive formal assessment of *DSM* PDs with tests such as the MCMI-III, although the most sensitive and accurate, can be a difficult, expensive, time-consuming endeavor. There has also been some conflict in clinical practice regarding the utility of the MCMI as far as validity in actual practice (Chick, Sheaffer, Goggin, et al., 1993). One such study of the MCMI's diagnostic efficiency statistics for each of the MCMI PD scales revealed overall low sensitivity, poor specificity, poor positive predictive power, and low diagnostic power, suggesting that the MCMI may have limited utility in identifying PDs in clinical settings (Chick et al.).

Most clinicians are interested in a screening tool that is rapid, accurate, free (if possible), and requires little or no training to use. This allows for portability, ease of support staff training, and rapid assessment. There are two types of screening instruments for PDs: clinician administered and self-report.

Clinician-Administered Screening Instruments

Clinical interviews are based on *DSM-IV-TR* criteria and are developed for screening purposes. Examples of clinical interviews include the Iowa Personality Disorder Screen (IPDS, with 11 diagnostic criteria); the Standardized Assessment of Personality–Abbreviated Scale (SAPAS, with 8 criteria); and the Freeman Quick Screening (FQS) for personality disordered behavior (Freeman, 2005). The Freeman instrument (Box 7.2) consists of 12 items that rate behaviors in terms of severity and impact on the patient's life. The FQS, in particular, is an instrument intended to yield a "yes" or "no" answer to the question, "Does this person have a personality disorder?"

In psychiatric samples across four studies, the brief interviews (i.e., the IPDS, SAPAS, and FQS) demonstrated sensitivities ranging from .69 to .96 and specificities ranging from .50 to .91 (Langbehn, Pfohl, Reynolds, et al., 1999; Moran, Leese, Lee, et al., 2003; Nurnberg, Seidman, Gelenberg, et al., 2000; Walters, Moran, Choudhury, et al., 2004). The vast majority of instruments currently used for screening purposes have at least 100 items with a specific diagnostic outcome. Therefore, the clinician must decide what questions need to be answered to formulate a diagnosis and then choose the screening instrument accordingly.

The Freeman Quick Screening for Personality Disordered Behavior

The FQS is a brief assessment scale specifically designed to identify global personality pathology for further attention and evaluation (Freeman, 2005) (Box 7.2). The FQS was correlated with the MCMI-II using a group of outpatient counseling

Box 7.2 • Freeman Quick Screening for Personality Disordered Behavior

Instructions: For each issue or area, rate the individual's behavior in terms of the severity or impact of that factor on the individual's life. Circle the appropriate rating.

The Individual's Behavior Is:	***Impact of Life Functioning***						
Compulsive (Actions appear "driven," and the individual is impelled to act)	Mild		Moderate			Severe	
Inflexible (Action/thoughts are rigid and unyielding)	1	2	3	4	5	6	7
Thoughtless (Responds impulsively and does not problem solve and consider alternatives)	1	2	3	4	5	6	7
Highly noticeable (Actions are readily observable by others)	1	2	3	4	5	6	7
Generally negative (Actions create difficulty in the individual's life)	1	2	3	4	5	6	7
Generally maladaptive (Actions are poorly suited to the individual's purpose, situation, or use)	1	2	3	4	5	6	7
Unusually extreme (Actions are +/− two standard deviations from mean)	1	2	3	4	5	6	7
Usually at odds with general community (Actions cause problems within the larger culture)	1	2	3	4	5	6	7
Energy consuming (Causes the individual significant strain or energy loss)	1	2	3	4	5	6	7
Self-consonant (Ego syntonic) (Actions/thoughts/feelings are internally consistent for the individual)	1	2	3	4	5	6	7

(Continued)

Box 7.2 • (Continued)

The Individual's Behavior Is:	***Impact of Life Functioning***
Interpersonally conflictual (Frequent problems with family, friends, colleagues, coworkers)	1 2 3 4 5 6 7
Personally discomforting (Patient reports distress because needs, goals, or wishes are not met)	1 2 3 4 5 6 7
	Total score:
Scores 50 and greater should be fully evaluated for PD.	
Comments:	

Reprinted with permission from Freeman, S. M., & Freeman, A. (2005). *Cognitive therapy in nursing practice* (p. 251). New York: Springer Publishing Company.

participants ($N = 59$) that had a score >25 on the instrument. This score suggested a high likelihood that a PD existed, but further investigation was indicated as to which PD(s) existed in the individual (Baughman, 2004).

The FQS rates an individual's behavior from adaptive to severe with potential impact on life function (Freeman and Diefenbeck, 2005). Behaviors assessed by the FQS (Box 7.3) coincide with the general criteria outlined in *DSM-IV-TR* for the diagnosis of PD (APA, 2000).

The clinician combines the scores from individual categories for the FQS total score. A total score exceeding 50 is considered indicative of a PD disorder, and the clinician is instructed to evaluate further for specific symptoms and category according to *DSM-IV-TR*. In a primary care practice, the patient can be referred at this point to a psychiatric or psychological specialist for further evaluation and counseling after medications are started for symptomatic relief, if indicated.

Self-Report Screening Instruments

Self-report instruments are pencil-and-paper instruments that an individual completes about herself to maximize efficiency and are developed largely by extracting a small subset of items from longer, structured diagnostic interviews. Self-report instruments are not usually intended as screening tools and require

Box 7.3 • Personality Attributes Measured by the Freeman Quick Screen

- Inflexible, rigid, unyielding
- Pervasively troubled
- Impulsive, impelled to act
- Interpersonal conflicts, distrustful, clingy, troubled relationships
- Socially inhibited
- Thoughtlessly acts without regard to consequences or effects on others
- Highly noticeable, actions are readily observed by others
- Emotionally unusual: restricted or excessive
- Personally uncomfortable and unsatisfying self-image that is unstable or inadequate
- Affectively unstable
- Perceptually distorted, unusual perceptions and interpretations
- Eccentric, behaviors are at odds with social norms of community

interpretation as well as a diagnostic interview. Self-report instruments range from 140 to 395 items and ask in an inclusive way about Axis II diagnostic features. The amount of time many of these instruments takes up, though, is inconsistent with the intended goal of finding a short but also valid instrument to use for initial screening.

The Psychiatric Diagnostic Screening Questionnaire

The Psychiatric Diagnostic Screening Questionnaire (PDSQ) is a brief, psychometrically strong, self-report scale designed to screen for the most common *DSM-IV* Axis I disorders encountered in outpatient mental health settings. The PDSQ was developed at the Rhode Island Hospital Department of Psychiatry with a subset of patients ($N = 630$) in an outpatient practice. The final version of the PDSQ consists of 126 yes/no questions assessing the symptoms of 13 *DSM-IV* disorders in five areas and is completed by the patient. The PDSQ is intended to be administered and scored in the office before the initial diagnostic evaluation. Based on the cutoffs resulting in a sensitivity of 90 percent, the mean negative predictive value of the PDSQ subscales is 97 percent, and the false-positive rate is 34 percent (Zimmerman and Mattia, 2001).

DSM-IV and ICD-10 Personality Questionnaire

The *DSM-IV* and ICD-10 Personality Questionnaire (DIP-Q) is a true/false self-report questionnaire designed to measure all ten *DSM-IV* and all eight ICD-10 PDs (Ottosson, Vikman-Adolfsson, Enerbäck, et al., 1995). The DIP-Q has 140 items in total, with 135 keyed to the PD diagnostic criteria (Ottosson, Grann, and Kullgren, 2005). The DIP-Q was tested by comparing results to those obtained from a structured expert clinical interview in a clinical sample of 138 individuals (Ottosson et al., 2005). When dimensional self-report and interview scores for the various PDs were compared, the intraclass correlations for the *DSM-IV*–specific disorders ranged from .37 to .87 (Ottosson et al., 2005). This self-report, similar to the PDSQ, takes approximately 20 to 30 minutes for the patient to complete and is scored by the office staff prior to the clinical evaluation.

Personality Disorder Diagnostic Clusters

According to *DMS-IV-TR*, Cluster A includes the "odd" or "eccentric" cluster and includes individuals with paranoid, schizoid, and schizotypal PDs. Individuals who meet the criteria for these disorders often manifest behaviors that include difficulty with close relationships, restricted emotions and expressiveness, and difficulty understanding the nuances inherent in subtle social cues. Paranoid individuals are suspicious of others and distrust motives, interpreting behaviors as a means to malign. Schizoid and schizotypal PDs are usually considered as schizophrenia spectrum disorders (Sass and Junemann, 2001). Use of second-generation antipsychotics may therefore be considered on a time-limited basis, but there are little empirical data to support this practice. There is similar lack of evidence in treatment of paranoid PD (Table 7.2).

Cluster B includes antisocial, borderline, histrionic, and narcissistic PDs and features patterns consistent with drama and lack of consideration of others' feelings, rights, or views. Very often, individuals in this cluster have patterns of unstable or broken relationships, impulsivity, and unstable affect and are prone to mood disorders, often as a result of the dissatisfaction with their lives. Individuals within this cluster with NPD, for example, tend to crave admiration and need (not want) to be the center of attention and feel special (first one to speak if a question is posed in a group or if there is a silent moment, etc.). Individuals with histrionic personality disorder (HPD) may behave provocatively, giggle, talk loudly, and dress to attract attention. Those with BPD may attract attention positively (flirting, similar to the HPD) or negatively (with suicidal gestures or actual attempts). Cluster B tends to cluster with mood disorders genetically, which

Table 7.2 • Personality Disorder Symptoms and Off-Label Uses

Personality Disorders	Target Symptoms and Syndromes	Medications Used "Off label"	Comments
Paranoid Schizoid Schizotypal	Brief psychotic symptoms	Antipsychotics	Distinguish brief psychosis associated with PDs from comorbid persistent psychosis
Borderline Narcissistic Antisocial Hostility	Irritability Histrionic Impulsivity Emotional lability Brief psychotic symptoms Suicidal and parasuicidal behaviors	Antipsychotics Lithium salts SSRIs Anticonvulsants Benzodiazepines Beta blockers Alpha-2 agonists Newer transdermal selegiline patch in low dose instead of oral MAOIs Last choice: Oral MAOIs	SSRIs and benzodiazepines may cause paradoxical worsening Intramuscular ziprasidone and olanzapine for acute agitation Educate patient about serious drug and diet interactions with MAOIs Consider newer transdermal patch with selegiline instead of MAOIs
Avoidant Dependent Obsessive Compulsive	Sadness Anxiety Social anxiety	SSRIs Beta blockers MAO inhibitors	Educate patient about serious drug and diet interactions with MAOIs

has treatment implications psychopharmacologically. Although the *DSM-IV-TR* notes that 75 percent of those with BPD are female and 50 to 75 percent of those with NPD are male, these statistics cannot be supported empirically in the literature at the time of this writing.

Cluster C includes the anxious types such as avoidant, dependent, and obsessive-compulsive personality disorders. Individuals with avoidant personality disorder (APD) often experience anxiety disorders and tend to be socially inhibited, suffer feelings of personal inadequacy, and are hypersensitive that others might be negatively evaluating them. The individual with DPD fears being left to care for oneself, clings, and fears separation. The individual with obsessive-compulsive personality disorder (OCPD) is concerned with order, mental control, doing things the "right way," neatness, and perfection. There is usually little room for flexibility, and they are wonderful "list makers."

Differential Diagnoses for Personality Disorder

Substance misuse disorder is the primary confounding factor in misdiagnosing PDs and personality disordered behavior, specifically antisocial PD and BPD (Marchesi, De Panfilis, Cantoni, et al., 2006). Box 7.4 outlines the parallel presentations that often confuse the diagnostic picture with substance misusing persons and persons with PDs (Freeman, 2005).

Box 7.4 • Commonalities Between Personality Disorder and Substance Use Disorders

1. Support system exhaustion (family, employment, financial, social)
2. Primary reactions and defenses are "other blaming"
3. Changes in behavior can usually be traced to early to mid teens
4. Progresses over time as behaviors and drug use escalates
5. Frequent exacerbation and remissions with frequent crises
6. Often many manipulative interactions
7. May be at risk for affective disorders
8. Inadequate/limited/poor problem-solving skills
9. Multiple failure experiences in all aspects of life; with substance use, there are the additional neurobiologic changes precipitated by the drug itself

From Freeman, S. M. (2005). CBT with substance misusing patients. In S. M. Freeman & A. Freeman (Eds.), *Cognitive behavior therapy in nursing practice* (pp. 113–144). New York: Springer Publishing Company.

Posttraumatic stress disorder (PTSD) may also be confused with PD due to the potential for substance abuse to mask or exacerbate the psychiatric symptoms (Frans, Rimmo, Aberg, et al., 2005; Galea, Vlahov, Tracy, et al., 2004; Gomez-Beneyto, Salazar-Fraile, Marti-Sanjuan, et al., 2006). Patients with a history of traumatic violence may present with impaired coping skills that can be confused with the symptoms of PD (Schumm, Hobfoll, and Keogh, 2004). In addition, individuals with PTSD have disturbances of thought, mood, and character, depending on the presenting problem and current level of stress, which also may mimic symptoms of PD (Gomez-Beneyto et al.).

TREATMENT OPTIONS

Among treatment options for PDs are psychotherapy, including cognitive behavioral therapy (CBT) and dialectical behavioral therapy (DBT); pharmacotherapy; and a combination of both (psychopharmacotherapy).

Psychotherapy

Psychological interventions include cognitive (changing of thinking patterns), behavioral (changing of behavior patterns), or a combination of both, as in CBT and DBT. In addition, there are a multitude of psychotherapeutic interventions that aim to treat PDs without the use of medications and instead use behavioral interventions such as relaxation training for times when an individual is feeling extremely anxious or behavioral interventions such as thought stopping when an individual is obsessing. It is important for the PCP to remember that severely disrupted individuals should be referred to a specialist.

Cognitive Behavior Therapy

CBT is a short-term, here-and-now–oriented psychotherapy that has been empirically demonstrated as effective for a variety of psychiatric disorders, including PD. It is known for its collaborative, structured, and educative focus, which reduces the individual's defensiveness, increases motivation for treatment, improves problem solving, and improves success in achieving goals (Beck and Reilly, 2006; Freeman, 2006).

Therapists trained in CBT assist individuals to modify their dysfunctional thinking, modify specific behaviors, and improve their emotional (and often physiologic) response. Progress is documented at each session, giving the individual the experiential validation of successes incrementally as they occur. This makes the CBT model ideal for a primary care setting because it is time sensitive and focuses on an empowerment model and individual control of emotion and behavior (Beck and Reilly, 2006; Freeman, 2006).

Dialectical Behavior Therapy

DBT is a modification of CBT that combines weekly individual CBT sessions with a primary therapist, weekly skills-training groups lasting 2.0 to 2.5 hours per session, and weekly supervision and consultation meetings for the therapists (Linehan, 1993). Individual therapy focuses primarily on motivational issues, including the motivation to stay alive and to stay in treatment. Group therapy teaches self-regulation and change skills as well as skills for self-acceptance and acceptance of others. Central principles include simultaneous focus on both acceptance and validation strategies and change strategies to achieve a synthetic (dialectical) balance in client functioning (Linehan). Another component of DBT is usually carried out in a group context, ideally by someone other than the individual therapist. In the skills-training groups, patients are taught skills considered relevant to their particular problems. There are four modules focusing in turn on four groups of skills: (a) core mindfulness skills, (b) interpersonal effectiveness skills, (c) emotion modulation skills, and (d) distress tolerance skills (Linehan).

Recently, studies have demonstrated that therapists who are trained in the full model of DBT can export the model outside of the academic treatment setting with equal efficacy in women with parasuicidal behaviors. These are the behaviors for which DBT was originally developed, although the model has been adapted for other self-harm behaviors since that time (Linehan, Comtois, Murray, et al., 2006).

Pharmacotherapy

In general, PT of PDs is symptom based, not diagnosis based (Freeman, 2005). PT can be especially helpful if the patient presents with an activated Axis I problem. As discussed previously, individuals do not necessarily present with Axis II pathology, and the patient's failure to respond to traditional treatment algorithms for Axis I disorders could, among many other variables, signal the presence of an Axis II disorder. Certain symptoms or manifestations of Axis II disorders that may be modified pharmacologically include mood lability, anxiety and inhibition, and disordered thinking and dissociation. No currently marketed psychotropic medication has Food and Drug Administration (FDA)-approved indication for treating PDs. The *DSM-IV-TR* classifies PD as discrete entities (categorical approach) rather than quantitative variations in temperament and characterologic traits (dimensional approach). Recent research, however, increasingly favors a dimensional approach to PD over a categorical one (Marcus, Lilienfeld, Edens, et al., 2006; Nestadt, Costa, Hsu, et al., 2006; Samuel and Widiger, 2006). Some of the dimensional approaches cut across the boundaries not only between various PDs but also between the Axis I and Axis II disorders (Simm and Clark, 2006; Flanagan and Blashfield, 2006).

In general, health care practitioners use the following general categories to offer support for the symptoms of PDs along with psychotherapy:

Antidepressants. The selective serotonin reuptake inhibitors (SSRIs) such as fluoxetine, sertraline, citalopram, paroxetine, nefazodone, and escitalopram; selective serotonin norepinephrine reuptake inhibitors (SNRIs) such as venlafaxine or duloxetine; and the newer antidepressant/antianxiety medication in transdermal patch form, selegiline, which increases all three targeted neurotransmitters (serotonin, norepinephrine, and dopamine) may be prescribed for the treatment of PD symptoms. The oral form of the monoamine oxidase inhibitors (MAOI) such as phenelzine and tranylcypromine were recommended at one time for the treatment of PDs but are rarely used any longer due to severe diet restrictions and potentially lethal side effects. Although selegiline is an MAOI, it is not as problematic in the patch formulation (Hori, 1998; Kapfhammer and Hippius, 1998).

Anticonvulsants. These medications may help to suppress impulsive and aggressive behavior. Most commonly prescribed are carbamazepine or valproic acid (Citrome, 1995; Wroblewski, Joseph, Kupfer, et al., 1997). Most recently, there is interest in topiramate due to its ability to decrease appetitive drives, which occurs in many patients with PDs who have eating disorders or substance use disorders. Topiramate is being studied as an aid in managing impulse-control problems as a primary medication (Dolengevich Segal, Rodriguez Salgado, Conejo Garcia, et al., 2006).

Antipsychotics. People with borderline and schizotypal PDs often have thought disorders. As a result, it makes sense to use antipsychotic medications such as risperidone, aripiprazole, and olanzapine to improve distorted thinking (Mobascher, Mobascher, Schlemper, et al., 2006; Nickel, Muehlbacher, Nickel, et al., 2006; Pascual, Madre, Puigdemont, et al., 2006).

Other medications. Anti-anxiety medications such as alprazolam and clonazepam and mood stabilizers such as anticonvulsants and lithium (Eskalith, Lithobid) help to relieve symptoms associated with PDs.

Medications for Cluster A: Paranoid, Schizoid, and Schizotypal Personality Disorders

Individuals in Cluster A rarely seek treatment due to their suspicious natures and tendency to avoid social contact. In the rare situation in which they may seek treatment, it is unlikely that they would consider psychotropic medication for their discomfort. Use of second-generation antipsychotics may be considered on a time-limited basis, but there are little empirical data to support this practice. There is similar lack of evidence in treatment of paranoid PD (Table 7.2).

Medications for Cluster B: Antisocial, Borderline, Histrionic, and Narcissistic Personality Disorders

Common targets of biologic treatments in Cluster B include affective dysregulation, impulsivity, cognitive-perceptual difficulties, and self-harm behaviors (Hilger, Barnas, snf Kasper, 2003; Mazaira, 2004). Limited evidence exists for efficacy of antidepressants, mood stabilizers, benzodiazepines, opiate antagonists, first-generation antipsychotics, and second-generation antipsychotics (Binks, Fenton, McCarthy, et al., 2006). There has been some evidence that anticonvulsants such as topiramate may be efficacious in reducing symptoms such as suicidal ideation, aggression, and mood lability in women categorized with a PD in Cluster B; however, such studies are early in their development (Loew, Nickel, and Muehlbacher, 2006).

A systematic search of 26 bibliographic databases related to treatment of BPD showed limited evidence because of paucity of randomized controlled trial data (Binks et al., 2006). Available evidence suggests some improvement in affective symptoms with antidepressants (Schmahl and Bohus, 2001). Weak evidence was noted for positive effect of antipsychotics and MAOIs on hostility. Adding a second-generation antipsychotic to DBT in a double-blind placebo-controlled trial reduced dropout rates in treating BPD (Soler, Pascual, Campins, et al., 2005). Similarly, minimal positive effect was noted from using divalproex (Depakote). In deciding about pharmacotherapy of mood symptoms in BPD, it is important to distinguish bipolar type II symptoms from true PD features. If a comorbid mood disorder is diagnosed, it should be treated as such, independent of the associated PD.

Medications for Cluster C: Avoidant, Dependent, and Obsessive-Compulsive Personality Disorders

Avoidant PD is often considered to be a part of the social anxiety spectrum (Denardin, Silva, Pianca, et al., 2004; Ralevski, Sanislow, Grilo, et al., 2005; Stein, Ono, Tajima, et al., 2004). It may therefore be worthwhile to use SSRI and

SNRI medications, which are commonly helpful in treating social anxiety disorder (Stein et al.).

Medications for Complex Symptoms

Acute decompensation symptoms such as psychosis and severe affective disturbances in PD may share biologic underpinnings with Axis I disorders. Additionally, PDs may share neurobiologic systems with other PDs within the same *DSM-IV-TR* cluster (Kendler, Czajkowski, Tambs, et al., 2006); therefore, it makes sense to choose an agent to treat these same symptoms. Aripiprazole (Abilify) is one of a growing list of atypical agents; however, at the time of this writing, it was the only partial dopamine agonist with relatively few risks for significant adverse effects employed in therapy for many psychiatric disorders. There are few studies evaluating aripiprazole in the treatment of BPD; however, one study found that in a group of individuals with BPD (43 women, 9 men), the drug appeared to be a safe and effective agent (Nickel et al., 2006). The study utilized structured rating scales and inventories for 8 weeks. Participants were evaluated for suicidality and parasuicidal injury as well as effect and side effects from the medication.

Psychopharmacotherapy Approaches

There are few guidelines for psychopharmacotherapy of PD, because studies are marred by a high frequency of dropouts, lack of compliance, short period of follow-up, differences in diagnostic procedures, comorbidity, and treatment traditions. A dimensional approach focusing on cognitive, affective, anxiety, and impulse dysfunction as well as a focus on target symptoms can make psychopharmacotherapy a useful adjunct to psychosocial programs (Ryden and Vinnars, 2002). There are interesting biotheoretical studies looking at alterations in the serotonin (5-HT) system, for example, focusing on dysregulation of systems that affect impulsive aggression and suicidal behavior, which are common features of BPD. One enzyme studied in the early 1980s, tryptophan hydroxylase (TPH), has two isoforms: TPH-1 and TPH-2. TPH-1, which is the rate-limiting enzyme in 5-HT biosynthesis, has been correlated to various psychiatric and behavioral disorders by gene polymorphism association studies (Zaboli, Gizatullin, Nilsonne, et al., 2006).

A bidimensional approach to psychopharmacotherapy of PD based on fear and anger traits has some biologic basis, because fear traits are influenced by the amygdala and the serotonergic, noradrenergic, and GABAergic systems, whereas anger is affected by nucleus accumbens, dopaminergic, and glutamatergic systems (Lara and Akiskal, 2006). Excessive fearfulness could therefore be modulated by antidepressants and antianxiety medications, while lack of fear could be modulated with lithium and alpha-2 presynaptic agonists. This may have implications in PT of Cluster B and Cluster C PDs. Dopaminergic antidepressants and psychostimulants could disinhibit anger, while anticonvulsant mood stabilizers could help with anger management (Schmahl and Bohus, 2001). These are broad generalizations, however, and much variability and contradictory responses are common in clinical situations. There is little evidence for or against this generalization in the literature. Table 7.2 provides more information on off-label medication usage for PD symptoms.

Crisis or Emergency Care Guidelines for Pharmacologic Treatment of Personality Disorders

Acute, moderate, or severe agitation with and without self-mutilation associated with an underlying PD is a common situation in emergency rooms. A recent survey of expert opinion in this area suggests that oral second-generation antipsychotics with and without a benzodiazepine are preferred agents (Allen, Currier, Carpenter, et al., 2005). If a rapid-acting agent is needed, intramuscular olanzapine alone receives more support than intramuscular ziprasidone (Geodon) alone (Allen et al., 2005). There is more support, however, for intramuscular ziprasidone alone or in combination with the benzodiazepine than for olanzapine plus a benzodiazepine. Intramuscular olanzapine should not be combined with intramuscular benzodiazepine for the fear of serious hypotension. When an initial intervention with a second-generation antipsychotic is unsuccessful, the addition of a benzodiazepine to the antipsychotic is recommended (Allen et al.).

MANAGING PROBLEM PATIENTS IN PRIMARY CARE SETTINGS

Hostile or Aggressive Individuals

Psychotic disorders, including mood disorders of psychotic intensity, are particularly apt to give rise to aggression. For these reasons, a careful medical and psychiatric history, physical examination, and indicated laboratory testing are mandatory in the evaluation of aggression (Freeman and Rathbun, 2005). Major psychiatric disturbances on Axis I of the *DSM* criteria may explain aggressive behavior and must be evaluated before an accurate diagnosis of Axis II problems becomes feasible. Definitive treatment of personality problems is usually facilitated by resolution of acute problems on Axis I.

Box 7.5 • Possible Causes of Impulsive or Aggressive Behavior

- Impulsivity is damage or immaturity of the connections between the limbic structures and the prefrontal cortex. Research suggests a healthy individual's prefrontal screening process takes less than half a second (Barratt, 1993; Davidson, 2000).
- Physical traumas that result in frontal lobe lesions such as anoxia, malnutrition, infection, irradiation, endocrine/metabolic disturbances, and poisonings are among the most common nongenetic causes of cerebral imperfections that may lead to impulsive and/or aggressive behaviors (Freeman and Rathbun, 2005). Poisoning includes the chronic use of mood-altering substances such as alcohol, cocaine, and amphetamine such as methamphetamine, etc.
- The effects of some mood-altering chemicals on aggression may be mediated by glutamate and GABA, while severe Axis I psychiatric disturbance is associated with abnormalities in serotonin, dopamine, and glutamate levels. Abuse of stimulants, especially cocaine and methamphetamine, produces aggressive effects through increasing both dopamine and norepinephrine levels.
- Nicotine has been found to have potent antiaggressive effects, possibly because of its influence on serotonin (Seth, Cheeta, Tucci, et al., 2002). The elimination of toxins such as alcohol, androgens, and stimulants is mandatory.

If the person demonstrates remorse after an aggressive action, the behavior may be amenable to change. If not, the behavior may meet the *DSM* criteria for antisocial PD and therefore may be modified temporarily through psychopharmacologic intervention. Normally, this requires careful monitoring if the individual has chronic and/or severely dangerous behaviors.

It is important to remember that impulsive behavior as well as aggressive behavior may have a biologic basis. Box 7.5 lists potential reasons for aggressive or impulsive behavior.

Getting the individual to her behavior as inappropriate may be the most challenging task. Individuals will not view anger as a problem and will not care how it affects others. In this frame of mind, it will not be easy to stop the behavior with typical coping methods, such as defensiveness. Any responses from the PCP

Box 7.6 • Examples of Therapeutic Statements for Dealing with Angry Patients

"It sounds like you have something very important for me to hear."

"This does not appear to be a very private setting, and it is difficult for me to hear you with your voice raised. Please sit here." (The patient is asked to go to a preselected area that is quieter and in view of other staff members. The PCP's back should be to the door or exit, and no weapons [obvious or nonobvious] are in easy reach of the patient.)

"This is disappointing for us as well."

"We may be able to find a way to get your wife to stop her complaining so you can enjoy your freedom." (This uses a "partnership perception" to get the individual to cease negative behaviors.)

that are "offense" or "defense" in posture will result in a continued offense or defense interaction. Lowered tones of voice, smiles, acceptance, firmness, and possibly apologies are helpful. Conflict resolution training for staff is beneficial. Box 7.6 lists some potential therapeutic statements that the PCP may use in dealing with an angry patient.

Medication Options

Most studies of PT for PDs have been conducted with individuals who have antisocial and borderline PDs, and partial positive results have been obtained using various classes of drugs for dealing with aggression and impulsive behaviors, including lithium, beta-blockers, carbamazepine, valproate, antipsychotic drugs, and SSRIs (Swann, 2003).

Topiramate is another medication to consider; it has been shown to reduce alcohol abuse (Johnson, 2003) and might also have benefits in impulsive aggression. If the individual is overweight, it might be useful to point out that topiramate can cause significant appetite suppression and weight loss. Hope for gain in cooperation may be accomplished through this avenue.

Dependent or Somatic Individuals

The adult or juvenile somatization patient may also describe symptoms that resemble fibromyalgia, chronic fatigue syndrome, and irritable bowel syndrome. This adult functions poorly in work or school, overuses medical services, and may report high rates of emotional distress such as depression and anxiety. The most commonly reported problem in pediatric care, recurrent abdominal pain, is equivalent to a somatization syndrome in children. The target for CBT in children or adolescents is stress-management techniques for their symptoms and to train parents not to reinforce illness behavior.

Treatment Goals

Regularly structured sessions, discouraging emergency visits, setting behavioral goals, and avoiding the pursuit of physical investigations and treatments provide a supportive, nonauthoritarian, medical psychotherapeutic framework (François, 2004). It is also valuable to work with the patient's spouse and family. They may be unwittingly involved in the patient's illness and behavior and harbor feelings and reactions that will have a positive or negative effect on the outcome.

The PCP should do the following:

1. Schedule regular appointments every 4 to 6 weeks.
2. Conduct a physical examination in the organ system relevant to the presenting complaint while calmly "talking" out loud as one would to a student or intern.
3. Avoid unnecessary diagnostic procedures, invasive treatments, and hospitalizations.
4. Avoid any negative or "parental" type statements such as, "Your symptoms are all in your head" or "Mrs. Jones, we've discussed this before. You need to stop worrying about your bowels and start getting out to Bingo like a good girl."
5. During each appointment, focus attention away from health and symptoms toward daily life, activities, and relationships.
6. Avoid inquiring about the presence of specific symptoms; however, if these are volunteered spontaneously, the response should be limited to general support, and a symptomatic line of inquiry should not be pursued.

Manipulative Individuals

The difficulties that occur as a result of individuals who are successful at manipulating staff are less of a problem with the patient than they are with the staff members. Splitting (setting up one person against another for the sake of "looking good" or achieving a manipulative goal) most often occurs with two particular

Box 7.7 • Avoiding Staff Splitting

Mrs. Smith frequently schedules with another provider if she does not receive the requested treatment or procedure that she was hoping for in her first visit for the initial complaint. When seen by the second provider, she states, "I am coming back in because I didn't understand what Dr. Jones told me about my blood tests. He speaks funny and is always so rushed! You always take your time with me and are so patient with my questions. This test I am supposed to be scheduled for, is that going to be in 2 weeks or in 3 weeks?"

In this scenario, the second provider may be flattered; however, he or she should check with Dr. Jones before proceeding further as a matter of office policy and professional courtesy. The following scenario demonstrates how the second provider could respond:

"Mrs. Smith, I understand now why you were confused. It appears that Dr. Jones did not schedule you for the test. Let me go over your blood tests, and I will be happy to answer any questions you have. I know that you may want more time, so if you want to schedule a second appointment when we are finished, in a week or two we can get together again to see how things are going."

Note: At no time did the second provider confront Mrs. Smith on her manipulation, as that would have been counterproductive. Instead, Mrs. Smith has been introduced to a new system of communication that will reduce this form of staff splitting.

types of PDs that often occur together: BPD and the NPD. Staff splitting can only occur if staff members allow it to happen. Granting of favors outside of department guidelines should be dealt with in a manner that is consistent with department disciplinary guidelines. If the action was not outside of guidelines and instead was miscommunication based, then communication among staff members may be the problem and should be addressed. Box 7.7 provides an example of how staff splitting can be avoided.

CONCLUSION

PDs are long-standing, pervasive, relatively rigid patterns of behaving and thinking that present across a wide range of social and personal situations (APA, 2000). Most individuals with PDs do not present for treatment for the PD;

rather, they desire relief for the depression or anxiety that results from other clinical problems (usually an Axis I disorder). Typically, individuals with a PD see their problems as caused by things other than themselves and independent of their behaviors. Most often, it is their significant other who pressures them into therapy or a medical problem that brings them to the health care provider. Very often, they are difficult individuals due to their very nature, characterized as "noncompliant" or "attention seeking," resulting in compromised medical care. A few of the more severe problems in these individuals may include impulsivity, instability of affect, clingy behaviors, dependent behaviors, unstable interpersonal relationships, and suicidal behaviors.

Clinicians often feel ill prepared to deal with individuals with PDs in a primary care practice. The best advice is this: First, do no harm. Keep realistic expectations in mind of what can be done at this level of care to avoid overtreatment, punishment, or abandonment (Adler, 2006). Second, protect yourself and the patient physically and emotionally. Have access to crisis management, and refer patients to knowledgeable, well-trained psychiatric/psychological clinicians. Therefore, it is necessary to get consultation, support, and help from others to manage the feelings and behavioral reactions engendered within ourselves (Adler).

Pharmacotherapeutic options are available as adjunctive or symptomatic treatments with no treatments having current FDA approval for primary use in PD. Many pharmacologic therapies and psychotherapies are used with success based on solid empirical evidence. These therapies are based on treatment of the symptoms associated with the PD rather the PD itself and are very successful at symptom reduction, thereby allowing for a more enjoyable quality of life for both the individual with the PD and her caregivers.

Resources for Providers

Beck, A. T., Freeman, A., & Davis, D. D. (2006). *Cognitive therapy of personality disorders* (2nd ed.). New York: Guilford Press.

Foa, E., Hembree, E., & Rothbaum, B. (2006). *Prolonged exposure therapy for PTSD: Emotional processing of traumatic experiences therapist guide*. New York: Oxford University Press.

Freeman, A., & Reineke, M. A. (2007). *Personality disorders in children and adolescents*. New York: John Wiley and Sons.

Freeman, S. M. (2007). Acute and chronic pain. In F. M. Dattilio & A. Freeman (Eds.), *Cognitive-behavioral strategies in crisis intervention* (3rd ed.). New York: Guilford Press.

Freeman, S. M., & Freeman, A. (2005). *Cognitive behavior therapy in nursing practice*. New York: Springer Publishers.

Freeman, S. M., & Story, M. (2007). Substance misuse. In F. M. Dattilio & A. Freeman (Eds.), *Cognitive-behavioral strategies in crisis intervention* (3rd ed.). New York: Guilford Press.

Freeman, Gilson, Freeman, et al. (2008). *Overcoming depression: A cognitive therapy approach for taming the depression BEAST: Therapist manual.* New York: Oxford University Press. In press.

Linehan, M. (2007). *Dialectical behavior therapy: Applications across disorders and settings.* New York: Guilford Press.

Websites for Providers

Academy of Cognitive Therapy: *www.academyofct.org*

American Psychiatric Association's Practice Guidelines: *www.psych.org/mainmenu/psychiatricpractice/practiceguidelines_1.aspx*

Medline Plus Personality Disorders Page: *www.nlm.nih.gov/medlineplus/personalitydisorders.html*

Mental Health America—Personality Disorder Factsheet: *www.mentalhealthamerica.net/go/information/get-info/personality-disorders*

National Institute of Mental Health: *http://nimh.nih.gov/publicat/index.cfm*

Psychology Information Online: *www.psychologyinfo.com*

Resources for Patients

National Alliance for the Mentally Ill (NAMI): *www.nami.org*

Treatments That Work series by Oxford University Press. (New York: Oxford University Press). Available for purchase online through *www.amazon.com* or *www.barnesandnoble.com*. Examples of titles:

Mastery of your anxiety and worry by David Barlow and Michelle Craske

Managing social anxiety: A cognitive behavioral approach by Debra Hope

Overcoming depression: A cognitive therapy approach for taming the depression BEAST client workbook by Freeman, Gilson, Freeman, and Yates. Oxford Univesity Press (In press).

References

Adler, D. A. (2006). Difficult patients with themselves and their caregivers. *Psychiatric Services, 57*(6), 767.

Allen, M. H., Currier, G. W., Carpenter, D., et al. (2005). Treatment of behavioral emergencies. *Journal of Psychiatric Practice, 11*(Suppl 1), 5–108; quiz 110–102.

American Psychiatric Association. (2000). *Diagnostic and statistical manual of mental disorders* (Revised 4th ed.). Washington, DC: Author.

Arntz, A. (1994). Treatment of borderline personality disorder: A challenge for behavioural therapy. *Behaviour Research and Therapy, 32*(4), 419–430.

Barratt, E. S. (1993). The use of anticonvulsants in aggression and violence. *Psychopharmacology Bulletin*. 29, 75–81.

Baughman, I. R. (2004). The Freeman Quick Screening for personality disorders. *Dissertation Abstracts*. Philadelphia College of Osteopathic Medicine, Philadelphia, PA, U.S.A.

Beck, J. S., & Reilly, C. (2006). Nurses integrate cognitive therapy treatment into primary care: Description and clinical application of a pilot program [Electronic Version]. *Medscape Nursing*, 6. Retrieved September 19, 2006, from *www.medscape.com/viewarticle/544402*.

Binks, C. A., Fenton, M., McCarthy, L., et al. (2006). Pharmacological interventions for people with borderline personality disorder. *Cochrane Database of Systematic Reviews* (1), CD005653.

Boggs, C., Morey, L., Shea, M., et al. (2005). Differential impairment as an indicator of sex bias in DSM-IV criteria for four personality disorders. *Psychological Assessment, 17*(4), 492–496.

Borjesson, K., Ruppert, S., & Bajedahl-Strindlund, M. (2005). A longitudinal study of psychiatric symptoms in primiparous women: Relation to personality disorders and sociodemographic factors. *Archives of Women's* [SF23]*Mental Health, 8*, 232–242.

Chick, D., Sheaffer, C. I., Goggin, W. C., et al. (1993). The relationship between MCMI personality scales and clinician-generated DSM-III-R personality disorder diagnoses. *Journal of Personality Assessment, 61*(2), 264–276.

Citrome, L. (1995). Use of lithium, carbamazepine, and valproic acid in a state-operated psychiatric hospital. *Journal of Pharmacologic Technologies, 11*(2), 55–59.

Davidson, R. J., Putnam, K. M., & Larson, C. L. (2000). Dysfunction in the neural circuitry of emotion regulation—a possible prelude to violence. *Science*. 289 (5479), 591–594.

Denardin, D., Silva, T. L., Pianca, T. G., et al. (2004). Is avoidant disorder part of the social phobia spectrum in a referred sample of Brazilian children and adolescents? *Brazilian Journal of Medical and Biological Research, 37*(6), 863–867.

Dolengevich Segal, H., Rodriguez Salgado, B., Conejo Garcia, A., et al. (2006). [Efficacy of topiramate in children and adolescent with problems in impulse control: preliminary results]. *Actas Espanolas de Psiquiatria, 34*(4), 280–282.

Feske, U. (2004). Clinical outcome of ECT in patients with major depression and comorbid borderline personality disorder. *American Journal of Psychiatry, 161*, 2073–2080.

Flanagan, E. & Blashfield, R. (2006). Do clinicians see Axis I and Axis II as different kinds of disorders? *Comprehensive Psychiatry*. Nov-Dec vol. 47 No 6 pps 496–502.

François, M. (2004). Somatization disorder: A practical review. *Canadian Journal of Psychiatry, 49*(10), 652–662.

Frans, O., Rimmo, P. A., Aberg, L., et al. (2005). Trauma exposure and post-traumatic stress disorder in the general population. *Acta Psychiatrica Scandinavica, 111*(4), 291–299.

Freeman, A. (2001). Cognitive-behavioral therapy for severe personality disorders. In S. G. Hofmann & M. C. Tompson (Eds.), *Treating chronic and severe mental disorders*. New York: Guilford Press (pp. 382–402).

Freeman, A., & Diefenbeck, C. (2005). Cognitive-behavioral therapy of personality disorders. In S. M. Freeman, & A. Freeman (Eds.), *Cognitive behavior therapy in nursing practice* (pp. 239–268). New York: Springer Publishing Company.

Freeman, A., & Reineke, M. A. (2007). *Personality disorders in children and adolescents*. New York: John Wiley and Sons.

Freeman, S. M. (2005). CBT with substance misusing patients. In S. M. Freeman & A. Freeman (Eds.), *Cognitive behavior therapy in nursing practice* (pp. 113–144). New York: Springer Publishing Company.

Freeman, S. M. (2006). Cognitive behavioral therapy in advanced practice nursing: An overview [Electronic Version]. *Medscape Nursing*, Topics in Advanced Practice Nursing eJournal. Retrieved October 19, 2006, from *www.medscape.com/viewarticle/545336*.

Freeman, S. M., & Rathbun, J. M. (2005). Integrating psychotherapy and medication. In F. Rotgers & M. Maniacci (Eds.), *Antisocial personality disorder: A practitioner's guide to comparative treatments for psychological disorders* (pp. 179–194). New York: Springer Publishing Company.

Galea, S., Vlahov, D., Tracy, M., et al. (2004). Hispanic ethnicity and post-traumatic stress disorder after a disaster: Evidence from a general population survey after September 11, 2001. *Annals of Epidemiology, 14*(8), 520–531.

Gomez-Beneyto, M., Salazar-Fraile, J., Marti-Sanjuan, V., et al. (2006). Posttraumatic stress disorder in primary care with special reference to personality disorder comorbidity. *British Journal of General Practice, 56*(526), 349–354.

Hahn, S. R., Kroenke, K., & Spitzer, R. L. (1996). The difficult patient: Prevalence, psycho-pathology, and functional impairment. *Journal of General Internal Medicine, 11*, 1–8.

Hilger, E., Barnas, C., & Kasper, S. (2003). Quetiapine in the treatment of borderline personality disorder. *World Journal Biological Psychiatry, 4*(1), 42–44.

Hirschfeld, R., Williams, J. B, Spitzer, R. L., et al. (2000). Development and Validation of a Screening Instrument for Bipolar Spectrum Disorder: The Mood Disorder Questionnaire. *American Journal of Psychiatry*. 157:11. (November, 2000). 1873–1875.

Hori, A. (1998). Pharmacotherapy for personality disorders. *Psychiatry and Clinical Neurosciences, 52*(1), 13–19.

Johnson, B. (2003). Psychological Addiction, Physical Addiction, Addictive Character, a Nosology of Addictive Disorders. *Canadian J. Psychoanalysis*, 11:135–160.

Kapfhammer, H. P., & Hippius, H. (1998). Special feature: Pharmacotherapy in personality disorders. *Journal of Personality Disorders, 12*(3), 277–288.

Kendler, K. S., Czajkowski, N., Tambs, K., et al. (2006). Dimensional representations of DSM-IV Cluster A personality disorders in a population-based sample of Norwegian twins: A multivariate study. *Psychological Medicine, 36*(11), 1583–1591.

Koekkoek, B., van Meijel, B., & Hutschemaekers, G. (2006). Difficult patients in mental health care: A review. *Psychiatric Services* 57(6), 795–802.

Langbehn, D. R., Pfohl, B. M., Reynolds, S., et al. (1999). The Iowa Personality Disorder Screen: Development and preliminary validation of a brief screening interview. *Journal of Personality Disorders, 13*, 75–89.

Lara, D. R., & Akiskal, H. S. (2006). Toward an integrative model of the spectrum of mood, behavioral and personality disorders based on fear and anger traits: II. Implications for neurobiology, genetics and psychopharmacological treatment. *Journal of Affective Disorders, 94*(1–3), 89–103.

Linehan, M. M. (1993). *Cognitive behavioral treatment of borderline personality disorder*. New York: Guilford Press.

Linehan, M. M., Comtois, K. A., Murray, A. M., et al. (2006). Two-year randomized controlled trial and follow-up of dialectical behavior therapy vs therapy by experts for suicidal behaviors and borderline personality disorder. *Archives of General Psychiatry, 63*(7), 757–766.

Loew, T. H., Nickel, M. K., & Muehlbacher, M. (2006). Topiramate improves psychopathological symptoms and quality of life in women with borderline personality disorder. *Journal of Clinical Psychopharmacology, 26*, 61–66.

Loffler-Stastka, H., Ponocny-Seliger, E., Meissel, T., et al. (2006). Gender aspects in the planning of psychotherapy for borderline personality disorder. *Wiener Klinische Wochenschrift, 118*(5–6), 160–169.

Marchesi, C., De Panfilis, C., Cantoni, A., et al. (2006). Personality disorders and response to medication treatment in panic disorder: A 1-year naturalistic study. *Progress in Neuro-Psychopharmacology and Biological Psychiatry, 30*(7), 1240–1245.

Marcus, D. K., Lilienfeld, S. O., Edens, J. F., et al. (2006). Is antisocial personality disorder continuous or categorical? A taxometric analysis. *Psychological Medicine, 36*(11), 1571–1581

Mazaira, S. (2004). [Pharmacological treatment of borderline personality disorder]. *Vertex, 15*(58), 303–308.

McCue, J. D. (1982). The effects of stress on physicians and their medical practice. *New England Journal of Medicine, 306*, 458–463.

Millon, T., & Davis, R. D. (1997). The MCMI-III: Present and future directions. *Journal of Personality Assessment, 68*(1), 69–85.

Mobascher, A., Mobascher, J., Schlemper, V., et al. (2006). Aripiprazole pharmacotherapy of borderline personality disorder. *Pharmacopsychiatry, 39*(3), 111–112.

Moran, P., Leese, M., Lee, T., et al. (2003). The Standardised Assessment of Personality–Abbreviated scale (SAPAS): Preliminary validation of a brief screen for personality disorder. *British Journal of Psychiatry, 183*(3), 228–232.

Nestadt, G., Costa, P. T. Jr., Hsu, F. C., et al. (2006). The relationship between the five-factor model and latent Diagnostic and Statistical Manual of Mental Disorders, Fourth Edition personality disorder dimensions. *Comprehensive Psychiatry, 49*(1), 98–105.

Nickel, M., Muehlbacher, M., Nickel, C., et al. (2006). Aripiprazole in the treatment of patients with borderline personality disorder: A double-blind, placebo-controlled study. *American Journal of Psychiatry, 163*(5), 833–839.

Nurnberg, H. G., Seidman, S. N., Gelenberg, A. J., et al. (2002). Depression, antidepressant therapies and erectile dysfunction: Clinical trials of sildenafil citrate in treated and untreated patients with depression. *Urology, 60*(Suppl. 2B), 58–62.

Ottosson, H., Grann, M., & Kullgren, G. (2005). Test-Retest Reliability of a Self-Report Questionnaire for DSM-IV and ICD-10 personality disorders. *European Journal of Psychological Assessment, 16*(1), 53–58.

Ottosson M., Vikman-Adolfsson K., Enerbäck S., et al. (1995). Growth hormone inhibits lipoprotein lipase activity in human adipose tissue. *Journal of Clinical Endocrinology Metabolism, 80*, 936–941.

Pascual, J. C., Madre, M., Puigdemont, D., et al. (2006). [A naturalistic study: 100 consecutive episodes of acute agitation in a psychiatric emergency department]. *Actas Espanolas de Psiquiatria, 34*(4), 239–244.

Ralevski, E., Sanislow, C. A., Grilo, C. M., et al. (2005). Avoidant personality disorder and social phobia: Distinct enough to be separate disorders? *Acta Psychiatrica Scandinavica, 112*, 208.

Ryden, G., & Vinnars, B. (2002). [Pharmacological treatment of borderline personality disorders. Several options for symptom reduction but nothing for the disorder per se.]. *Lakartidningen, 99*(50), 5088–5094.

Samuel D. B., & Widiger T. A. (2006) Differentiating normal and abnormal personality from the perspective of the DSM. In S. Strack (Ed.), *Differentiating normal and abnormal personality* (2nd ed.; pp. 165–183). New York: Springer.

Sass, H., & Junemann, K. (2001). Affective disorders, personality and personality disorders. *Nordic Journal of Psychiatry, 55*, 107–111.

Schmahl, C., & Bohus, M. (2001). [Symptom-focussed drug therapy in borderline personality disorder]. *Fortschritte der Neurologie- Psychiatrie, 69*(7), 310–321.

Schumm, J. A., Hobfoll, S. E., & Keogh, N. J. (2004). Revictimization and interpersonal resource loss predicts PTSD among women in substance-use treatment. *Journal of Traumatic Stress, 17*(2), 173.

Seth, P., Cheeta, S., Tucci, S., et al. (2002). Nicotinic-serotonergic interactions in brain and behavior. *Pharmacology, Biochemistry and Behavior, 71*, 795–805.

Simms, L. J., & Clark, L. A. (2006). The Schedule for Nonadaptive and Adaptive Personality (SNAP): A dimensional measure of traits relevant to personality and personality pathology. In Steven Strack (Ed.), *Differentiating normal and abnormal personality* (pp. 431–450). New York: Springer.

Soler, J., Pascual, J. C., Campins, J., et al. (2005). Double-blind, placebo-controlled study of dialectical behavior therapy plus olanzapine for borderline personality disorder. *American Journal of Psychiatry, 162*(6), 1221–1224.

Stein, D. J., Ono, Y., Tajima, O., et al. (2004). The social anxiety disorder spectrum. *Journal of Clinical Psychiatry, 65*(Suppl 14), 27–33; quiz 34–36.

Steinmetz, D., & Tabenkin, H. (2001). The "difficult patient" as perceived by family physicians. *Family Practice, 18*(5), 495–500.

Strand, S., & Belfrage, H. (2005). Gender differences in psychopathy in a Swedish offender sample. *Behavioral Sciences and the Law, 23*(6), 837–850.

Swann, A. C. (2003). Neuroreceptor mechanisms of aggression and its treatment. *Journal of Clinical Psychiatry, 64*(Suppl 4), 26–35.

Walters, P., Moran, P., Choudhury, P., et al. (2004). A comparison of informant and patient accounts of personality disorder. *International Methods of Psychiatric Research, 13*(1), 34–39.

Wroblewski, B. A., Joseph, A. B., Kupfer, J., et al. (1997). Effectiveness of valproic acid on destructive and aggressive behaviours in patients with acquired brain injury. *Brain Injury, 11*(1), 37–47.

Zaboli, G., Gizatullin, R., Nilsonne, A., et al. (2006). Tryptophan hydroxylase-1 gene variants associate with a group of suicidal borderline women. *Neuropsychopharmacology, 31*(9), 1982–1990.

Zimmerman, M., & Mattia, J. I. (2001). A self-report scale to help make psychiatric diagnoses: The Psychiatric Diagnostic Screening Questionnaire. *Archives of General Psychiatry, 58*, 787–794.

Zimmerman, M., Rothschild, L., & Chelminski, I. (2005). The prevalence of DSM-IV personality disorders in psychiatric outpatients. *American Journal of Psychiatry, 162*, 1911–1918.

Joan C. Urbancic

chapter 8

Severe and Persistent Mental Illness

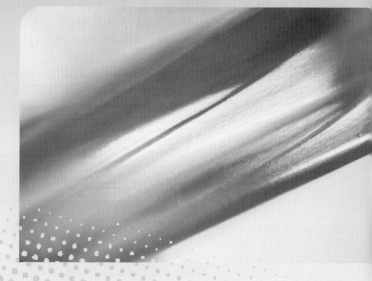

Mental illness is a very common phenomenon in men and women in the United States as well as the world. The U.S. Department of Health and Human Services (DHHS) reports that about 20 percent of Americans experience a mental disorder each year (U.S Department of Health and Human Services [DHHS], 1999). Of this 20 percent, from 5 to 7 percent of American adults and 5 to 9 percent of children have a *serious* mental illness (SMI). Half of the people with an SMI (approximately 2.6 percent of all adults) are even more handicapped and are referred to as the seriously and persistently mentally ill (SPMI). Among the population of older adults (over age 55 years), approximately 4 percent have SMI and another 1 percent have SPMI. These statistics do not include persons with severe cognitive disorders such as Alzheimer's disease. According to the World Health Organization, the combination of all SMIs accounts for more than 15 percent of the total burden of diseases from all causes (World Health Association [WHO], 2001).

Besides the great numbers of people with SMI, the costs of mental illness in the United States are staggering. According to the DHHS, the direct costs of services in 1996 were $69 billion, accounting for 7.3 percent of the total health spending (DHHS, 2001). Indirect costs of mental illness in 1990 were approximately $78.6 billion. In addition, Alzheimer's disease services cost $17.7 billion, and substance abuse treatment cost $12.6 billion (HDDS, 2001).

Despite the high prevalence and huge costs, the majority of persons with diagnosable disorders and severe mental illnesses are untreated or receive minimally adequate treatment (Wang, Demler, and Kessler, 2002). Because primary care providers (PCPs) are often the initial health care providers who people with SMIs encounter and depend on for treatment, PCPs need to recognize the importance of their diagnosing and treating the severely mentally ill in primary care settings but also referring these people, when necessary, to appropriate mental health professionals (WHO, 2001). The WHO recommends management and treatment of mental disorders in primary care settings because they afford the easiest access and can serve the greatest number of people (WHO). The WHO emphasizes that this role requires curricula that trains the PCP as well as ongoing refresher courses.

This chapter addresses serious and persistent mental illness with specific gender issues that relate to women with SPMI. Psychiatric and medical comorbidities will be discussed along with the psychological and social aspects of SPMI. Schizophrenia will be described as the prototypical SPMI followed by treatment of the acutely psychotic person in the primary care setting as well as referral. Medications and psychosocial treatment options are also discussed, as is the question of recovery among the SPMI.

DEFINING SERIOUS AND PERSISTENT MENTAL ILLNESS

According to Spollen (2003), the most commonly accepted definition of serious and persistent mental illness (SPMI) includes the following:

- A diagnosis of nonorganic psychosis
- Disability in both social and occupational realms
- Long-term mental illness and treatment

SPMIs include schizophrenia (discussed later as a prototypical SPMI); bipolar disorder; major depression; severe anxiety disorders; and in some arenas, substance use dependence and personality disorders. Pomerantz (1999) has argued that most of the major diagnostic categories of the *Diagnostic and Statistical Manual of Mental Disorders* (*DSM-IV-TR*) qualify as chronic and relapsing disorders, including those noted as eating disorders, attention deficit disorder, somatoform disorders, and sexual and gender identity disorders. The one exception cited by Pomerantz is adjustment disorder.

Prior to the Community Mental Health Centers Act in 1963, people who were institutionalized because of mental illness were identified as the chronically mentally ill (CMI) (Spollen, 2003). With the implementation of the Act and the introduction of antipsychotic medications, the care of the CMI moved from hospitals to the community. At that time, it became clear that many patients were able to function independently and therefore were no longer viewed as CMI. The term *chronically mentally ill* also reflected a pessimistic and pejorative view, so it gradually was replaced with the terms *serious and persistent mental illness* or *serious mental illness* (Spollen).

There is no single profile, pattern, diagnosis, or course for SPMI. The one commonality is the disabling nature of the mental illness with frequent relapses over the long term so that daily functioning is seriously compromised.

Access to Care

People with SPMI are often lost to the mental health system and are unable or unwilling to access and use available mental health resources. In many instances, they do not accept the reality of their mental illness and, therefore, refuse any treatment that may be offered. Even with adherence to treatment methods, their illness may have exacerbations that require emergency services and hospitalization. The illness also leaves them vulnerable to a host of medical and social problems such as poor nutrition related to or resulting from poverty, substance abuse, homelessness, interpersonal violence, and exposure to infectious diseases including HIV, sexually transmitted diseases (STDs), and tuberculosis. They are also at risk for hypertension, type 2 diabetes, and morbid obesity (Hoffman, Ahl, Meyers, et al., 2005; Nemeroff, Conley, and Newcomer, 2007; Newcomer, Buckley, and Correll, 2007).

Wang, Berglund, and Kessler (2000) reported that only 14.3 percent of patients with mental disorders received care that was based on evidenced-based practice. Of the patients with the most severe and disabling mental disorders, only 25 percent received guideline-concordant treatment. Although being white, female, and severely ill and having health insurance were the strongest predictors of receiving appropriate care, Wang and colleagues concluded that an epidemic of untreated and poorly treated mental disorders is the standard today, especially for vulnerable groups such as the nation's uninsured and underinsured.

According to Mechanic (2002), the main barriers to access to care by people with SPMIs are limited knowledge of services, inadequate insurance coverage, and stigma. Mechanic views the current state of mental health care services as a major health crisis but admits that more efforts are being directed toward improving care and educating the public about mental illness and available services.

Currently, the main sources of treatment for SPMI are inpatient hospitals and community outpatient centers. However, many people with SPMIs receive medication and support from their PCPs, who are able to track both mental and physical health treatment responses over time and limit negative outcomes such as hospitalization, job loss, and suicide (Jackson, 2006). However, much more involvement is needed for this population because so many remain undiagnosed and untreated. Therefore, PCPs have the opportunity to intervene holistically by treating both the physical and mental disorders of their patients who fall through the cracks of the health system.

Treating Serious and Persistent Mental Illness

In the past, SPMI was thought to take a gradual, deteriorating course. Recent studies, however, show that with treatment, one half to two thirds of people with SPMI significantly improve and/or recover (Ciompi, 1988; Fisher, 2006; Harding, 2003; Harding and Zahniser, 1994).

Until recently, the primary treatment for persons in the United States with SPMI consisted mainly of medications. Today, medication is only one component in the treatment plan for achieving functional status in people with SPMI. A wide variety of psychosocial interventions for this population include connecting to community resources, developing social support systems, assisting with job searches and housing, and initiating psychosocial rehabilitation. PCPs may be the only health providers with whom the person with SPMI has contact. PCPs can successfully prescribe antipsychotic medications, but it is critical to go beyond medication therapy and actively connect patients to all the available resources the community may offer.

Culture and Serious and Persistent Mental Illness

Because the United States, Canada, and most other countries have vastly diverse populations, it is critical that all health care providers appreciate cultural differences in values, beliefs, and mental health presentations among their patients. To assist health care providers, the *DSM-IV-TR* includes a new emphasis on the influence of culture on diagnosis and a glossary of culture-bound syndromes (American Psychiatric Association [APA], 2000). Many studies describe these cultural differences. Of particular interest are differences in the diagnosis and treatment of mental illnesses among various ethnic and racial populations. These differences often result in disparities for the persons involved (DHHS, 2001). For example, compared with European Americans or Latinos, black patients were systematically more often diagnosed as having a schizophrenic disorder. Latinos were systematically diagnosed as having major depression despite higher levels of self-reported psychotic symptoms (Minsky, Vega, Miskimen, et al., 2003; Strakowski, Keck, and Arnold, 2003). The researchers indicated that more studies are needed to understand these outcomes and suggested that self-selection, cultural bias due to the clinician's lack of cultural competence, culturally determined expression of symptoms, and inaccurate application of *DSM-IV* criteria are possible explanations (APA, 1994).

SERIOUS AND PERSISTENT MENTAL ILLNESS AND RELATED PROBLEMS

Not only must people with SPMI cope with the illness itself, but they must also deal with problems that may be triggered by the disabling effect of the illness. Such problems include comorbidities such as substance dependence; nutritional abnormalities; and socioeconomic difficulties such as homelessness, poverty, and stigma.

Psychiatric Comorbidities

The most common comorbidities in the population with SPMI are substance use disorders (SUD). In 2002, an estimated 7 to 10 million adults met the criteria for co-occurring serious mental disorder and substance dependence in the United States (Epstein, Barker, Vorburger, et al., 2002). SUD is estimated to affect approximately 50 percent of patients with schizophrenia. Alcohol and cannabis are the most typically used substances. Cocaine and amphetamines have been reported to worsen psychotic symptoms in persons with SPMI and to initiate symptoms in those who are not psychotic. Methamphetamine use reportedly presents as paranoid schizophrenia with effects that extend for months and may recur during periods of stress. The longer the duration of use, the greater the likelihood of psychosis; with preexisting psychosis, the patient may become resistant to treatment. Among the SPMI population, those with SUDs typically have poorer psychosocial outcomes than those without SUDs (Nasrallah and White, 2006). Patients with the dual diagnosis of a mental illness and SUD have higher rates of hospitalization, are more difficult to treat, and have a more severe disease trajectory. They are often homeless and more prone to violence than the person who has SPMI and does not depend on substances (Nasrallah and White).

Smoking is a serious problem for the population with SPMI. Approximately 70 percent of patients in the Clinical Antipsychotic Trials of Intervention Effectiveness (CATIE) study were reported to be current smokers (Lieberman, 2006). In general, persons with mental illnesses smoke 34 to 44 percent of all cigarettes in the United States (Newcomer et al., 2007).

Another potentially hazardous substance is excessive use of caffeinated beverages. Some researchers found a positive relationship between the amount of caffeine consumed and positive symptoms of psychosis (e.g., hallucinations and delusions). However, a decrease in negative symptoms (e.g., impoverishment of thought, lack of goal-directed behavior, and flat affect) has also been reported (Nasrallah and White, 2006).

Another very common psychiatric comorbidity among patients with the SPMI schizophrenia is depressive disorders (risk as high as 81 percent) (Nasrallah and White, 2006). Obsessive-compulsive disorder is also fairly common in the severely mentally ill, with a prevalence of approximately 9 percent. Finally, some medical conditions may present as schizophrenialike-psychoses including Wilson's disease, metachromatic leukodystrophy, basal ganglia calcification, and systemic lupus erythematosus (Nasrallah and White).

Medical Comorbidities

People with SPMI are at high risk for acquiring a multitude of medical problems, including dental and vision problems. As well, they have higher morbidity and mortality rates than the average person. Much of this may be caused by lack of accessibility due to being uninsured (Mechanic, 2002).

In particular, women, substance abusers, and the elderly are at greatest risk for undiagnosed physical health problems. However, health problems are often caused by environmental conditions such as homelessness and lack of nutrition or medication side effects that go unrecognized. Generally, health care providers tend to focus on the mental illnesses before the medical problems. This is a situation that is very appropriate for PCPs to address, because they often are the only professionals with whom the severely mentally ill person may have contact.

Metabolic Syndrome and Coronary Artery Disease

In recent years, much evidence has been generated indicating that people who are severely mentally ill are at great risk for a host of medical problems. Of particular concern is the metabolic syndrome, which is a cluster of at least three of the following cardiovascular risk factors: obesity, dyslipidemia, hypertension, insulin resistance, and impaired glucose control. The feared outcome of this syndrome is coronary artery disease. Black women and Mexican Americans are at high risk for metabolic syndrome, but it occurs twice as often in persons with SMI than the general population. The impact of metabolic syndrome is reflected by cardiovascular disease being the primary cause of early death in persons with SMIs. The consequence is a life span shortened by 25 to 30 years as compared to the general population.

Emphysema and Bronchitis

Because most people with SPMI are heavy smokers, many have severe emphysema and chronic bronchitis as well. Newcomer, Buckley, and Correll (2007) claim that health professionals are failing patients with SMIs because when patients with SMI or SPMI have a medical problem, they receive less care and more substandard care than the general population.

Human Immunodeficiency Virus

Treisman (2007) asserts that people with psychiatric illnesses are at high risk for HIV, and when they test positive for HIV, they often adhere poorly to their HIV medication regimen. When men have a severe psychiatric illness, they tend to lose their sexual drive early in their disease. This is not the case for women, which places them at greater risk for STDs than men and at risk for unwanted pregnancies as well (Seeman, 2000). Women's increased risk for HIV may also be related to poverty and the use of sexual favors to obtain food and shelter (Perese and Perese, 2003).

In one study, two thirds of women with SPMI had not used condoms during sexual intercourse in the past 3 months, and more than two thirds had sex with multiple partners (Randolph, Pinkerton, Somlai, et al., 2007). The HIV prevalence among people with SPMI is approximately 6 percent nationally. While these numbers are very disturbing, studies demonstrate that educational interventions are effective in decreasing unprotected sexual behavior among people with SPMI (Kalichman, Malow, Devieux, et al., 2005; Treisman, 2007). Most importantly, effective treatment for the psychiatric illness results in improved patient HIV outcomes and a decrease in HIV transmission.

Psychological Aspects of Serious and Persistent Mental Illness

Because of their psychotic symptoms, persons with SPMI have cognitive problems that affect their ability to solve problems, make decisions, express their thoughts and feelings, and manage their activities of daily living. Often, they have paranoid delusions that preclude them from trusting others and seeking assistance for their mental health problems. Moreover, impaired communication, lack of social skills, and poor hygiene may create barriers to developing relationships with others (Brady and McCain, 2005). Thus, they often live in isolation that tends to increase their low self-esteem, sense of worthlessness, and loneliness. Consequently, people with SPMI are frequently depressed and at high risk for suicide.

Social Problems Related to Serious and Persistent Mental Illness

Some people with SPMI cannot function independently in the community because of their inability to care for themselves and find employment. Without employment, they are poverty bound and often homeless.

Often, they do not adhere to their medication regimen and must be rehospitalized because of acute exacerbations of their disease. Side effects of medications are one of the main reasons for therapeutic nonadherence. However, patients may also lose their prescriptions, lack the funds needed to get the prescriptions filled, or may believe that they do not require medications and refuse to take them. Because medication adherence is such a major problem in treating people with SPMI, many treatment programs conduct educational programs for patients and their families to learn about their medications in order to self-manage their medications. Despite the problems mentioned, many people with SPMI are able to manage their self-care and live independently in the community with proper resources and support.

Involvement with the Criminal Justice System

People with SPMI have a 64 percent greater chance of being arrested and going to jail than persons who commit the same crimes but are not mentally ill (Bazelon Center for Mental Health Law). The situation for people with SPMI may be compounded because of their disordered behavior, homelessness, substance dependence, and lack of mental health services. The increase in criminal justice involvement with persons with SPMI reflects the deinstitutional process between 1975 and 1985. Police, corrections officials, families, and communities are increasingly frustrated by the repeated criminalization of the mentally ill (Lamb, Weinberger, and Gross, 2004). Most people agree on the need for improved mental health services for the mentally ill, particularly for those with comorbid substance dependencies. However, while some communities are beginning to collaborate by developing programs conjointly with the criminal justice system and the public mental health system, no major changes have occurred as yet (Bazelon Center for Mental Health Law).

SPECIFIC GENDER ISSUES IN WOMEN WITH SERIOUS AND PERSISTENT MENTAL ILLNESS

Men and women with SPMI experience many of the same problems. However, besides the typical medical problems such as hypertension, obesity, diabetes, asthma, heart disease, irritable bowel syndrome, infectious diseases, substance abuse and interpersonal violence, women with SPMI often have specific gender problems as well as differences in the course and outcome of their psychiatric disease. Among women with schizophrenia, premorbid functioning is better than that of men; their first episode of illness occurs later (4 to 6 years), and they recover faster. While these factors predict superior outcomes for women, these advantages disappear when a woman is older than 45 years. Late onset of the disease occurs twice as often in women as men, and the symptoms and course are also more severe at this time (Riecher-Rossler, 2004). Women also require lower doses of antipsychotic medication than men (Seeman, 2000).

Hyperprolactinemia

Excess prolactin can theoretically be caused by the psychiatric illness and its stressful consequences, but it may also be caused by psychotropic medications. First-generation antipsychotics (FGAs) are known to block dopamine receptors, thereby increasing the serum level of prolactin. While the second-generation atypical antipsychotic agents have less affinity for dopamine, risperidone (Risperdal) is the one exception. Weiden and Buckley (2007) reported that risperidone has an even greater affinity for dopamine receptors than the FGAs, while aripiprazole (Abilify) seems to have the least affinity. Outcomes related to elevated prolactin levels in women include amenorrhea, breast engorgement and galactorrhea, vaginal dryness, and sexual dysfunction. Excess prolactin may also cause a decrease in bone density, leading to osteoporosis. With the use of the selective serotonin reuptake inhibitor (SSRI) antidepressants comes an increased risk for sexual dysfunction because of their serotonin effects.

Another side effect of excess prolactin resulting from psychotropic medication is the secondary suppression of physiologic estrogen. Long-term use of some antipsychotic medications may result in partial *iatrogenic early menopause* with increased risk for osteoporosis, cardiovascular disease, and cognitive disturbances. Both prolactin and estrogen levels should be measured if hyperprolactinemia is suspected. PCPs should consider switching to an antipsychotic with prolactin-sparing properties and/or adding estrogen as an adjunct if estrogen deficiency is present. Once prolactin levels are normalized, women may begin to have normal periods again, with the potential for an unplanned pregnancy. The switching of antipsychotic medications may further complicate matters because of potential teratogenic effects (Riecher-Rossler, 2004). For all of these reasons, consultation with an obstetrician is recommended.

Women with SPMI have reported serious distress from menopause-related problems that may be aggravated by hyperprolactinemia. Nonetheless, their complaints are frequently overlooked by PCPs. In a study by Friedman, Sajatovic, Schuermeyer, et al. (2005), women with severe psychiatric illnesses reported distressing vasomotor, physical, sexual, and psychosocial symptoms related to their menopause. This was especially the case for women with depression. The Friedman study supports claims that persons with SPMI are often not receiving appropriate medical care.

Interpersonal Violence

While both men and women with SPMI are at very high risk for being victims of interpersonal violence, women are much more likely to be victims of sexual abuse, while men are more likely victims of physical abuse. Very often, the women have histories of childhood sexual and physical abuse and revictimization as adults. As adults, women with SPMI are often victimized by males who also have severe mental illnesses (Seeman, 2002).

The sexual and physical victimization occurs in all settings, including health care. Disabled women and pregnant women with SPMI are at the greatest risk for interpersonal violence because they are perceived as weak and vulnerable. Furthermore, their cognitive impairment may leave them unable to protect themselves, so they are often exploited and abused. While some women may welcome the sexual advances of men, Seeman (2002) questions whether a woman with SPMI is capable of giving true consent. Because of the frequency and potentially severe psychological long-term effects of abuse, it is imperative to obtain a complete history of abuse so that interventions future prevention strategies can be implemented.

Breast Cancer Risk

Women with SPMI are at increased risk for breast cancer because of their greater incidence of obesity, smoking, alcohol use, and antidepressants. According to a study by Halbreich, Shen, and Panaro (1996), women with SPMI have an incidence of breast cancer 3.5 times greater than women at high risk and 9.5 times greater than women in general. While obesity is a risk for men and women with SPMI, the prevalence of obesity in women is higher than in men (Daumit, Clark, Steinwachs, et al., 2003).

Motherhood and Serious and Persistent Mental Illness

Although most of the literature on motherhood is specific for women with schizophrenia, most of the following discussion applies to women with SPMI as well. Approximately 50 percent of women with schizophrenia become mothers, which is similar to the rates among the general female population. However, women with schizophrenia and other SPMIs are at risk for being unable to adequately care for their children. Interactional skills and negative symptoms (especially blunt or flat affect) can interfere with bonding, maternal awareness, and competence. For women with mood disorders, maternal bonding is also a challenge. If the woman is psychotic, she may have hallucinations and delusions that may distort her perceptions and place her children in life-threatening danger.

Medication during pregnancy is a complicated process because of potential adverse effects to the developing fetus as well as balancing the psychiatric needs of the woman. Therefore, referral to an obstetrician is critical for both mother and child. The postpartum period is another challenge for the mother and child, as this is the time for bonding, and excessive medication to control psychosis may cause drowsiness and prevent the woman from interacting with her infant.

Being a single mother is also common with the SPMI population along with minimal education and few, if any, work skills. Therefore, finances are major problems as well as interaction with destructive male partners and severe substance abuse. Approximately one third of women with SPMI lose custody of their children. Children of women with schizophrenia have greater developmental and behavioral problems than children from healthy mothers, but it is not clear to what degree genetics versus adverse childhood events affect these outcomes. Therefore, when women with SPMI become parents, the challenge becomes twofold, as the therapeutic needs of the woman and the best interests of her child must both be considered (Riecher-Rossler, 2004).

PROTOTYPICAL SERIOUS AND PERSISTENT MENTAL ILLNESS: SCHIZOPHRENIA

This section focuses primarily on schizophrenia because other major mental health disorders that can become severe and persistent are addressed in other chapters throughout this text. However, because schizophrenia is the prototype for the SPMI, much of what is covered under schizophrenia may have application to the other major severe and persistent mental health disorders.

Assessment and Diagnosis

Schizophrenia occurs in 1 percent of people across cultures and gender. It affects males and females equally. While men usually exhibit signs of the disease in their late teens or early 20s, women generally do not exhibit signs until their late 20s or early 30s. Studies indicate that schizophrenia has a bimodal age of onset for women, as evidenced by a second peak later in life, while men have a strictly unimodal age of onset. Women seem to have better premorbid functioning than men, and they typically exhibit more positive symptoms while men exhibit more negative symptoms of mental illness (APA, 2000).

Some researchers have suggested that estrogen has a neuroprotective function in women, as evidenced by the second peak of onset in women with the onset of menopause and lower estrogen levels. Younger women seem to have a less severe course of the disease, but after menopause, the course of the disease becomes more severe (Riecher-Rossler, 2004). More research is needed to determine if estrogen therapy would be helpful to reduce negative symptoms and the need for higher doses of antipsychotic medication.

People with schizophrenia have a 10 percent suicide risk, with 20 percent to 40 percent making at least one attempt. More men than women commit suicide (Pomerantz, 2006). The public often has an image of the typical schizophrenic person as being violent. But the violent patient represents only a subgroup, characterized by young males who reject medication and have a history of violence and substance abuse (APA, 2000). Most people with schizophrenia are not more violent than the general population.

Researchers conclude that the most important risk factor is a family history of schizophrenia (Tienari, Wynne, Sorri, et al., 2004; Wahlberg, Wynne, Hakko, et al., 2004). There are no diagnostic laboratory tests for schizophrenia, but recent neurophysiologic imaging research has found significant differences in people with schizophrenia compared with control groups. Neuropsychological testing has also revealed deficits in cognitive functioning among persons with schizophrenia, including memory, attention, psychomotor skills, and inability to change the response set (rigid thinking) (APA, 2000).

Symptoms of Schizophrenia

According to the *DSM-IV-TR*, schizophrenia is a mental disorder with a constellation of signs and symptoms that impairs social and occupational functioning (APA, 2000). It consists of both negative and positive symptoms. It endures for at least 6 months and has at least 1 month of at least two of the following active symptoms: delusions, hallucinations, disorganized speech, grossly disorganized or catatonic behaviors, and negative symptoms. Only one of the mentioned active symptoms is required if the person has hallucinations with voices conversing with one other or one voice with a running commentary on the person or bizarre delusions. Bizarre or extreme delusions are characteristic of schizophrenia, although not always present. These four types of symptoms are known as positive symptoms, and they may preclude people from performing even simple daily living activities. However, positive symptoms usually respond well to antipsychotic medications.

Negative symptoms include flat or inappropriate affect, poverty of speech (alogia), lack of motivation, loss of interest in goal-directed activities (avolition), and social withdrawal. The negative symptoms are more resistant to treatment than the positive ones and are more difficult to assess than positive ones because they exist on a continuum and can be ascribed to a variety of causes besides schizophrenia. These causes include depressive symptoms, medication side effects, and chronic lack of environmental stimulation. According to the *DSM-IV-TR*, the best test of negative symptoms is their enduring nature over time (APA, 2000).

Schizophrenia is also known as a formal thought disorder (disorganized thinking), but because the concept is so difficult to operationalize, the *DSM-IV-TR* uses the concept of disorganized speech in its definition (APA, 2000). Disorganized speech can range from rapidly changing topics (loose associations) to a jumble of words know as *word salad.* Catatonic motor behaviors, in which there is a significant decrease in reactivity to surroundings, may also be present. However, catatonic symptoms are not unique to schizophrenia and may develop because of medical conditions and medication-induced movement disorders, such as neuroleptic-induced Parkinson's disease. Before diagnosing a person with schizophrenia, the clinician must rule out the possibility of symptoms being caused by a medication, substance abuse, or a medical condition (Box 8.1).

Box 8.1 • *DSM-IV-TR* Criteria for Schizophrenia

DSM

A. Characteristic symptoms
   Two or more of the following significantly present during a 1-month period (or less if successfully treated):
   1. Delusions
   2. Hallucinations
   3. Disorganized speech (e.g., frequent derailment or incoherence)
   4. Grossly disorganized or catatonic behavior
   5. Negative symptoms

B. Social/occupational dysfunction
   Since the onset of symptoms, one or more major areas such as work, interpersonal relations, or self-care are markedly below the presymptom level

C. Duration
   Persistent continuous signs of disturbance for at least 6 months with at least 1 month of symptoms (or less if successfully treated) that meet Criterion A

D. Substance/general medical condition exclusion
   Cannot be due to direct physiologic effects of a substance (e.g., a drug of abuse, a medication) or a general medical condition.

From the American Psychiatric Association (2000). *Diagnostic and statistical manual of mental disorders* (Revised 4th ed.). Washington, DC: Author.

There are five subtypes of schizophrenia, and a person's diagnosis in a particular subtype may change over time. The types include the following:

- *Paranoid.* Distinguished by persecutory or grandiose delusions or both. However, delusions relating to jealousy, religion, or somatization may also be present. Hallucinations are commonly reflective of the delusional content. Onset for paranoid schizophrenia is later in life, and prognosis is better than the other types of schizophrenia.
- *Disorganized* (previously known as hebephrenic). Consists of odd and disorganized speech and behavior and flat or inappropriate affect. Disorganized behavior prevents performance of simple activities of daily living. Onset of the disease is earlier and characterized by chronic course of deterioration without significant remissions.
- *Catatonic.* Features at least two of the following: (a) motor immobility, (b) excessive, purposeless motor behavior, (c) extreme negativism or mutism (unresponsive to any instructions), (d) voluntary bizarre posturing or movements, and (e) echolalia (senseless repeating of another person's words).
- *Undifferentiated.* Meets the criteria for schizophrenia but does not meet the more specific criteria to be categorized as paranoid, disorganized, or catatonic.
- *Residual.* Diagnosed when the person has no positive psychotic symptoms although at least two negative symptoms persist. Residual schizophrenia may be a transition period between an active episode and complete remission, or it may remain continuously for long periods without any acute episodes (APA, 2000).

Differential Diagnosis

Alternative diagnoses may need to be considered when schizophrenia is suspected. Because of racial and ethnic disparities and many other possible diagnoses, a close relative or friend can be extremely helpful in confirming the diagnosis. The diagnosis of schizophrenia often changes over time. According to Schultz, North, and Shields (2007), the most common diagnostic changes are from schizophrenia to bipolar or organic disorders. Conversely, organic disorders, psychotic disorders, and major depression diagnoses are most commonly changed to schizophrenia. Table 8.1 examines some of the differential diagnoses between schizophrenia and alternatives. Much of this information has application to other SPMIs characterized by psychotic symptoms.

Table 8.1 • Differential Diagnosis of Schizophrenia

Differential Diagnosis	Distinguishing Characteristics
Psychotic disorder due to a medical condition	Brain tumors, hypoglycemia, electrolyte imbalance, sepsis, hepatic encephalopathy, Wilson's disease, and systemic lupus erythematosus; symptoms abate with treatment of medical condition
Medication-induced psychosis	Narcotics, anxiolytics, steroids, anticholinergics, anticonvulsants
Delirium	Much shorter duration
Brief psychotic episode	Psychotic behavior lasting <1 month
Mood disorder with psychotic features	Major depression and manic symptoms do not occur concurrently with active phase of schizophrenia
Schizophreniform disorder	Psychotic symptoms for at least 1 month but <6 months
Schizotypal personality disorder	Long-term pattern of avoiding social and interpersonal contacts; no delusions or hallucinations
Schizoaffective disorder	Differentiation may be difficult; requires a major depression, manic or mixed episode with Criteria A symptoms of schizophrenia including hallucinations, delusions, disorganized speech, and negative thinking
Substance use disorder	Cocaine and amphetamines associated with psychotic symptoms; withdrawal from substances can also cause hallucinations and delusions

From Schultz, S.H., North, S.W., & Shields, C.G. (2007). Schizophrenia: A review. *American Family Physician, 75*(12), 1821–1829.

THE ACUTELY PSYCHOTIC PATIENT IN THE PRIMARY CARE SETTING

Acutely psychotic patients are not typically seen in the primary care setting, so the management of their care in such a situation can be very challenging. A few years ago, it was typical to use haloperidol (Haldol) as a first-line treatment, often with lorazepam (Ativan). Today, however, there is a wider array of medications from which to choose, with atypical antipsychotic or SGA in intramuscular (IM) form being preferred regardless of whether the illness is a first episode or a relapse.

The PCP will need to determine from the patient or family which, if any, antipsychotic medication the patient has been taking. This is especially important because sometimes patients become very agitated and/or aggressive from their medication. Thus, their aggression may be the result of akathisia. They also may have extrapyramidal side effects (EPS) and other movement disorders from a current antipsychotic, with the potential for these symptoms to increase in severity with a larger dose or other antipsychotic. To avoid such potential side effects, atypical SGAs are the first-line choice of medications for the acutely psychotic patient (Buckley, 2005).

Most acutely psychotic patients will respond in a similar fashion to antipsychotic medications regardless of their diagnosis. Lorazepam 2 mg has effectively been combined with antipsychotic medication. It is available in IM form, as are ziprasidone and olanzapine.

According to Allen (2005), the expert consensus guideline indicates that lorazepam alone is preferred when no diagnosis is available or when there is a substance abuse disorder, delirium, or conduct disorder. With schizophrenia or mania, atypical antipsychotic monotherapy is preferred. Haloperidol either alone or in combination with lorazepam is usually not recommended.

PCPs need to calm the agitated, distressed patient while minimizing any danger to the patient, staff, and others as well as themselves. Security personnel must be available if there is any possibility of escalating behavior and/or inability to control and calm the patient. Despite their psychotic, agitated state, patients always need to be treated with respect and dignity and given as many choices in their treatment as possible. Many times, they will have a preference in medication. Despite appropriate medication, some patients will not stabilize and will require emergency medical services support for transport to the nearest emergency department. Hospitalization must be considered if the patient is a harm to self or others, if she is unable to take the prescribed medication and perform self-care, and if there is no reliable person to whom the patient may be released until she stabilizes.

REFERRALS TO MENTAL HEALTH PROFESSIONALS

While PCPs may effectively prescribe medication for patients with SPMI, it is recommended that patients be referred to psychiatric professionals if they are a danger to themselves or to others, are not stabilized on their medications, are nonadherent to medication therapy, or if they need resources and social support from mental health agencies.

Pregnant and postpartum women with SPMI should also be referred for specialty care. Other reasons for referrals include lack of confidence by PCPs in diagnosing, prescribing antipsychotic medication, and managing care; barriers to continuity of care for the patients between primary care and psychiatric care; and time constraints that preclude providing the care needed for the patient with SPMI.

TREATMENT OPTIONS

Medication Therapy

Persons with mental illness have been treated with antipsychotic medication since the 1950s, when chlorpromazine (Thorazine), an FGA, was introduced. Generally, the FGAs are referred to as neuroleptics and are known for increasing the risk for EPS (e.g., tremor, slurred speech, decreased muscle tone) and other movement disorders as compared with the second-generation antipsychotics (SGAs), also known as atypical antipsychotics. Some researchers have reported that the advantages of the atypical antipsychotics were probably due to the much higher doses of FGAs that were used in clinical trials (Geddes, Freemantle, Harrison, et al., 2000). Nevertheless, evidence suggests that atypical antipsychotics carry only a minimal risk for EPS. The exception is risperidone, which is associated with a mild risk (Lehman, Lieberman, and Dixon, 2004). In recent years, the atypical antipsychotics have become the standard of care and currently remain so. Unfortunately, these agents produce other side effects, such as sedation, weight gain, and increased glucose and lipid levels, which contribute to the risk of metabolic syndrome and cardiovascular disease.

With both FGAs and SGAs, women typically require lower doses than men, even when body weight is considered. Research is inconsistent about whether or not women are more vulnerable to neurologic side effects such as tardive dyskinesia, akathisia, and acute dystonias. However, women do appear more susceptible to weight gain, cardiovascular problems, and hyperprolactinemia (Lehman, Lieberman, and Dixon, 2004).

Regardless of which medication is used, there is general agreement that delaying the administration of antipsychotics may have lifetime negative effects for the patient. Therefore, it is incumbent on the PCP to begin treatment if psychiatric services are unavailable. Furthermore, PCPs can be very helpful in supporting medication adherence in patients, because poor adherence may lead to relapse and self-neglect, rehospitalization costs, and neurotoxicity with progressive loss of gray matter (Cahn, Hulshoff Pol, Lems, et al., 2002).

Despite the significant improvements in the side effects profile of the atypical antipsychotics, nonadherence among people with SPMI remains a major problem.

In the CATIE study, Lieberman, Stroup, McEvoy, et al. (2005) reported that 74 percent of patients discontinued or switched their antipsychotic medication within 18 months of initiating the therapy. There was no difference between FGAs and SGAs on patient adherence. Among all of the antipsychotics, olanzapine (Zyprexa) had the highest discontinuation rate from side effects. Reasons for discontinuation or switching were lack of efficacy; intolerable side effects such as weight gain, EPS, and excessive sedation; and sexual side effects. As well, some patients discontinued their medications because they lacked insight into their disease and believed that they did not need medication.

The first lesson learned from the CATIE study was that atypical antipsychotics are not a homogeneous group of medications, as they have different efficacy, safety, and tolerability profiles. Second, there is no simple formula for determining which drug will work the best for a particular person. Switching medications may be required, and that can also be a challenge since differences among medications can be subtle and doses uncertain.

When prescribing an antipsychotic, the provider needs to work with patients to determine what aspects of their life situation prevent them from accomplishing their goals. Many times, social affiliation is the most important goal for them, so the treatment needs to focus on that goal. For example, a medication that is oversedating or one that impacts sexual function may interfere with the goal of social affiliation. Often, patients with negative symptoms will not complain about such side effects, and they will suffer in silence for many years without realizing that improvements can be made. Therefore, it is important to ask patients about possible side effects and work to diminish them by lowering doses or switching to another medication (Lieberman, Stroup, McEvoy, et al., 2005).

Side Effects

In general, all of the FGAs cause significant weight gain and movement disorders to some degree. With the SGAs, weight gain varies from minimal to none with both aripiprazole and ziprasidone (Geodon) to significant gain with clozapine and olanzapine. Weight gain is a serious problem, as it places patients at risk for becoming obese and in turn leads to chronic diseases including hypertension, dyslipidemia, and type 2 diabetes. Ultimately, these chronic disorders increase the probability of cardiovascular disease, which is a leading cause of mortality in schizophrenia.

This process is particularly troublesome with patients who have SPMI, because they are often unaware of their medical status, do not function sufficiently to seek medical treatment, or have no access to medical care. This lack of medical care is reflected in statistics showing that persons with SMIs served by

Table 8.2 • ADA/APA Consensus on Antipsychotic Drugs and Obesity and Diabetes Monitoring Protocol*

	Initial	4 Weeks	8 Weeks	12 Weeks	3 Months	12 Months	5 Years
Personal/Family history	X	—	—	—	—	X	—
Weight (BMI)	X	X	X	X	X	—	—
Waist circumference	X	—	—	—	—	X	—
Blood pressure	X	—	—	X	—	X	—
Fasting glucose	X	—	—	X	—	X	X
Fasting lipid profile	X	—	—	X	—	X	←X

BMI, body mass index.
*More frequent assessments may be warranted based on clinical status.
From ADA/APA Consensus Conference (2004). *Diabetes Care, 27,* 596–601.

the U.S. public mental health system live 25 years *less* on average than the general population (Newcomer et al., 2007). Therefore, it is critical that PCPs provide the total medical care that is needed when caring for those with SPMI.

The American Psychiatric Association/American Diabetes Association consensus guidelines (APA/ADA, 2004) recommend that before patients begin antipsychotic therapy, the following protocol should be followed: (a) personal family disease history, (b) weight (body mass index [BMI]), (c) waist circumference (WM), (d) blood pressure, (e) fasting glucose, and (f) fasting lipid profile (Table 8.2). BMI of 25.0 to 24.9 is categorized as overweight, while a BMI >30 is obese. The BMI may not be a reliable measure for the elderly, people with high muscle mass, people <5 feet tall, and certain racial and ethnic groups. WM is used today as a measure of abdominal obesity. For men, it is defined as WM >40 inches and >35 inches for women. Taken together, the BMI and the WM can be helpful tools to predict cardiometabolic risk (Conley and Newcomer, 2007).

Choosing Between First- and Second-Generation Antipsychotics

There has been widespread belief that the SGAs were superior medications compared with the FGAs for treating schizophrenia. Some researchers have claimed that unlike the FGAs, the SGAs have a neuroprotective effect on the brain and actually promote neurogenesis and cell survival (Lieberman, Tollefson,

Cecil, et al., 2005; Molina, 2005). However, in the CATIE study and the Commentary on Cost Utility of the Latest Antipsychotic Drugs in Schizophrenia Study (CutLASS) from Great Britain, the FGAs were as effective and well tolerated as the SGAs (Jones, Barnes, and Davies, 2006). The perceived superiority of the SGAs may have been the result of using high doses of haloperidol (Haldol; the comparator SGA) and/or the overrepresentation of more treatment-resistant patients in the earlier SGA studies. The results of these two large government studies may signal a return to greater use of the FGAs for schizophrenia and other people with SPMI, especially in the public health sector where budgets are often very tight (Nagy, 2007). In these environments, resources for interventions have been sacrificed to cover the cost of the more expensive SGAs.

However, the CATIE study was not without criticism, particularly regarding methodology. One of the main criticisms was the exclusion of patients with tardive dyskinesia to the FGA (e.g., perphenazine) group, thus introducing a distinct selection bias in the sample. Other concerns were the low generalizability because of the nature of the sample, inclusion of treatment-resistant patients, low percentage of females, and questionable doses of antipsychotics relative to one another (Essock, 2006; Essock, Covell, Davis, et al., 2006; Meltzer and Bobo, 2006). Regardless of study outcomes, researchers agree that the SGAs are a most heterogeneous group of drugs with various efficacy, safety, side effects, and psychosocial improvement profiles. Besides the differences among the SGAs, there are also significant individual differences in clinical response to them. Lieberman (2006) emphasized these individual differences when he stated that equivalency in the CATIE does not mean identical response. He also emphasized that while the FGAs deserve continued consideration for use, they cannot replace the SGAs. Table 8.3 identifies the FGAs currently available in the United States. Table 8.4 summarizes the multiple variations of side effects among the atypical antipsychotic agents. Table 8.5 lists the starting and maintenance doses for the SGAs.

Psychomotor Side Effects of Antipsychotics

Many patients seen in primary care settings have successfully been treated with FGAs for years, whereas other patients may be switched to FGAs in the future based on the CATIE study and CUtLASS as well as the higher costs of SGAs. Therefore, PCPs must be aware of the increased possibility of physical motor disorders associated with the FGAs, as they are a common medical finding among patients with SPMI and a serious factor in nonadherence to medication. The disorders can also result in psychosocial and occupational dysfunction. Although the FGAs are known for a higher incidence of movement disorder

Text continues on page 278.

Table 8.3 • Antipsychotics Currently Available in the United States

Medication Class	Medication	Year Approved by FDA	Usual Effective Dose	Monthly Cost*
Dopamine (D2) antagonists (high potency)	Perphenazine (Trilafon†)	1957	16 mg bid	$83–$93
	Trifluoperazine (Stelazine†)	1959	6 mg bid	$150–$234
	Fluphenazine (Prolixin†)	1960	2.5 mg bid	$45–$54
	Haloperidol (Haldol	1967	5 mg tid	$9–$88
	Thiothixene (Navane)	1967	10 mg tid	$37–$60 (generic)
	Fluphenazine decanoate (Prolixin Decanoate†)	1972	25 mg IM q3wk	$5–$15
	Haloperidol decanoate (Haldol Decanoate)	1986	100 mg IM q4wk	$19–$53 (generic)
Dopamine (D2) antagonist (mid potency)	Molindone (Moban)	1974	25 mg tid	$271
	Loxapine (Loxitane)	1975	50 mg bid	$154 (generic)
Dopamine (D2) antagonists (low potency)	Chlorpromazine (Thorazine†)	1957	100 mg tid	$6–$103
	Thioridazine (Mellaril†)	1962	100 mg tid	$15–$62
Atypical (mixed neuroreceptor antagonists [low affinity D2 antagonists, high-affinity 5 HT2A antagonists])				
	Clozapine (Clozaril)	1989	125 mg bid	$407 (brand); $266–$284 (generic)
	Risperidone (Risperdal)	1993	4 mg × 1 daily	$317
	Olanzapine (Zyprexa)	1996	10 mg × 1 daily	$353
	Quetiapine (Seroquel)	1997	200 mg bid	$397
	Ziprasidone (Geodon)	2001	40 mg bid	$315
	Aripiprazole (Abilify)	2002	20 mg × 1 daily	$490

*Estimated cost to pharmacist: Medical Economics (2006). These costs are based on 2006 data and may be significantly different by the time of publication.

†Brand no longer available in the United States.

From Schultz, S.H., North, S.W., & Shields, C.G. (2007). Schizophrenia; A review. *American Family Physician, 75*(12), 1821–1829.

Table 8.4 • Summary of Side Effects of Atypical Antipsychotics*

Antipsychotic Medication	Extrapyramidal Symptoms/ Tardive Dyskinesia (EPS/TD)	Prolactin	Weight (Wt.)	Glucose	Lipids	Sedation	Hypotension	Anticholinergic
Clozapine (Clozaril)	o	o	+++	+++	+++	+++	+++	+++
Risperidone (Risperdal)	+	+++	++	++	++	+	+	oo
Olanzapine (Zyprexa)	o	o	+++	+++	+++	+	+	++
Quetiapine (Seroquel)	o	o	++	++	++	++	++	o
Ziprasidone (Geodon)	o	+	o	o	o	o	o	o
Aripiprazole (Abilify)	o	o	o	o	o	+	o	o

o, no risk or rarely causes side effects at therapeutic doses; +, mild or occasionally causes side effects at therapeutic doses; ++, sometimes causes side effects at therapeutic doses; +++, frequently causes side effects at therapeutic doses.

From Lehman, A.F., Lieberman, J. A., & Dixon, L. B. (2004). Practice guidelines for the treatment of patients with schizophrenia (2nd ed.). *American Journal of Psychiatry, 161*(Suppl 2), 63–72.

Table 8.5 • Recommended Doses for Atypical Antipsychotics

Antipsychotic Medications	Half-Life (hr) (Mean)	Starting Dose (Total mg/day)	Average Dose Range 1st Episode	Average Dose Range Recurrent Episode	Average Maintenance Dose (mg/day)	Routes of Administration
Clozapine (Clozaril)	10-105 (16)	25-50	150-300	400-600	400	Oral
Risperidone (Risperdal)	3-24 (15)	1-2	2-4	3-6	3-6	Oral, depot
Olanzapine (Zyprexa)	20-70 (30)	5-10	10-20	15-30	10-20	Oral, IM
Quetiapine (Seroquel)	4-10 (7)	50-100	300-600	500-800	400-800	Oral
Zyprasidone (Geodon)	4-10	40-80	80-120	120-200	120-160	Oral, IM
Aripiprazole (Abilify)	(75-96)	10-15	10-30	15-30	15-30	Oral

From Lieberman, J. A., & Tasman, A. (2006). *Handbook of psychiatric drugs.* West Sussex, England: John Wiley and Sons Ltd.
Source: Adapted from Lieberman & Tasman, 2006.

than the SGAs, among the the SGAs, risperidone has a mild potential to cause movement disorders.

Typically, movement disorders occur in the first days or weeks when medication is begun with exception of tardive dyskinesia, which can occur months or years after the initiation of antipsychotic medication. A useful tool to monitor tardive dyskinesia is the Abnormal Involuntary Movement Scale, which can be accessed at *http://www.atlantapsychiatry.com/forms/AIMS.pdf*. The neuroleptic-induced motor disorders include the following (APA, 2000; Schultz et al., 2007):

- *Tardive dyskinesia*. A chronic nervous system disorder distinguished by involuntary jerking movements of the face, tongue, jaw, and extremities. The prevalence in persons on long-term neuroleptics is approximately 20 to 30 percent, with no gender differences except for a possible increase in menopausal women. Symptoms must persist for at least a month for diagnosis. Symptoms may be worse on withdrawal, and treatment is not satisfactory. Prevention is the focus particularly using lowest possible dose of psychotropic medication.
- *Neuroleptic-induced parkinsonism*. Includes a coarse tremor, shuffling gait, muscular rigidity (cogwheel or leadpipe), and akinesia (a decrease in spontaneous facial and body movements). Treatment consists of antiparkinsonian medications.
- *Acute dystonia*. Painful muscle spasms that may involve the tongue, face, neck, and back; they usually occur early in administration of medication. Treatment is antiparkinsonian medications, which are both diagnostic and effective.
- *Akathisia*. Motor restlessness as evidenced by pacing, foot swinging, rocking movements, and inability to sit or stand still for a few minutes. Patients will report feelings of restlessness. Treatment consists of reducing or changing medication and using antiparkinsonian medications. Propanolol (Inderal) or benzodiazepines (e.g., Valium) may be useful.
- *Neuroleptic malignant syndrome (NMS)*. A serious medical response to psychotropic medication requiring emergency room treatment. Usually, the patient has a complete recovery from NMS but in a few cases can be fatal. NMS is characterized by severe muscle rigidity and an elevated temperature. The NMS diagnosis requires at least two symptoms among the following: diaphoresis, dysphagia, tremor, incontinence, tachycardia, labile blood pressure, and changes in the level of

consciousness. Laboratory data indicate leukocytosis and an elevated creatine level. Treatment consists of immediately discontinuing the medication and administering dantrolene (Dantrium) or bromocriptine (Parlodel).

Switching Antipsychotic Medications

The main reason for switching antipsychotic medication is the lack of efficacy, but one cannot be certain that improved efficacy will result with a new medication. Therefore, the change requires frank discussion with the patient and a careful weighing of the risks and benefits. The other main reason for switching antipsychotic medications is adverse effects. These include all of the side effects identified in Table 8.4. However, switching itself can cause a multitude of problems, including dopamine psychosis and cholinergic rebound. When switching from a more sedating antipsychotic to a less sedating one, rebound activation (insomnia) may occur. In the past, it was common practice to quickly discontinue one medication and immediately begin the second. Today, it is clear that most switch-emergent adverse events can be significantly reduced if a gradual cross-taper method of switching is used (Buckley, 2007).

The dopaminergic, muscarinic, and histaminic tracts are associated with adverse effects that may require switching medications. They are also associated with withdrawal-emergent adverse effects. Antipsychotics with high dopamine D2 affinity can result in EPS and high prolactin levels (hyperprolactinemia). Antipsychotics with affinity for muscarinic receptors may trigger adverse effects related to cognition, memory, motor activity, and sleep. Finally, antipsychotics with a high affinity for histamine (H1) will generally induce more weight gain, type 2 diabetes, and sedative effects. Therefore, it is very helpful to consider the receptor-binding profiles of antipsychotics that are involved in the switch in order to minimize adverse effects and optimize the transition (Buckley, 2007).

Many medication switches fail because of poor planning and lack of consideration for the impact of withdrawal symptoms. Because of a high risk for withdrawal symptoms, Lambert (2007) recommends using the *abrupt switch* only when the patient's side effects are severe. Patients need close monitoring with this type of switch.

The *gradual cross-taper switch* involves an immediate but gradual taper of the initial antipsychotic agent over 2 weeks while gradually increasing the new medication. This method carries a low risk of adverse withdrawal effects but a higher risk of relapse because the patient has a longer period of time on subtherapeutic doses of the new medication. The *cross-taper switch* involves decreasing the initial medication over *N* [a determined number of] weeks while simultaneously increasing the new medication over *N* days. This is the most commonly used method of switching and seems to be the safest way to prevent relapse (Lambert, 2007).

Psychosocial Treatments

Many psychosocial treatments with strong research support exist for schizophrenia and other severe mental illnesses. These include cognitive behavioral therapy (CBT), self-management training, family psychoeducation, family group therapy, assertive community treatment (ACT), skills training, vocational rehabilitation, and self-help groups. Psychosocial treatments are critical once the patient's psychotic symptoms abate and the patient becomes stable on medication. In recent years, treatment has focused more on rehabilitation. This approach requires commitment, trained professionals, and support of the community.

Weight Control

Because persons with SPMI often do not have nutritional options and many of their medications promote weight gain, PCPs must educate and support weight control efforts. Patients who do not have the financial option of eating more fruits and vegetables can avoid fatty foods, learn to eat smaller portions, and develop a daily routine of exercise.

Because they may have minimal social support systems, patients with SPMI need assistance in identifying potential new support systems. Often, they have access to churches, social agencies, and self-help groups that are welcoming and supportive. Some organizations may offer nutrition and exercise classes. Increasing socialization and decreasing isolation can be an important factor in improving self-esteem and, ultimately, the motivation for self-improvement and health.

Cognitive Behavioral Therapy

In the past, mental health professionals believed that patients with schizophrenia and other SPMIs could not benefit from CBT. However, in recent years, research studies reported positive outcomes with CBT for patients with schizophrenia, bipolar disorder, and major depression (Butler, Chapman, Forman, et al., 2006). In a meta-analysis, Rector and Beck (2001) reported that CBT improved both negative and positive symptoms of schizophrenia. Most of the schizophrenia studies were conducted in the United Kingdom and included treatment-resistant patients (Temple & Ho, 2005; Turkington, Kingdon, and Weiden, 2006). While CBT is effective, it is not used often because of a lack of professionals with the needed preparation and skills. Beck (2005) recommends that CBT be taught to nurses and other health care professionals because of its great potential to address myriad mental health disorders. Beck offers a three-tiered, graded training program in which professionals can progress from one level to another as desired.

Family Therapy

Family therapy can be conducted with groups of families or with a single family. This modality is highly effective in educating and supporting families with members who have SPMI. Research indicates that people with schizophrenia are very sensitive to environments that are rejecting, highly emotional, critical, and overly involved. Family therapy can be very productive in addressing these issues. Research studies examining outcomes of family interventions have documented a reduction in relapse rates and improvement in symptoms (Huxley, Rendall, and Sederer, 2000).

Community-Based Treatment Programs

Community-based treatment programs, also known as intensive case management, continuous treatment teams, and programs for ACT, have been quite successful in supporting high-risk patients and preventing relapse and rehospitalization. They also reduce arrests, homelessness, and emergency room visits. Although ACT programs are expensive, they are cost-effective. The ACT program consists of an interdisciplinary team of mental health professionals who work closely together to deliver services to patients in their own settings.

The treatment focus is on rehabilitation and services both for the patients and their families. Services include medications, housing, food, clothing, basic living skills, and vocational training. The ACT program has demonstrated its effectiveness with extensive research for the past 20 years. It has become a model for comprehensive treatment for people with SPMI and is strongly supported by the National Alliance for the Mentally Ill (NAMI) and other mental health advocacy agencies.

Another provider resource is the series of nine modules developed by Dr. Robert Lieberman of UCLA. The modules are focused on daily living challenges, including symptom control and medications. The modules were developed for professional use in a small group format and include a series of learning activities that correspond to each module. The modules can be found at *www.psychrehab.com/*. Clubhouses are a variation on the rehabilitation model. While the ACT programs are provider based, the clubhouse model was originally developed as a self-help organization and remains member rather than provider focused. Some other mutual support groups are based on the 12-step model. Refer to the Resources for Patients section for websites.

The National Alliance for the Mentally Ill

NAMI is best known as a support organization for families of people with SPMI. Local chapters offer a free 12-week Family-to-Family education program that is conducted by families for families.

THE QUESTION OF RECOVERY

In the past, most clinicians would agree that full recovery from severe mental illness was unlikely. But recently, multiple studies have demonstrated that with treatment, one half to two thirds of people with SPMI significantly improve and/or recover (Ciompi, 1988; Fisher, 2006; Harding, 2003; Harding and Zahniser, 1994). These researchers define complete recovery as being free of symptoms of mental illness, being medication free, living independently, working and being able to relate to others, and not being noticed for odd or unusual behavior. Fisher emphasizes that recovery is not synonymous with remission or rehabilitation.

Fisher (2006), a psychiatrist who had been diagnosed as schizophrenic, has studied recoveries of others as well as his own and is a member of the White House New Freedom Commission on Mental Health and executive director of the National Empowerment Center (NEC). The Commission is very positive, and its vision statement foresees a future when all people with a mental illness will recover. This organization's main goal is to transform the mental health system from one that is currently maintenance and symptom reducing to a recovery-oriented approach that is consumer and family focused. The Commission also recommends that consumers and families be actively involved in mental health training, policy development, service evaluation, and service delivery. The Commission distinguishes between recovery and rehabilitation versus remission. Remission refers to the absence of symptoms, and rehabilitation refers to improvement in functioning; however, with both of these concepts, the person remains mentally ill. In contrast, recovery involves regaining a full life. The Commission claims that recovery entails not just the mental illness itself but emancipation from the role of the consumer of the mental health system.

The NEC has been studying people who have recovered from severe mental illness and has published two qualitative studies that focus on major principles of how people recover. These principles include trusting self and others and valuing self-determination as well as having a belief in one's potential and recovery. The

Center also emphasized the critical importance of connecting with another human on a deep emotional level so that one's feelings and thoughts are validated. This requires being treated with dignity and respect. Finally, having life goals and a sense of purpose are also critical to recovery. Based on the outcomes of these qualitative studies, the NEC has developed a model that describes how people become severely mentally ill and how they recover (Fisher, 2006).

The NEC has also developed the Personal Assistance in Community Existence (PACE) educational program in the hope that it will facilitate the transformation of the mental health culture from institutional thinking to recovery thinking (Ahern and Fisher, 2001a; Ahern and Fisher, 2001b).

CONCLUSION

Providing mental and medical health services to patients with SMI and SPMI in primary care practice is a great challenge to PCPs. Furthermore, this challenge extends beyond the person with the mental illness to the families who are also suffering from the impact of the disease and require education and support. Despite significant improvements in medications and psychosocial treatments, many patients with SMI and SPMI are not being diagnosed and treated for their diseases, while some remain treatment resistant. PCPs are in a position to significantly impact the care of the SMI because of their access to them and the potential to make a diagnosis, begin early treatment, and support the patient and family. PCPs can also connect the patient and her family to community resources, particularly those that provide psychosocial interventions. Research demonstrates that medications and psychosocial interventions must be integrated for optimal success in the treatment of people with SMI and SPMI. Although much more research is needed to address the needs of the treatment-resistant patient, PCPs can make a difference for many patients who otherwise may never be diagnosed and treated.

Resources for Patients

American Academy of Family Physicians: *http://familydoctor.org*

Depression and Bipolar Support Alliance: *www.dbsalliance.org*

Emotions Anonymous: *www.emotionsanonymous.org*

International Center for Clubhouse Development: *www.iccd.org/default.asp*

National Alliance on Mental Illness: *www.nami.org*

National Empowerment Center: *www.medscape.com/viewarticle/496394*

Recovery, Inc.: *www.recovery-inc.com*

Recovery Circles: *www.recoverycircles.org*

Schizophrenics Anonymous: *www.sanonymous.com*

References

ADA/APA Consensus Conference. (2004). *Diabetes Care, 27*, 596–601.

Ahern, L., & Fisher, D. (2001a). Recovery at your own PACE (Personal Assistance in Community Existence). *Journal of Psychosocial Nursing and Mental Health Services, 39*, 22–32.

Ahern, L., & Fisher, D. (2001b). *PACE/Recovery Curriculum*. National Empowerment Center, Inc., Lawrence, MA. Retrieved July 8, 2007, from *www.power2u.org*.

Allen, M. H. (2005). Considering consumer choice during management of behavioral emergencies. Management of behavioral emergencies and the use of atypical antipsychotics. *The Postgraduate Institute of Medicine*. Retrieved August 30, 2007, from *www.medscape.com/viewprogram/4733_pnt.*

American Psychiatric Association. (1994). *Diagnostic and statistical manual of mental disorders* (4th ed.). Washington, DC: Author.

American Psychiatric Association. (2000). *Diagnostic and statistical manual of mental disorders* (Revised 4th ed.). Washington, DC: Author.

Bazelon Center for Mental Health Law. Fact sheet #1: Criminal justice system involvement of people with serious mental illness. Retrieved August 9, 2007, from *www.bazelon.org/decrim.html.*

Beck, A. T. (2005). The current state of cognitive therapy: A 40-year retrospective. *Archives of General Psychiatry, 62*, 953–959.

Brady, N., & McCain, G. C. (2005). Living with schizophrenia: A family perspective. *Online Journal of Issues in Nursing, 10*(1). Retrieved July 6, 2007, from *www.medscape.com/viewarticle/ 499269_print.*

Buckley, P. (2005). Atypical antipsychotics for acute stabilization of agitation and beyond: Implications for long-term. Management of behavioral emergencies and the use of atypical antipsychotics. *The Postgraduate Institute of Medicine*. Retrieved August 30, 2007, from *www. medscape.com/viewprogram/4733_pnt.*

Buckley, P. F. (2007). The art and science of switching antipsychotic medications. *Journal of Clinical Psychiatry, 68*(Suppl 6), 4–9.

Butler, A. C., Chapman, J. E., Forman, E. M., et al. (2006). The empirical status of cognitive-behavioral therapy: A review of meta-analyses. *Clinical Psychology Review, 26*, 17–31.

Cahn, W., Hulshoff Pol, H. E., Lems, E. B., et al. (2002). Brain volume changes in first-episode schizophrenia: A 1-year follow-up study. *Archives of General Psychiatry, 59*, 1002–1010.

Ciompi, L. (1988). *Psyche and schizophrenia*. Cambridge, MA: Harvard University Press,

Conley, R. R., & Newcomer, J. W. (2007). Weight gain with the atypicals: How to screen, monitor and intervene. *Neuroscience CME*. Retrieved August 30, 2007, from *http://www.neurosciencecme. comcmea.asp?ID=217&email=true*.

Daumit, G. L., Clark, J. M., Steinwachs, D. M., et al. (2003). Prevalence and correlates of obesity in a community sample of individuals with severe and persistent mental illness. *Journal of Nervous Mental Disorders, 191*(12), 799–805.

Epstein, J., Barker, P., Vorburger, M., et al. (2002). Serious mental illness and its co-occurrence with substance use disorders, 2002. *SAMHSA, Office of Applied Studies*. Retrieved August 12, 2007, from *www.oas.samhsa.gov/CoD/CoD.htm*.

Essock, S. M. (2006). Enhancing generalizability: Stepping up to the plate. *Psychiatric Services, 57*, 141.

Essock, S. M., Covell, N. H., Davis, S. M., et al. (2006). Effectiveness of switching antipsychotic medications. *American Journal of Psychiatry, 163*, 2090–2095.

Fisher, D. (2006). *Recovery from schizophrenia: From seclusion to empowerment*. Retrieved July 6, 2007, from *www.medscape.com/viewprogram/5097_pnt*.

Friedman, S. H., Sajatovic, M., Schuermeyer, I. N., et al. (2005). Menopause-related quality of life in chronically mentally ill women. *International Journal of Psychiatric Medicine, 35*(3), 259–271.

Geddes, J., Freemantle, N., Harrison, P., et al. (2000). Atypical antipsychotics in the treatment of schizophrenia: A systematic overview and meta-regression analysis. *British Medical Journal, 321*, 1371–1376.

Halbreich, U., Shen, J. , & Panaro, V. (1996). Are chronic psychiatric patients at increased risk for developing breast cancer? *American Journal of Psychiatry, 153*(4), 559–560.

Harding, C. (2003). Changes in schizophrenia across time. In C. Cohen (Ed.), *Schizophrenia into later life*. Washington, DC: American Psychiatric Association (pp. 19–42).

Harding, C. M., & Zahniser, J. H. (1994). Empirical correction of seven myths about schizophrenia with implications for treatment for serious mental illness. *Acta Psychiatrica Scandinavica, 90*, 140–148.

Hoffman, V. P., Ahl, J., Meyers, A., et al. (2005). Wellness intervention for patients with serious and persistent mental illness. *Journal of Clinical Psychiatry, 66*(12), 1576–1579.

Huxley, N. A., Rendall, M., & Sederer, L. (2000). Psychosocial treatments in schizophrenia: A review of the past 20 years. *Journal of Nervous Mental Disorders, 188*, 187–201.

Jackson, W. C. (2006). Schizophrenia in the era of Medicare Part D. *Consultations in Primary Care Supplement, 46*(7), 1–36.

Jones, P. B., Barnes, T. R. E., & Davies, L. (2006). Randomized controlled trial of the effect on quality of life of second- vs first-generation antipsychotic drugs in schizophrenia: Cost utility of the latest antipsychotic drugs in schizophrenia study (CUtLASS I). *Archives of General Psychiatry, 63*, 1079–1087.

Kalichman S., Malow R., Devieux J.A., et al. (2005). HIV risk reduction for substance using seriously mentally ill adults: Test of the information-Motivation-Behavior Skills (IMB) Model. *Community Mental Health Journal, 41*, 277–290.

Lamb, H. R., Weinberger, L. E., & Gross, B. H. (2004). Mentally ill persons in the criminal justice system: Some perspectives. *Psychiatric Quarterly, 75*(2), 107–126.

Lambert, T. (2007). Switching antipsychotic therapy: What to expect and clinical strategies for improving therapeutic outcomes. *Journal of Clinical Psychiatry, 68*(Suppl 6), 10–13.

Lehman, A. F., Lieberman, J. A., & Dixon, L. B. (2004). Practice guidelines for the treatment of patients with schizophrenia (2nd ed.). *American Journal of Psychiatry, 161*(Suppl 2), 63–72.

Lieberman, J. A. (2006). Interpreting the results of the CATIE study. *Psychiatric Services, 57*, 139.

Lieberman, J. A., Stroup, T. S., McEvoy, J. P., et al. (2005). Effectiveness of antipsychotic drugs in patients with chronic schizophrenia. *New England Journal of Medicine, 353*, 1209–1223.

Lieberman, J. A., & Tasman, A. (2006). *Handbook of psychiatric drugs*. West Sussex, England: John Wiley and Sons Ltd.

Lieberman, J. A., Tollefson, G. D., Cecil, C., et al. (2005). Antipsychotic drug effects on brain morphology in first-episode psychosis. *Archives of General Psychiatry, 62*, 361–370.

Mechanic, D. (2002). Removing barriers to care among persons with psychiatric symptoms. *Health Affairs, 21*, 137–147.

Medical Economics. (2006). *The red book*. Montvale, NJ: Medical Economics Data.

Meltzer, H. Y., & Bobo, W. V. (2006). Interpreting the efficacy findings in the CATIE study: What clinicians should know. *CNS Spectrum, 11*(7 Suppl 7), 14–24.

Minsky, S., Vega, W., Miskimen, T., et al. (2003). Diagnostic patterns in Latino, African American, and European American psychiatric patients. *Archives of General Psychiatry, 60*, 637–644.

Molina, V. (2005). Structural effects of atypical antipsychotics: Implications for the meaning of cortical volume deficit in schizophrenia. *European Journal of Psychiatry, 19*. Retrieved August 3, 2007, from *http://scielo.isciii.es/scielo.php?pid=S0213-61632005000400004&script=sci_arttext.*

Nagy, M. (2007). What is the latest scoop on typical vs atypical antipsychotics? *Medscape Psychiatry and Mental Health*. Retrieved August 1, 2007, from *www.medscape.com/view/article/548208.*

Nasrallah, H. A., & White, R. F. (2006). Treatment resistant schizophrenia. *Medscape CME/CE.* Retrieved July 5, 2007, from *www.medscape.com/viewprogram/5464_pnt.*

Nemeroff, C., Conley, R. R., & Newcomer, J. W. (2007). Weight gain with the atypicals: How to screen, monitor, and intervene. *Neuroscience CME activities*. Retrieved March 30, 2007, from *www.neurosciencecme.com/cmea.asp?ID=217&email=true.*

Newcomer, J. J., Buckley, P. F., & Correll, C. U. (2007). Metabolic considerations in the treatment of schizophrenia. *PsychForum-Round Series*. Retrieved July 11, 2007, from *www.medscape.com/viewprogram/7352_pnt.*

Perese, E. F., & Perese, K. (2003). Health problems of women with severe mental illness. *Journal of American Academy of Nurse Practitioners, 15*(5), 212–218.

Pomerantz, J. M. (1999). Behavioral health matters: Managed care's treatment of chronic and relapsing disease. *Drug Benefit Trends, 11*, 2–5.

Pomerantz, J. M. (2006). Difficulties in treating schizophrenia. *Consultant, 46*(Suppl), 6–14.

Randolph, M. E., Pinkerton, S. D., Somlai, A. M., et al. (2007). Severely mentally ill women's HIV risk: The influence of social support, substance use, and contextual risk factor. *Community Mental Health, 43*(1), 33–47.

Rector, N. A., & Beck, A. T. (2001). Cogitive behavioral therapy for schizophrenia: An empirical review. *Journal of Nervous Mental Disorders, 189*, 278–287.

Riecher-Rossler, A. (2004). Schizophrenia in women. *Medscape and 2nd World Congress on Women's Mental Health*. Retrieved July 27, 2007, from *www.medscape.com/viewarticle/473295.*

Schinnar, S., Rothbard, A., Kanter, R., et al. (1990). An empirical literature review of definitions of severe and persistent mental illness. *American Journal of Psychiatry, 147*, 1602–1608.

Schultz, S. H., North, S. W., & Shields, C. G. (2007). Schizophrenia: A review. *American Family Physician, 75*(12), 1821–1829.

Seeman, M. (2000). Women and schizophrenia. *Medscape General Medicine, 2*(2). Retrieved January 17, 2007, from *www.medscape.com/viewarticle/308915.*

Seeman, M. V. (2002). Single-sex psychiatric services to protect woman. *Medscape General Medicine, 4*(3). Retrieved July 6, 2007, from *www.medscape.com/viewarticle/440095_print.*

Spollen, J. J. (2003). Perspectives in serious mental illness. *Medscape Psychiatry and Mental Health, 8*(1). Retrieved January 16, 2007, from *www.medscape.com?viewarticle/455449_print.*

Strakowski, S. M., Keck, P. E., & Arnold, L. M. (2003). Ethnicity and diagnosis in patients with affective disorders. *Journal of Clinical Psychiatry, 64*, 747–754.

Temple, S., & Ho, B. (2005). Cognitive therapy for persistent psychosis in schizophrenia: A case controlled clinical trial. *Schizophrenia Research, 74*, 195–199.

Tienari, P., Wynne, L. C., Sorri, A., et al. (2004). Genotype-environment interaction in schizophrenia-spectrum disorder. Long-term follow-up study of Finnish adoptees. *British Journal of Psychiatry, 184*, 216–222.

Treisman, G. J. (2007). Adherence, psychiatric disorders and HIV. *Medscape CME/CE.* Retrieved August 12, 2007, from *www.medscape.com/viewprogram/6727_pnt.*

Turkington, D., Kingdon, D., & Weiden, P. J. (2006). Cognitive therapy for schizophrenia. *American Journal of Psychiatry, 163*, 365–373.

U.S. Department of Health and Human Services (HDDS). (1999). *Mental health: A report of the Surgeon General—Executive Summary.* Rockville, MD: Substance Abuse and Mental Health Services Administration, Center for Mental Health Services, National Institute of Mental Health. Retrieved May 12, 2007, from *www.surgeongeneral.gov/library/mentalhealth/chapter2/sec2_1.html.*

U.S. Department of Health and Human Services (HDDS). (2001). *Mental health: Culture, race, and ethnicity. A supplement to mental health: A report of the surgeon general.* Rockville, MD: Substance Abuse and Mental Health Services Administration, Center for Mental Health Services, National Institute of Mental Health. Retrieved July 5, 2007, from *www.surgeongeneral.gov/library/mentalhealth/cre/execsummary-1.html.*

Wahlberg, K. E., Wynne, L. C., Hakko, H., et al. (2004). Interaction of genetic risk and adoptive parent communication deviance: Longitudinal prediction of adoptee psychiatric disorders. *Psychological Medicine, 34*, 1531–1541.

Wang, P. S., Berglund, P., & Kessler, R. C. (2000). Recent care of common mental disorders in the United States. Prevalence and conformance with evidenced-based recommendations. *Journal of General Internal Medicine, 15*(5), 284–292.

Wang, P. S., Demler, O., & Kessler, R. C. (2002). Adequacy of treatment for serious mental illness in the United States. *American Journal of Public Health, 92*, 92–98.

Weiden, P. J., & Buckley, P. F. (2007). Reducing the burden of side effects during long-term antipsychotic therapy: The role of switching medications. *Journal of Clinical Psychiatry, 68* (Suppl 6), 14–23.

World Health Organization (WHO). (1999). *World health report 1999—Making a difference.* Retrieved July 6, 2007, from *www.who.int/whr/1999/en/index.html.*

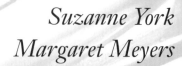

Suzanne York
Margaret Meyers

chapter 9

Chronic Diseases and Depression

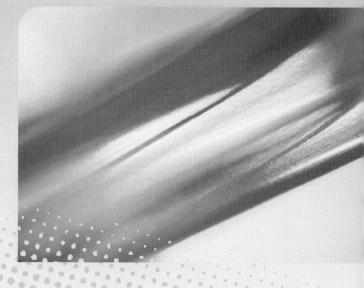

The relationship between chronic disease and depression is complex and one that we are only beginning to understand. Evidence suggests that chronic disease predisposes people to depression, and depression predisposes people to certain chronic diseases. Furthermore, treatment of chronic disease may influence the risk for and course of depression, while treatment of depression can influence the risk for and course of chronic disease.

In women more than in men, depression appears to be a stronger predictor of chronic disease (Table 9.1). One example of this is that some data suggest that depression is implicated in osteoporosis, which affects women at a much greater rate than men. A study by Misra, Papakostas, and Klibanski (2004) indicated that patients diagnosed with depression should be monitored for the development of bone thinning.

Finally, medications used to treat one disorder can interact with medications for the other. In this chapter, we will discuss the relationship of depression to chronic diseases such as cardiovascular disease (CVD), diabetes, cancer, and chronic pain syndromes.

ASSOCIATION BETWEEN CHRONIC DISEASE AND DEPRESSION

There is a strong, well-documented association between chronic disease and depression (Gagnon and Patten, 2002; Patten, Beck, Kassam, et al., 2005). Chronic illnesses predispose people to depression because of the subsequent disability as well as the disease process itself. Cancer, stroke, heart conditions, chronic obstructive pulmonary disease, diabetes mellitus, hypertension, and arthritis all substantially increase depressive symptoms (Brown, Majumdar, Newman, et al., 2006; Schnittker, 2005).

Chronic Disease Predisposes to Depression

As the number of comorbid illnesses increase, so do the rates of depression and decreased functional status (Charlson and Peterson, 2002). Therefore, a history of chronic disease should increase the suspicion of depression by the primary care provider (PCP) in those presenting with symptoms and also increase the screening of asymptomatic individuals. In the absence of depression, chronic disease is also implicated in worsening existing suicidal ideation (Goodwin, Kroenke, Hoven, et al., 2003). Therefore, asking about suicidal ideation, even in the absence of diagnosed depression, is important.

Table 9.1 • Gender Differences in the Relationship of Depression to Chronic Disease

Chronic Disease	Findings: Women	Findings: Men	Citation
Cancer	Depression associated with cancer	Depression only associated if had feeling of hopelessness	Schnieder & Chiriboga (2005)
	Major depression only associated with breast cancer	Major depression not associated with cancer	Gallo, Armenian, Ford, et al. (2000)
	Increased markers of cancer-related oxidative DNA damage related to depression	Increased markers of cancer-related oxidative DNA damage NOT related to depression (related to other measures)	Irie, Asami, Nagata, et al. (2001)
Metabolic syndrome (precursor to diabetes)	Metabolic syndrome twice as likely if had history of major depression	No significant difference	Kinder, Carnethon, Palaniappan, et al. (2004)
Diabetic complications (peripheral neuropathy)	Correlation at higher depression scores	No significant difference	Geringer, Perlmuter, Stern, et al. (1988)
Cardiovascular disease	Those with coronary artery disease (CAD) and a history of major depression were more likely to be female, have higher depression scores, and be younger	Those with CAD and a history of major depression were less likely to be male	Freedland, Carney, Lustman, et al. (1992)

The main mediators for chronic disease contributing to depression appear to be the severity of disability and symptoms related to the chronic disease (Gottlieb, Khatta, Friedman, et al., 2004; Ludman, Kato, Russo, et al., 2004). In heart failure, for example, social factors and health status, but not severity of disease, are predictive of depression (Havranek, Spertus, Masoudi, et al., 2004). In diabetic neuropathy, those symptoms that were perceived as being unpredictable, restricting activities of daily living (ADLs), and changing social self-perception contributed more to depression (Vileikyte, Leventhal, Gonzalez, et al., 2005). Additionally, those who develop illnesses earlier in life have more depressive symptoms (Gottlieb et al.; Okamura, Yamawaki, Akechi, et al., 2005) than those who do not.

There is also evidence that some diseases have a direct effect on causing depression. Stroke and cerebrovascular disease appear to have a causative role in depression that is only partially explained by the level of disability and symptoms. Prospective studies show that those with risk factors for cerebrovascular disease or documented lesions in the basal ganglia on magnetic resonance imaging have greater rates of depression (Kim, Stewart, Kim, et al., 2006; Mast, Yochim, MacNeill, et al., 2004; Whyte, Mulsant, Vanderbilt, et al., 2004). These physical changes in the brain could cause neurochemical changes that are the basis for the development of depression. In diabetes, a lower serotonin synthesis rate was seen in children with type 1 diabetes compared with children without diabetes (Manjarrez, Herrera, Leon, et al., 2006).

Depression Predisposes to Chronic Disease

Depression increases the risk of developing certain chronic illnesses such as myocardial infarction (MI), cerebrovascular disease, diabetes, cancer, and chronic pain. In addition, depression has been implicated in increasing the risk of heart failure (Abramson, Berger, Krumholz, et al., 2001) and Alzheimer's disease (Steffens, Plassman, Helms, et al., 1997).

The mechanisms for these effects are both behavioral/psychological and physiologic. In the behavioral/psychological realm, depression increases chronic disease by decreasing adherence to treatment regimens and exercise and increasing smoking, obesity, and alcohol use. In the physical realm, depression increases platelet activity, inflammatory markers, and cortisol as well as alters autonomic nervous system tone and immune function.

Interestingly, depression does not appear to cause a delay in seeking treatment or change patient decision making regarding treatment (Rozniatowski, Reich, Mallet, et al., 2005). However, symptom reporting may differ based on depression. In fact, in diabetics, symptom reporting appears to have more to do with depressive symptoms than with blood sugar control.

CHALLENGES OF DRUG TREATMENTS FOR CHRONIC DISEASE AND DEPRESSION

Medications given for chronic medical illnesses may cause depression, although less than was previously believed (Kotlyar, Dysken, and Adson, 2005; Patten and Lavorato, 2001).

Influence of Chronic Disease Medications on Depression

A number of medications have been associated with depression or depressive symptoms, including doxorubicin/cyclophosphamide (Okamura et al., 2005), sedative-hypnotics (Patten, Williams, and Love, 1996), and opioid analgesics (Patten and Lavorato, 2001). Patients on corticosteroid therapy have more depressive symptoms, especially those who have a personal or family history of depression (Patten, 2000).

Evidence for an association between depression and calcium channel blockers (Patten and Lavorato, 2001) and angiotensin-converting enzyme (ACE) inhibitors (Patten, Williams, and Love, 1996) is mixed.

Moreover, a literature review by Patten and Barbui (2004) found that certain medications caused or were associated with depressive symptoms, but there was no evidence that the studied medications caused major depression (Box 9.1).

Box 9-1 • Medications as Causative Agents of Depressive Symptoms
Corticosteroids
Contraceptive implants
Gonadotropin-releasing hormone agonists
Histamine-2 blockers
HMG-CoA reductase inhibitors
Interferon alpha and beta
Interleukin-2
Mefloquine
Tamoxifen

Medications as Causes of Depressive Symptoms

Information on how medications cause depressive symptoms is sparse. Some studies indicate that medications such as corticosteroids, the interferons, and tamoxifen have a relationship to depressive symptoms. For example, corticosteroids may increase memories of stressful experiences and therefore increase depressive symptoms (Peeters and Broekkamp, 1994). There appears to be a predisposition in some patients to depression from interferon (Capuron, Raison, Musselman, et al., 2003) associated with an exaggerated hypothalamic-pituitary-adrenal (HPA) response to the administration of interferon alpha. Both interleukin-2 and interferon alpha appear to cause depressive symptoms, possibly because these medications cause a drop in serum tryptophan levels (an amino acid that is a precursor of serotonin) (Capuron, Ravaud, Neveu, et al., 2002). Lower levels of serotonin in the brain are associated with depression. Another drug that may cause depressive symptoms is tamoxifen, which down-regulates serotonin and norepinephrine (Thompson, Spanier, and Vogel, 1999).

Monitoring for depressive symptoms in patients taking these medications is advisable. Whether the depressive symptoms are caused by the medication or only associated with it, these medications become identifiable risk factors for depressive illness.

Benefits of Drug Treatment

There is some evidence that treating depression can help in preventing or controlling chronic diseases. For example, adequately treating depression decreases insulin resistance, which is a precursor to diabetes (Weber-Hamann, Gilles, Lederbogen, et al., 2006), and therefore may decrease the costs associated with diabetes care (Simon, Katon, Lin, et al., 2007). Adherence to antidepressant drug regimens is associated with increased adherence to treatment regimens for comorbid disease and resultant reduced total medical costs (Katon, Cantrell, Sokol, et al., 2005).

Complications and Side Effects of Drug Treatment

There are potential complications associated with antidepressant medications. Table 9.2 lists some of these complications. Consult a *Physicians' Desk Reference* or other reliable reference for a more complete listing of potential complications.

The potential for complications underlines the importance of being familiar with the side effects of specific medications and their ability to cause or

Table 9-2 • Side Effects of Medications Used in Treatment of Depression

Class of Medication (Specific Medication)	Side Effect	Citation
Selective serotonin reuptake inhibitors (paroxetine, sertraline)	Upper gastrointestinal bleeding	Dalton, Sorensen, & Johansen (2006)
	Hepatotoxicity	Carvajal Garcia-Pando, Garcia del Pozo, Sanchez, et al. (2002) Fabian, Amico, Kroboth, et al. (2003)
	Hyponatremia, hypoglycemia	Pollak, Mukherjee, & Fraser (2001)
Tricyclic antidepressants	Hepatotoxicity	Carvajal Garcia-Pando et al.
Lithium as well as certain mood stabilizers and antipsychotics	Changes in bone metabolism and prolactin levels	Misra, Papakostas, & Klibanski (2004)
Atypical antipsychotics	Metabolic syndrome and diabetes mellitus	Newcomer (2007)

exacerbate other problems. It also emphasizes the importance of communication among mental health and PCPs. Additionally important is recognizing that treatment can be further complicated by untoward interactions among multiple medications and nutritional supplements as well—for instance, those mediated by interference with the cytochrome P-450 isoforms (Hemeryck and Belpaire, 2002).

It is wise to obtain a complete list of a patient's medications, including over-the-counter preparations and supplements, and to consult with a pharmacist or current drug reference resource regarding possible interactions.

EFFECTS OF DEPRESSION ON SELECTED COMMON CHRONIC CONDITIONS

Cerebrovascular Disease

Cerebrovascular disease, such as stroke, is associated with increased rates of depression in older adults. In a study by Steffens, Helms, Krishnan, et al. (1999), lesions of the basal ganglia were associated with increased depressive symptoms. In one prospective longitudinal epidemiologic survey, stroke predicted depressive symptoms 2 years later with an odds ratio of 6 to 3 (Whyte et al., 2004). This increased risk of depression could be partially caused by decreases in executive functioning caused by the stroke (Mast et al., 2004). Depression is also an independent risk factor for stroke because it increases the risk of stroke by 2.5 times over 10 to 13 years (Larson, Owens, Ford, et al., 2001).

Cardiovascular Disease

Major depression rates in individuals with a CVD, such as coronary artery disease (CAD), are estimated to be 15 to 23 percent, and most patients with a recent MI or unstable angina along with depression do not receive treatment for their depression (Glassman, O'Connor, Califf, et al., 2002). Because symptoms of depression are often similar to those of the chronic disease, patients are likely to be unaware of their depression because they believe their symptoms are related to the disease. For these reasons, patients with depression associated with CAD are unlikely to be screened or treated for depression (Glassman et al.; Goldstein, 2006).

Depression is also a risk factor for ischemic heart disease, even in those without diagnosed cardiac disease (Goldstein 2006; Lett, Blumenthal, Babyak, et al., 2004; Roose, Glassman, and Seidman, 2001; Wassertheil-Smoller, Shumaker, Ockene, et al., 2004). Patients with a history of depression are four times as likely to have an MI as those without depression (Chapman, Perry, and Strine, 2005). Persons with severe depression are at greater risk for MI and heart failure. They are at greater risk for undergoing balloon angioplasty and coronary artery bypass surgery, and they are twice as likely to develop CAD than those without depression (Gottlieb et al., 2004; Stein, Carney, Freedland, et al., 2000). Although it is more likely for depression to increase the risk of CAD in men rather than women, the Women's Health Initiative Observation Study found that depression is a risk factor for CVD in postmenopausal women who had not been previously diagnosed with CVD (Goldstein, 2006; Wassertheil-Smoller et al., 2004).

Results of a study by Suarez (2006) supported other research that found the risks of CAD and type 2 diabetes are associated with severity of depressive symptoms. Depression also changes responses to stress testing. Patients with higher depression scores develop anginal pain sooner, and this pain has a longer duration on stress testing (Krittayaphong, Light, Golden, et al., 1996). This response appears to be mediated through change in depressed patients' beta-endorphin responses.

Depression also increases mortality in those who experience a cardiac event (Lett et al., 2004; Thomas, 2006). Post-MI patients who are also depressed have more cardiac complications and are at increased risk for death (Chapman, Perry, and Strine, 2005). The Cardiovascular Health Study found that risk for CVD and death increased by 40 to 60 percent in persons with a higher depression score on screening (Goldstein, 2006). This finding was supported in other studies including the Established Populations for the Epidemiologic Studies of the Elderly and the first National Health and Nutrition Examination Survey (NHANES; Goldstein, 2006).

Mechanisms

Several mechanisms may explain the relationship between depression and CVD. Depression decreases adherence to treatment and is related to decreased exercise, increased smoking and alcohol use, nonadherence to medication regimens, and obesity (Lett et al., 2004). These lifestyle factors increase the risk of CVD.

The mechanism of CVD induced by depression may also be related to increased platelet activation (Roose et al., 2001), which has been associated with depression in otherwise healthy people. Antidepressant selective serotonin reuptake inhibitors (SSRIs) may decrease platelet reactivity, thereby reducing the risk for cardiac disease (Goldstein, 2006; Lett et al., 2004). Research has also shown an association between depression and inflammatory markers, such as soluble intercellular adhesion molecule that may affect endothelial function and thereby contribute to CVD (Lesperance, Frasure-Smith, Theroux, et al., 2004).

In a study by Stein, Carney, Freedland, et al. (2000), altered cardiac autonomic tone, a risk factor for mortality in cardiac disease, was found in medically well patients with depression. Increased sympathetic tone and decreased vagal tone raise the risk of ventricular fibrillation (Goldstein, 2006). Moreover, sympathetic nervous system hyperactivity is linked to hypertension (Lett et al., 2004). There is also evidence of increased malignant arrhythmias in patients who have depression (Whang, Albert, Sears, et al., 2005).

Depression is frequently associated with elevated plasma cortisol levels and an imbalance in the HPA axis. HPA axis dysregulation is related to truncal obesity, increased heart rate, hypercholesterolemia, and hypertension, which are additional risk factors for CAD (Lett et al., 2004; Roose et al., 2001).

Treatment

Evidence on the effect of treating depression in CAD is mixed. Studies have not demonstrated a direct relationship between improvement of depressive symptoms and improved morbidity or mortality from cardiac disease (Thomas, 2006;

Wassertheil-Smoller et al., 2004). In the case of coronary artery bypass grafting, studies have not shown a direct relationship between increased death or rehospitalization when patients are on SSRIs before the surgery (Xiong, Jiang, Clare, et al., 2006). However, several studies do show decreased risk of death and reinfarction for those with CAD treated with SSRI antidepressants (Taylor, Youngblood, Catallier, et al., 2005; Writing Committee for the ENRICHD Investigators, 2003).

The SSRIs are the preferred pharmacologic treatment for patients with depression and CVD because of they are not associated with cardiac side effects (Thomas, 2006). The SADHART trial found that the SSRI sertraline (Zoloft) improved scores on measures of depression in post-MI patients with unstable angina (Glassman et al., 2002). Tricyclic antidepressants should be avoided, as studies have shown increased cardiac-related mortality with their use (Thomas, 2006). Nonpharmacologic treatment, such as cognitive behavioral therapy (CBT), also has been shown to have a positive effect on depressive symptoms associated with chronic disease (Lett et al., 2004; Thomas, 2006). In patients with CAD, brief telephone counseling sessions were also found to improve depression (McLaughlin, Aupont, Bambauer, et al., 2005) (Box 9.2).

Box 9.2 • Key Points on Depression and Cardiovascular Disease

- Individuals with cardiovascular disease (CVD) should be screened for depression.
  - As many as 23% of patients with cardiac disease may also be depressed.
- Depression should be considered a risk factor for CVD.
  - Patients with a history of depression are four times as likely to have a myocardial infarction and are twice as likely to develop coronary artery disease.
- Current evidence indicates that selective serotonin reuptake inhibitors (SSRIs) are the preferred pharmacologic treatment for patients with depression and CVD.
  - Tricyclic antidepressants should be avoided, as studies have shown increased cardiac-related mortality with their use.
- In patients with CVD, study findings are mixed regarding a direct relationship between improved mood and better health and longer life.

Diabetes

Depression is more prevalent in persons with diabetes than in the general population. In fact, diabetes doubles the odds of depression, and the odds are higher for women than for men (Anderson, Freedland, Clouse, et al., 2001). Although the causative relationship is not clear, we do know that depression in diabetic patients increases the risk for complications of diabetes, while treatment of depression improves control of blood glucose levels. There appears to be a correlation between depressive scores and elevated hemoglobin A1c (HgbA1c) measures, and diabetic symptoms and complications are more strongly related to depression than to blood glucose levels (Winocour, Main, Medlicott, et al., 1990). In a 2004 study with 4,000 diabetic patients, Ludman, Katon, Russo, et al. (2004) found that those diagnosed with major depression ($N = 487$) reported significantly more diabetes symptoms than participants without depression.

Women with diabetes are significantly more likely to suffer from depression in diabetes than men (Chapman et al., 2005). In a study by Suarez (2006), the greater the severity of depressive symptoms in women, the higher the glucose level, as disclosed by fasting blood glucose tests.

Being diabetic increases the risk of initial diagnosis, recurrence, and duration of depression (Anderson et al., 2001; Lustman, Anderson, Freedland, et al., 2000). Although little research has been done on how psychosocial factors impact the development of depression in people with diabetes, empirical data suggest that factors such as perception of illness intrusiveness, social support, and coping may be mediators. Other mediators appear to be increased disability and decreased functioning as a result of diabetic complications (discussion to follow). However, trials of antihyperglycemic agents have shown that improvements in blood glucose control correspond to improvements in depression, which could support a biochemical mechanism (Lustman et al.).

Although depression can occur secondary to the onset of diabetes, depression is also a risk factor for the development of diabetes (Brown et al., 2005; Regenold and Marano, 2005). In a 6-year, multisite longitudinal study of 11,615 adults, participants that scored in the highest quartile for depressive symptoms at baseline had a relative hazard of 1.5 of developing type 2 diabetes over the study period compared with those who scored in the lowest quartile at baseline (Golden, Williams, Ford, et al., 2004). These results remained after controlling for stress-associated lifestyle factors, demographics, and metabolic covariates. A similar 8-year study of 2,764 men in Japan found that those with moderate or severe depressive symptoms had a 2.3 times higher risk of developing diabetes in the follow-up period (Kawakami, 1999).

Mechanisms

According to Talbot and Nouwen (2000), depression may increase the risk of type 2 diabetes as a result of biochemical changes that increase insulin resistance and reduce glucose uptake. These changes weaken an important metabolic balance; the relationship between depression and type 1 diabetes was not as clear. Other studies indicate that hypercortisolism secondary to depression can lead to insulin resistance (Saydah, Brancati, Golden, et al., 2003) or that HPA dysregulation and hypercortisolism may be a common pathway in obesity, metabolic syndrome, diabetes, and mood disorders. Another model suggests that there is a common pathway resulting from central nervous system dysregulation that leads to depression and affects insulin sensitivity, possibly through a neuroendocrinologic pathway leading to diabetes (Okamura, 1999).

Regardless of the direction of the relationship, depression decreases adherence to the diabetic treatment regimen, leading to poor glycemic control, increased complications, and impaired quality of life (Anderson et al., 2001; Ciechanowski, Katon, Russo, et al., 2003; Lustman and Clouse, 2005; Whittemore, Melkus, and Grey, 2004). Maintenance of glycemic control is one key to preventing the complications of diabetes, and according to the meta-analysis done by Lustman, Anderson, Freedland, et al. (2000), treatment of depression could significantly increase the proportion of subjects in good control as measured by HgbA1c. In addition to affecting blood glucose levels, depression adversely affects other risk factors for diabetic complications such as blood pressure and cholesterol levels.

Behavior associated with depression, like lack of physical activity and poor diet, not only leads to the development of diabetes but also contributes to complications in diabetes (Saydah et al., 2003) in both type 1 and 2 diabetes. Depression can increase the risks of complications (possibly through regimen nonadherence), or increased complications could increase the rates of depression (deGroot, Anderson, Freedland, et al., 2001). The direction of this relationship has not been fully established. However, there is evidence that certain aspects of self-care are not affected by depression, including home blood glucose monitoring and foot inspections and examinations. Screenings for microalbuminuria and retinopathy are also not related to depression, as these activities are more dependent on initiation by the patient's medical provider (Lin, Katon, Korff, et al., 2004).

Complications of diabetes, such as neuropathy, appear to increase the risk of depression. This relationship is mediated by perceptions of the symptom as unpredictable and not controlled with treatment and the restrictions the complication causes in activities of daily living and change in social self-perception

(Evans, Charney, Lewis, et al., 2005). Diabetic patients with major depression report more neuropathic symptoms even after controlling for the severity of their disease (Ciechanowski et al., 2003; Ludman et al, 2004).

Treatment

Although the relationship between diabetes and depression has long been known, depression is often not diagnosed or treated adequately. Fewer than 25 percent of people with diabetes and depression are diagnosed and treated for their depression (Chapman et al., 2005). As in other chronic conditions, part of this is due to the fact that depression may be expected to accompany a chronic and life-changing disease.

Little published research is focused specifically on treatment of depression in diabetes. Treatment of depression in diabetes with CBT and SSRIs does lead to improved glycemic control, decreased health care costs, and improved quality of life for these patients (Chapman et al., 2005; Whittemore et al., 2004). Psychotherapy alone can be an effective treatment for depression accompanying diabetes. In a controlled trial of CBT, researchers found a decrease in HgbA1c measures for those who received CBT (Regenold and Marano, 2005). Tricyclic antidepressants may improve depression and therefore indirectly improve diabetes but they also have a hyperglycemic effect.

The most promising pharmacotherapeutic agents for depression in diabetes are the SSRIs. Fluoxetine (Prozac) was found to reduce depressive symptoms and HgbA1c measures (although it did not reach statistical significance) in a randomized, double-blind, placebo-controlled trial by Lustman, Anderson, Freedland, et al. (2000). However, care must be taken when using SSRIs in

Box 9.3 • Key Points on Depression and Diabetes

- Depression is more prevalent in persons with diabetes, and depression is a risk factor for diabetes.
- Depression in diabetes increases the risk for complications, while treatment of depression improves control of blood glucose levels.
- Persons with diabetes should be screened for depression, and persons who are depressed may need to be screened for diabetes.
- The most promising pharmacotherapeutic agents for depression in patients with diabetes are the selective serotonin reuptake inhibitors.

diabetic patients because hypoglycemia can occur in patients taking insulin or sulfonylurea oral hypoglycemics. Daily blood glucose monitoring is important. The serotonin norepinephrine reuptake inhibitors (SNRIs) have not been studied in patients with diabetes and depression; however, SNRIs are indicated for treating neuropathy and are thought not to cause weight gain (Regenold and Marano, 2005). Studies indicate that depression in diabetic patients may be less responsive to treatment, so more aggressive therapies may be required to achieve results (Whittemore et al., 2004). Frequent follow-up and screening is essential to monitor for effective therapy (Box 9.3).

Cancer

Research indicates that nearly 50 percent of patients admitted for cancer treatment have psychiatric disorders, with as many as 25 percent reporting severe depressive symptoms (Burgess, Cornelius, Love, et al., 2005; Chapman et al., 2005; Chochinov, 2006). Depression is significant in terminally ill patients because it is associated with a desire for hastened death (Mystakidou, Rosenfeld, Parpa, et al., 2005).

In women with cancer, depression is related to performance status and history of depression but not to stage of illness (Burgess et al., 2005). For cancer patients with pain, pain predicts depression and depression, in turn, influences pain perception (Speigel, Sands, and Koopman, 1994; Tennen, Affleck, and Zautra, 2006). Pain also appears to increase rates of depression. In a study by Wong-Kim and Bloom (2005), women who had breast cancer and experienced severe side effects, pain, low self-esteem, and low emotional support were more likely to become depressed. In another study, patients with depression and a desire to hasten death were more likely to be experiencing pain and to have little social support (Chochinov, 2006). Depression associated with chronic pain may decrease the patient's ability to benefit from treatment and rehabilitation (Pallant and Bailey, 2005). In addition to psychosocial contributors to depression, cytokines may be a biochemical way that cancer increases depression (Illman, Corringham, Robinson, et al., 2005).

While depression appears to predispose individuals to certain specific cancers, including breast cancer in women (Carney, Jones, Woolson, et al., 2003; Schneider and Chiriboga, 2005)), there does not appear to be an increase in overall cancer rates in persons with preexisting depression (Aro, De Koning, Schreck, et al., 2005).

Depression may also be important in the prognosis of cancer. One study of 133 patients in the United Kingdom showed that depressive symptoms were more highly correlated with mortality than stage of disease in patients with lung cancer (Buccheri, 1998), but this finding has not been supported by other studies.

Mechanisms

A model for depression in relation to an increased risk for certain cancers includes reduction in natural killer cell activity, down regulation of interferon, and increased tumor necrosis factor levels (Garland, Lavelle, Doherty, et al., 2004). There is evidence of a lack of cortisol suppression in depressed patients receiving treatment with the corticosteroid dexamethasone (France and Krishnan, 1985). This dysregulation of the HPA axis could impair immune system function and therefore predispose patients to developing cancer.

Treatment

In terminal illness, the misperception that depression is natural with such a diagnosis leads to underdetection and treatment of depression (Chapman et al., 2005). Although treatment of depression in cancer patients has not been widely studied with randomized, placebo-controlled trials, a limited number of studies have found that treatment of depression in persons with cancer can decrease symptoms of depression, decrease pain, and improve immune function (Chapman et al.). With screening and intervention, depression in terminal illness or chronic pain can be treated successfully.

Once depression is diagnosed, supportive therapy can increase adaptive coping. Group psychotherapy is effective in improving quality of life and for reducing depression as well as physical symptoms (Chochinov, 2006). Counseling and use of support groups may prevent major depression (Wong-Kim and Bloom, 2005) (Box 9.4).

Box 9.4 • Key Points on Depression and Cancer

- Up to 25% of patients diagnosed with cancer may also be depressed.
- Treatment of depression in persons with cancer can decrease pain and desire for hastened death and increase benefits from treatment and rehabilitation.
- Counseling and support groups may be used to treat or prevent major depression.

Chronic Pain

Chronic pain and depression are clearly associated. Chronic back pain appears to precede depression in 50 percent or more of cases (Polatin, Kinney, Gatchel, et al., 1993). The odds ratio for having a major depressive disorder increased from 2.15 in those with a nonpainful medical condition to 4.39 in those with a chronic painful physical condition and up to 6.07 in those who have both. Having constant pain is an independent factor in the development of depression (Ohayon and Schatzberg, 2003).

Depression also changes how pain is experienced and described but does not necessarily lower the pain threshold. Depressed people use different types of words to describe their pain, rate their pain as more severe in the late evening and at bedtime, and report more disability from social and recreational activities (Doan and Wadden, 1989). Patients with increased psychopathology also have a decreased response to opioid analgesics (Wasan, Davar, and Jamison, 2005). The information on the effect of depression on decreasing or increasing the pain threshold is mixed (Sherman, LeResche, Huggins, et al., 2004; Suarez-Roca, Pinerua-Shuhaibar, et al., 2003) and may be dependent on the type of noxious stimulus. One meta-analysis of the studies indicates that overall, patients with depression actually have higher pain thresholds (Dickens, McGowan, and Dale, 2003).

Mechanisms

One model, which addresses the cause of depression in chronic pain, shows disability as a mediating factor. Depression and perceived disability are positively associated (Tschannen, Duckro, Margolis, et al., 1992). Another study showed that increased cerebrospinal fluid levels of prolactin (but not monoamine activity) correlated with depression in chronic pain patients (Alaranta, Hurme, Lahtela, et al., 1983). It is not clear if cortisol is a mediator of this relationship (McBeth, Chiu, Silman, et al., 2005).

Treatment

Antidepressants have been shown to help in chronic pain syndromes, including neurogenic pain and pain after stroke, independent of their effect on the depression (Shimodozono, Kawahira, Kamishita, et al., 2002). While electroconvulsive therapy does improve depression scores, it is unclear if it has an effect on the pain threshold (Schreiber, Shmueli, Grunhaus, et al., 2003) (Box 9.5).

Box 9.5 • Key Points on Depression and Chronic Pain

- Chronic pain and depression are clearly associated.
- Patients with depression have a higher pain threshold and a decreased response to opioid analgesics.
- Antidepressants have been shown to help patients with chronic pain syndromes.

ASSESSMENT OF DEPRESSION IN PATIENTS WITH CHRONIC MEDICAL COMORBIDITIES

Table 9.3 presents information on various screening tools for depression. While effective, these screens are time-consuming and not practical for routine screening in a busy primary care practice. However, even shorter screening tools have been shown to be effective in medically ill patients (Jefford, Mileshkin, L., Richards, K., et al., 2004). Sometimes, just asking one to two questions regarding sadness and loss of interest can have as much impact as longer, more time-consuming screens (Huffman, Smith, Blais, et al., 2006). It appears that overall, the choice of tool is not as important as getting the screening accomplished. A positive screen then needs a more thorough investigation for diagnosis.

CONCLUSION

There are several important points to remember regarding depression and chronic disease. First and foremost, diagnosing and properly treating depression saves lives, not only through suicide prevention but also from conditions such as heart attacks and strokes. Depression can lead to increased risk for medical illnesses, and conversely, medical disorders can lead to increased risk for depression. It is clear that there is a biologic link between depression and chronic disease with mechanisms that have yet to be elucidated. Despite extensive evidence for this association, research clearly indicates that depression is most often undiagnosed, and even when diagnosed, it is undertreated. For successful medical outcomes, diagnosing and treating depression must be done in tandem with treating the medical disorder.

Table 9.3 • Depression Screening Tools in Medically Ill Patients

Screening Tool	Number of Items	Medical Condition Where Tested	Outcomes	Citation
CES-D Center for Epidemiologic Studies Depression Scale	20	Elderly with physical illness, cognitive decline, or anxiety Chronic pain	Need to use cut off of 19 instead of 16 No increased false positives	Beekman, Deeg, Van Limbeet, et al. (1997) Turk & Okifuji (1994)
BDI Beck Depression Inventory	21	Diabetes	Used and validated	Lustman & Clouse (2004)
Brief ZSDS Brief Zung Self-Rating Depression Scale	11	Cancer Chronic fatigue syndrome	Useful Performed badly	Dugan, McDonald, Passik, et al. (1998) Farmer, Chubb, Jones, et al. (1996)
DCS Depressive Cognition Scale	8	Type 2 diabetes	Useful	Zauszniewski, Chung, Krafcik, et al. (2001)
HADS–D The Hospital Anxiety and Depression Scale–Depression	7	Chronic pain patients	Performed well	Pallant & Bailey (2005)
PHQ-9 Patient Health Questionnaire	9	General illness	Patient-administered questionnaire Positive results can be followed-up with clinical interview	Kroenke, Spitzer, & Williams (2001)

Treating depression also assists patients in self-managing their chronic medical conditions by promoting patients' interest in their own care. Besides medication, psychotherapy, such as CBT, can also assist patients in minimizing their fears and negative thinking. CBT has demonstrated effectiveness in patients with a wide range of chronic illnesses, including stroke, CAD, breast cancer, and chronic pain.

Finally, communication with all members of the care team is vital. Members of the team must be knowledgeable about all aspects of their patients' health and medications to avoid complications from antidepressants and interactions with other medications. Such an approach will facilitate optimal health outcomes for patients and greater satisfaction for providers.

Resources for Patients

American Diabetes Association: *http://diabetes.org/type-2-diabetes/depression.jsp*
Information about depression and common concerns related to diabetes

Depression and Bipolar Support Alliance: *http://ndmda.org*
Information about mood disorders, depression, and other illnesses (diabetes, heart disease, cancer, and others)

National Foundation for Depressive Illness (iFred): *www.ifred.org/facts/medical.html*
Information about depression and medical illness

Psychology Information Online: *www.psychologyinfo.com/depression/medical.html*
Information about depression and medical disorders

References

Abramson, J., Berger, A., Krumholz, H. M., et al. (2001). Depression and risk of heart failure among older persons with isolated systolic hypertension. *Archives of Internal Medicine, 161*(14), 1725–1730.

Alaranta, H., Hurme, M., Lahtela, K., et al. (1983). Prolactin and cortisol in cerebrospinal fluid: Sex-related associations with clinical and psychological characteristics of patients with low back pain. *Psychoneuroendocrinology, 8*(3), 333–341.

Anderson, R. J., Freedland, K. E., Clouse, R. E., et al. (2001). The prevalence of comorbid depression in adults with diabetes: A meta-analysis. *Diabetes Care, 24*(6),1069–1078.

Aro, A. R., De Koning, H. J., Schreck, M., et al. (2005). Psychological risk factors of incidence of breast cancer: A prospective cohort study in Finland. *Psychological Medicine, 35*(10), 1515–1521.

Beekman, A. T., Deeg, D. J., Van Limbeek, J., et al. (1997). Criterion validity of the Center for Epidemiologic Studies Depression scale (CES-D): Results from a community-based sample of older subjects in the Netherlands. *Psychological Medicine, 27*(1), 231–235.

Brown, L. C., Majumdar, S. R., Newman, S. C., et al. (2005). History of depression increases risk of type 2 diabetes in younger adults. *Diabetes Care,* May; 28(5):1063–1067.

Brown, L. C., Majumdar, S. R., Newman, S. C., et al. (2006). Type 2 diabetes does not increase risk of depression. *Canadian Medical Association Journal, 175*(1), 42–46.

Buccheri, G. (1998). Depressive reactions to lung cancer are common and often followed by a poor outcome. *European Respiratory Journal, 11*(1), 173–178.

Burgess, C., Cornelius, V., Love, S., et al. (2005). Depression and anxiety in women with early breast cancer: Five year observational cohort study. *British Medical Journal, 330*(7493), 702. Epub February 4, 2005.

Capuron, L., Raison, C. L., Musselman, D. L., et al. (2003). Association of exaggerated HPA axis response to the initial injection of interferon-alpha with development of depression during interferon-alpha therapy. *American Journal of Psychiatry, 160*(7), 1342–1345.

Capuron, L., Ravaud, A., Neveu, P. J., et al. (2002). Association between decreased serum tryptophan concentrations and depressive symptoms in cancer patients undergoing cytokine therapy. *Molecular Psychiatry,* 7(5), 468–473.

Carney, C. P., Jones, L., Woolson, R. F., et al. (2003). Relationship between depression and pancreatic cancer in the general population. *Psychosomatic Medicine, 65*(5), 884–888.

Carvajal Garcia-Pando, A., Garcia del Pozo, J., Sanchez, A. S., et al. (2002). Hepatotoxicity associated with the new antidepressants. *Journal of Clinical Psychiatry, 63*(2), 135–137.

Chapman, D. P., Perry, G. S., & Strine, T. W. (2005). The vital link between chronic disease and depressive disorders. *Preventing Chronic Disease,* 2(1), A14. Epub December 15, 2004.

Charlson, M., & Peterson, J. C. (2002). Medical comorbidity and late life depression: What is known and what are the unmet needs? *Biological Psychiatry, 52*(3), 226–235.

Chochinov, H. M. (2006). Dying, dignity, and new horizons in palliative end-of-life care. *CA: A Cancer Journal for Clinicians, 56*(2), 84–103.

Ciechanowski, P. S., Katon, W. F., Russo, J. E., et al. (2003). The relationship of depressive symptoms to symptom reporting, self-care and glucose control in diabetes. *General Hospital Psychiatry, 25*(4), 246–252.

Dalton, S. O., Sorensen, H. T., & Johansen, C. (2006). SSRIs and upper gastrointestinal bleeding: What is known and how should it influence prescribing? *CNS Drugs, 20*(2), 143–151.

deGroot, M., Anderson, R., Freedland, K. E., et al. (2001). Association of depression and diabetes complications: A meta-analysis. *Psychosomatic Medicine, 63*(4), 619–630.

Dickens, C., McGowan, L., & Dale, S. (2003). Impact of depression on experimental pain perception: A systematic review of the literature with meta-analysis. *Psychosomatic Medicine, 65*(3), 369–375.

Doan, B. D., & Wadden, N. P. (1989). Relationships between depressive symptoms and descriptions of chronic pain. *Pain, 36*(1), 75–84.

Dugan, W., McDonald, M. V., Passik, S. D., et al. (1998). Use of the Zung Self-Rating Depression Scale in cancer patients: Feasibility as a screening tool. *Psycho-Oncology,* 7(6), 483–493.

Evans, D. L., Charney, D. S., Lewis, L., et al. (2005). Ketter mood disorders in the medically ill: Scientific review and recommendations. *Biological Psychiatry, 58*(3), 175–189. Review.

Fabian, T. J., Amico, J. A., Kroboth, P. D., et al. (2003). Paroxetine-induced hyponatremia in the elderly due to the syndrome of inappropriate secretion of antidiuretic hormone (SIADH). *Journal of Geriatric Psychiatry and Neurology, 16*(3), 160–164.

Farmer, A., Chubb, H., Jones, I., et al. (1996). Screening for psychiatric morbidity in subjects presenting with chronic fatigue syndrome. *British Journal of Psychiatry, 168*(3), 354–358.

France, R. D., & Krishnan, K. R. (1985). The dexamethasone suppression test as a biologic marker of depression in chronic pain. *Pain, 21*(1), 49–55.

Freedland, K. E., Carney, R. M., Lustman, P. J., et al. (1992). Major depression in coronary artery disease patients with vs. without a prior history of depression. *Psychosomatic Medicine, 54*(4), 416–421.

Gagnon, L. M., & Patten, S. B. (2002). Major depression and its association with long-term medical conditions. *Canadian Journal of Psychiatry, 47*(2), 149–152.

Gallo, J. J., Armenian, H. K., Ford, D. E., et al. (2000). Major depression and cancer: The 13-year follow-up of the Baltimore Epidemiologic Catchment Area sample (United States). *Cancer Causes and Control, 11*(8), 751–758.

Garland, M. R., Lavelle, E., Doherty, D., et al. (2004). Cortisol does not mediate the suppressive effects of psychiatric morbidity on natural killer cell activity: A cross-sectional study of patients with early breast cancer. *Psychological Medicine, 34*(3), 481–490.

Geringer, E. S., Perlmuter, L. C., Stern, T. A., et al. (1988). Depression and diabetic neuropathy: A complex relationship. *Journal of Geriatric Psychiatry and Neurology, 1*(1), 11–15.

Glassman, A. H., O'Connor, C. M., Califf, R. M., et al.; Sertraline Antidepressant Heart Attack Randomized Trial (SADHEART) Group. (2002). Sertraline treatment of major depression in patients with acute MI or unstable angina. *Journal of the American Medical Association, 288*(6), 701–709.

Golden, S. H., Williams, J. E., Ford, D. E., et al. (2004). Depressive symptoms and the risk of type 2 diabetes: The atherosclerosis risk in communities study. *Diabetes Care, 27*(2), 429–435.

Goldstein, M. M. (2006). Depression—An independent risk factor for cardiovascular disease. *Journal of the American Academy of Physician Assistants, 19*(9), 40–42, 44, 46.

Goodwin, R. D., Kroenke, K., Hoven, C. W., et al. (2003). Major depression, physical illness, and suicidal ideation in primary care. *Psychosomatic Medicine, 65*(4), 501–505.

Gottlieb, S. S., Khatta, M., Friedman, E., et al. (2004). The influence of age, gender, and race on the prevalence of depression in heart failure patients. *Journal of the American College of Cardiology, 43*(9), 1542–1549.

Havranek, E. P., Spertus, J. A., Masoudi, F. A., et al. (2004). Predictors of the onset of depressive symptoms in patients with heart failure. *Journal of the American College of Cardiology, 44*(12), 2333–2338.

Hemeryck, A., & Belpaire, F. M. (2002). Selective serotonin reuptake inhibitors and cytochrome P-450 mediated drug-drug interactions: An update. *Current Drug Metabolism, 3*(1), 13–37.

Huffman, J. C., Smith, F. A., Blais, M. A., et al. (2006). Rapid screening for major depression in post-myocardial infarction patients: An investigation using beck depression inventory II items. *Heart, 92*(11), 1656–1660. Epub April 27, 2006.

Illman, J., Corringham, R., Robinson, D. Jr., et al. (2005). Are inflammatory cytokines the common link between cancer-associated cachexia and depression? *Journal of Supportive Oncology, 3*(1), 37–50.

Irie, M., Asami, S., Nagata, S., et al. (2001). Psychosocial factors as a potential trigger of oxidative DNA damage in human leukocytes. *Japanese Journal of Cancer Research, 92*(3), 367–376.

Jefford, M., Mileshkin L., Richards, K., et al. (2004). Rapid screening for depression—validation of the Brief Case-Find for Depression (BCD) in medical oncology and palliative care patients. *Br J Cancer. Aug* 31; 91(5):900–906.

Katon, W., Cantrell, C. R., Sokol, M. C., et al. (2005). Impact of antidepressant drug adherence on comorbid medication use and resource utilization. *Archives of Internal Medicine, 165*(21), 2497–2503.

Kawakami, N. (1999). Depressive symptoms and occurrence of type 2 diabetes among Japanese men. *Diabetes Care, 22*(7), 1071–1076.

Kim, J. M., Stewart, R., Kim, S. W., et al. (2006). Vascular risk factors and incident late-life depression in a Korean population. *British Journal of Psychiatry, 189*, 26–30.

Kinder, L. S., Carnethon, M. R., Palaniappan, L. P., et al. (2004). Depression and the metabolic syndrome in young adults: Findings from the Third National Health and Nutrition Examination Survey. *Psychosomatic Medicine, 66*(3), 316–322.

Kotlyar, M., Dysken, M., & Adson, D. E. (2005). Update on drug-induced depression in the elderly. *American Journal of Geriatric Pharmacotherapy, 3*(4), 288–300.

Krittayaphong, R., Light, K. C., Golden, R. N., et al. (1996). Relationship among depression scores, beta-endorphin, and angina pectoris during exercise in patients with coronary artery disease. *Clinical Journal of Pain, 12*(2), 126–133.

Kroenke, K., Spitzer. R. L. Williams, J. B. (2001). The PHQ-9: Validity of a brief depression severity measure. *Journal of General Internal Medicine 16*(9), 606–613.

Larson, S. L., Owens, P. L., Ford, D., et al. (2001). Depressive disorder, dysthymia, and risk of stroke: Thirteen-year follow-up from the Baltimore Epidemiologic Catchment Area study. *Stroke, 32*(9), 1979–1983.

Lesperance, F., Frasure-Smith, N., Theroux, P., et al. (2004). The association between major depression and levels of soluble intercellular adhesion molecule 1, interleukin-6, and C-reactive protein in patients with recent acute coronary syndromes. *American Journal of Psychiatry, 161*(2), 271–277.

Lett, H. S., Blumenthal, J. A., Babyak, M. A., et al. (2004). Depression as a risk factor for coronary artery disease: Evidence, mechanisms, and treatment. *Psychosomatic Medicine, 66*(3), 305–315.

Lin, E. H., Katon, W., Korff, M., et al. (2004). The relationship of depression and diabetes self-care, medication adherence, and preventive care. *Diabetes Care, 27*(9), 2154–2160.

Ludman, E. F., Katon, W., Russo, J., et al. (2004). Depression and diabetes symptom burden. *General Hospital Psychiatry, 26*(6), 430–436.

Lustman, P. J., Anderson, R. J., Freedland, K. E., et al. (2000). Depression and poor glycemic control: A meta-analytic review of the literature. *Diabetes Care, 23*(7), 934–942.

Lustman, P. J., & Clouse, R. E. (2004). Section III: Practical considerations in the management of depression in diabetes. *Diabetes Spectrum, 17*(3), 160–166.

Lustman, P. J., & Clouse, R. E. (2005). Depression in diabetic patients: The relationship between mood and glycemic control. *Journal of Diabetes and Its Complications, 19*(2), 113–122.

Manjarrez, G., Herrera, R., Leon, M., et al. (2006). A low brain serotonergic neurotransmission in children with type 1 diabetes detected through the intensity dependence of auditory-evoked potentials. *Diabetes Care, 29*(1), 73–77.

Mast, B. T., Yochim, B., MacNeill, S. E., et al. (2004). Risk factors for geriatric depression: The importance of executive functioning within the vascular depression hypothesis. *Journals of Gerontology. Series A, Biological Sciences and Medical Sciences, 59*(12), 1290–1294.

McBeth, J., Chiu, Y. H., Silman, A. J., et al. (2005). Hypothalamic-pituitary-adrenal stress axis function and the relationship with chronic widespread pain and its antecedents. *Arthritis Research and Therapy*, 7(5), R992–R1000. Epub June 17, 2005.

McLaughlin, T. J., Aupont, O., Bambauer, K. Z., et al. (2005). Improving psychologic adjustment to chronic illness in cardiac patients. The role of depression and anxiety. *Journal of General Internal Medicine*, *20*(12), 1084–1090.

Misra, M., Papakostas, G. I., & Klibanski, A. (2004). Effects of psychiatric disorders and psychotropic medications on prolactin and bone metabolism. *Journal of Clinical Psychiatry*, *65*(12), 1607–1618; quiz 1590, 1760–1761.

Mystakidou, K., Rosenfeld, B., Parpa, E., et al. (2005). Desire for death near the end of life: The role of depression, anxiety and pain. *General Hospital Psychiatry*, *27*(4), 258–262.

Newcomer, J. W. (2007). Metabolic considerations in the use of antipsychotic medications: A review of recent evidence. *Journal of Clinical Psychiatry*, *68*(1), 20–27.

Ohayon, M. M., & Schatzberg, A. F. (2003). Using chronic pain to predict depressive morbidity in the general population. *Archives of General Psychiatry*, *60*(1), 39–47.

Okamura, F. (1999). Insulin resistance in patients with depression and its changes in the clinical course of depression: A report on three cases using the minimal model analysis. *Internal Medicine*, *38*(3), 257–260.

Okamura, M., Yamawaki, S., Akechi, T., et al. (2005). Psychiatric disorders following first breast cancer recurrence: Prevalence, associated factors and relationship to quality of life. *Japanese Journal of Clinical Oncology*, *35*(6), 302–309. Epub June 16, 2005.

Pallant, J. F., & Bailey, C. M. (2005). Assessment of the structure of the Hospital Anxiety and Depression Scale in musculoskeletal patients. *Health and Quality of Life Outcomes*, *19*(3), 82.

Patten, S. B. (2000). Exogenous corticosteroids and major depression in the general population. *Journal of Psychosomatic Research*, *49*(6), 447–449.

Patten, S. B., & Barbui, C. (2004). Drug-induced depression: A systematic review to inform clinical practice. *Psychotherapy and Psychosomatics*, *73*(4), 207–215.

Patten, S. B., Beck, C. A., Kassam, A., et al. (2005). Long-term medical conditions and major depression: Strength of association for specific conditions in the general population. *Canadian Journal of Psychiatry*, *50*(4), 195–202.

Patten, S. B., & Lavorato, D. H. (2001). Medication use and major depressive syndrome in a community population. *Comprehensive Psychiatry*, *42*(2), 124–131.

Patten, S. B., Williams, J. V., & Love, E. J. (1996). Self-reported depressive symptoms following treatment with corticosteroids and sedative-hypnotics. *International Journal of Psychiatry in Medicine*, *26*(1), 15–24.

Peeters, B. W., & Broekkamp, C. L. (1994). Involvement of corticosteroids in the processing of stressful life-events. A possible implication for the development of depression. *Journal of Steroid Biochemistry and Molecular Biology*, *49*(4–6), 417–427.

Polatin, P. B., Kinney, R. K., Gatchel, R. J., et al. (1993). Psychiatric illness and chronic low-back pain. The mind and the spine—Which goes first? *Spine*, *18*(1), 66–71.

Pollak, P. T., Mukherjee, S. D., & Fraser, A. D. (2001). Sertraline-induced hypoglycemia. *Annals of Pharmacotherapy*, *35*(11), 1371–1374.

Regenold, W. T., & Marano, C. M. (2005). Sweet sorrow: The relationship between depression and diabetes mellitus. *Psychiatric Times*, *23*(5), 20–23.

Roose, S. P., Glassman, A. H., & Seidman, S. N. (2001). Relationship between depression and other medical illnesses. *Journal of the American Medical Association, 286*(14), 1687–1690.

Rozniatowski, O., Reich, M., Mallet, Y., et al. (2005) Psychosocial factors involved in delayed consultation by patients with head and neck cancer. *Head Neck.* Apr; 27(4):274–280.

Saydah, S. H., Brancati, F. L., Golden, S. H., et al. (2003). Depressive symptoms and the risk of type 2 diabetes mellitus in a US sample. *Diabetes/Metabolism Research Review, 19*(3), 202–208.

Schneider, M. G., & Chiriboga, D. A. (2005). Associations of stress and depressive symptoms with cancer in older Mexican Americans. *Ethnicity and Disease, 15*(4), 698–704.

Schnittker, J. (2005). Chronic illness and depressive symptoms in late life. *Social Science in Medicine, 60*(1), 13–23.

Schreiber, S., Shmueli, D., Grunhaus, L., et al. (2003). The influence of electroconvulsive therapy on pain threshold and pain tolerance in major depression patients before, during and after treatment. *European Journal of Pain,* 7(5), 419–424.

Sherman, J. J., LeResche, L., Huggins, K. H., et al. (2004). The relationship of somatization and depression to experimental pain response in women with temporomandibular disorders. *Psychosomatic Medicine, 66*(6), 852–860.

Shimodozono, M., Kawahira, K., Kamishita, T., et al. (2002). Reduction of central poststroke pain with the selective serotonin reuptake inhibitor fluvoxamine. *International Journal of Neuroscience, 112*(10), 1173–1181.

Simon, G. E., Katon, W. J., Lin, E. H., et al. (2007). Cost-effectiveness of systematic depression treatment among people with diabetes mellitus. *Archives of General Psychiatry, 64*(1), 65–72.

Spiegel, D., Sands, S., & Koopman, C. (1994). Pain and depression in patients with cancer. *Cancer, 74*(9), 2570–2578.

Steffens, D. C., Helms, M. J., Krishnan, K. R., et al. (1999). Cerebrovascular disease and depression symptoms in the cardiovascular health study. *Stroke, 30*(10), 2159–2166.

Steffens, D. C., Plassman, B. L., Helms, M. J., et al. (1997). A twin study of late-onset depression and apolipoprotein E epsilon 4 as risk factors for Alzheimer's disease. *Biological Psychiatry,41*(8), 851–856.

Stein, P. K., Carney, R. M., Freedland, K. E., et al. (2000). Severe depression is associated with markedly reduced heart rate variability in patients with stable coronary artery disease. *Journal of Psychosomatic Research, 48*(4–5), 493–500.

Suarez, E. C. (2006). Sex differences in the relation of depressive symptoms, hostility, and anger expression to indices of glucose metabolism in nondiabetic adults. *Health Psychology, 25*(4), 484–492.

Suarez-Roca, H., Pinerua-Shuhaibar, L., Morales, M. E., et al. (2003). Increased perception of post-ischemic paresthesias in depressed subjects. *Journal of Psychosomatic Research, 55*(3), 253–257.

Talbot, F., & Nouwen, A. (2000). A review of the relationship between depression and diabetes in adults: Is there a link? *Diabetes Care, 23*(10), 1556–1562.

Taylor, C. B., Youngblood, M. E., Catellier, D., et al.; ENRICHD Investigators. (2005). Effects of antidepressant medication on morbidity and mortality in depressed patients after myocardial infarction. *Archives of General Psychiatry, 62*(7), 792–798.

Tennen, H., Affleck, G., & Zautra, A. (2006). Depression history and coping with chronic pain: A daily process analysis. *Health Psychology, 25*(3), 370–379.

Thomas, R. J. (2006). Behavioral cardiology: Where the heart and head meet. *Business Briefing, US Cardiology.*

Thompson, D. S., Spanier, C. A., & Vogel, V. G. (1999). The relationship between tamoxifen, estrogen, and depressive symptoms. *Breast Journal, 5*(6), 375–382.

Tschannen, T. A., Duckro, P. N., Margolis, R. B., et al. (1992). The relationship of anger, depression, and perceived disability among headache patients. *Headache, 32*(10), 501–503.

Turk, D. C., & Okifuji, A. (1994). Detecting depression in chronic pain patients: Adequacy of self-reports. *Behaviour Research and Therapy, 32*(1), 9–16.

Vileikyte, L., Leventhal, H., Gonzalez, J. S., et al. (2005). Diabetic peripheral neuropathy and depressive symptoms: The association revisited. *Diabetes Care, 28*(10), 2378–2383.

Wasan, A. D., Davar, G., & Jamison, R. (2005). The association between negative affect and opioid analgesia in patients with discogenic low back pain. *Pain, 117*(3), 450–461.

Wassertheil-Smoller, S., Shumaker, S., Ockene, J., et al. (2004). Depression and cardiovascular sequelae in postmenopausal women. The Women's Health Initiative (WHI). *Archives of Internal Medicine, 164*(3), 289–298.

Weber-Hamann, B., Gilles, M., Lederbogen, F., et al. (2006). Improved insulin sensitivity in 80 nondiabetic patients with MDD after clinical remission in a double-blind, randomized trial of amitriptyline and paroxetine. *Journal of Clinical Psychiatry, 67*(12), 1856–1861.

Whang, W., Albert, C. M., Sears, S. F. Jr., et al.; TOVA Study Investigators. (2005). Depression as a predictor for appropriate shocks among patients with implantable cardioverter-defibrillators: Results from the Triggers of Ventricular Arrhythmias (TOVA) study. *Journal of the American College of Cardiology, 45*(7), 1090–1095.

Whittemore, R., Melkus, G. D., & Grey, M. (2004). Self-report of depressed mood and depression in women with type 2 diabetes. *Issues in Mental Health Nursing, 25*(3), 243–260.

Whyte, E. M., Mulsant, B. H., Vanderbilt, J., et al. (2004). Depression after stroke: A prospective epidemiological study. *Journal of the American Geriatric Society, 52*(5), 774–778.

Winocour, P. H., Main, C. J., Medlicott, G., et al. (1990). A psychometric evaluation of adult patients with type 1 (insulin-dependent) diabetes mellitus: Prevalence of psychological dysfunction and relationship to demographic variables, metabolic control and complications. *Diabetes Research, 14*(4), 171–176.

Wong-Kim, E. C., & Bloom, J. R. (2005). Depression experienced by young women newly diagnosed with breast cancer. *Psycho-Oncology, 14,* 564–573.

Writing Committee for the ENRICHD Investigators. (2003). Effects of treating depression and low social support on clinical events after myocardial infarction: The enhancing recovery in coronary heart disease patients. *Journal of the American Medical Association, 289,* 3106–3116.

Xiong, G. L., Jiang, W., Clare, R., et al. (2006). Prognosis of patients taking selective serotonin reuptake inhibitors before coronary artery bypass grafting. *American Journal of Cardiology, 98*(1), 42–47. Epub May 5, 2006.

Zauszniewski, J. A., Chung, C., Krafcik, K., et al. (2001). Psychometric testing of the depressive cognition scale in women with type 2 diabetes. *Journal of Nursing Measurement, 9*(1), 61–72.

Carla J. Groh
Joan C. Urbancic
Shane LaGore
Ann Whall

chapter 10

Mental Health Issues for Older Women

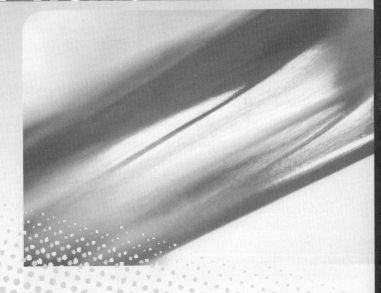

In 2003, there were 21 million women aged 65 years and older living in the United States, representing 13.5 percent of the total female population (U.S. Department of Health and Human Services [DHHS], 2005). Older women represent the largest single group of health care users (Blow, 2000). They accounted for more than 134,488 office visits to physicians in 2004, with most of these visits to primary care providers (PCPs) (Hing, Cherry, and Woodwell, 2006). As women age, they are confronted with myriad social and economic issues that impact their physical and mental health. Older women are twice as likely to live alone than older men (40 percent vs. 19 percent, respectively) (DHHS), and a significant portion live in poverty. For women aged 65 to 74 years, the poverty rate is 10.6 percent; for women 75 years and older, the rate is 14.3 percent (DHHS).

These socioeconomic issues often exacerbate many of the normal age-related declines of physiologic, cognitive, and physical functions and exacerbate the symptoms of existing disease. Therefore, it is important that PCPs understand the unique health needs of older women so that they can provide appropriate care to this growing patient population. This chapter will focus on the psychiatric comorbidities most often experienced by older women seen in primary care settings: depression, suicide, anxiety, substance abuse, and the dementias.

DEPRESSION AND OLDER WOMEN

Depression is widespread in late life and is estimated to affect 17 to 37 percent of older persons seen in primary care settings: 30 percent are diagnosed with major depression, and the remainder experience subsyndromal symptoms (Alexopoulos, 2000; Lyness, Heo, Datto, et al., 2006). Depression in older women can be divided into early-life onset (before age 65 years) or late-life onset (after age 65 years). By definition, early-life major depression begins in early adulthood, tends to be chronic, and continues into late adulthood (Lapid and Rummans, 2003). Late-life depression occurs more frequently in the context of medical illness, has a high rate of cognitive impairment, and is often associated with cerebrovascular abnormalities (Lapid and Rummans). Comorbid conditions may be more prominent in late-life depression compared with early-life depression, with anxiety, somatic complaints, memory loss, and/or cognitive impairment being the most prominent presenting symptoms (Lapid and Rummans). Geriatric depression is a remitting and relapsing disorder. A poor prognosis in depressed community-dwelling older adults is associated with several factors, including chronic limiting diseases, functional limitations, pain or cognitive impairment, older age, *female* gender, and lack of social support (Steunenberg, Beekman, Deeg, et al., 2007).

Specific gender differences for depressive symptoms have been reported. One study found that elderly depressed women tended to have more symptoms than depressed men, including appetite problems and sadness, while men were more often agitated (Kockler and Heun, 2002). A second study, however, reported that men had more severe vegetative signs and suicidal ideations compared with women (Lavretsky, Lesser, Wohl, et al., 1999).

Assessment

Diagnosing depression in the elderly is often a challenge for the health care provider. Estimates of major depression in older adults living in the community range from <1 percent to about 5 percent but rises to 13.5 percent in those who require home health care and to 11.5 percent in hospitalized patients (Hybels and Blazer, 2003). Subsyndromal depression, defined as when symptoms that do not meet the full diagnostic criteria, is especially common among older adults. It is estimated that 8 to 20 percent of older adults in the community and up to 37 percent in primary care settings suffer from subsyndromal depression (DHHS, 1999), which is associated with an increased risk of developing major depression if not treated. Despite the high prevalence, only 10 percent of the elderly are diagnosed and treated for their depression. Reasons for this lack of attention include the belief that depression is a normal part of aging, denial by patients because of shame and stigma fears, and atypical presentations. Further, depressive symptoms in older adults are often comorbid with psychiatric, neurologic, and medical disorders.

The clinical presentation of depression is similar in younger and older adults, with some noted differences (Box 10.1). Although the clinical presentation of subsyndromal depression varies from person to person, there are common presentations that could alert the PCP to possible depression (Alexopoulos, 2000) (Box 10.2).

Psychiatric Disorders

The common psychiatric comorbidities of depression in older adults include anxiety and substance abuse. Generalized anxiety or panic symptoms include tremors, body aches and pains, fatigability, restlessness, palpitations, dizziness, faintness, nausea and vomiting, frequent urination, facial flushing, insomnia, and dyspnea. The somatic focus of anxiety symptoms may be mistakenly ascribed to

Box 10.1 • Differences in Depressive Symptoms Between Older and Younger Adults

Common Traits of Older Adults

More somatic complaints

Minimization of the presence of depressed mood

More hypochondriacal symptoms (occur in about 65% of elderly persons with depression)

More psychotic delusional depression (e.g., guilt, nihilism, persecution, jealousy)

More pronounced agitation or retardation, or both, especially with psychotic delusions

medical illnesses and easily missed in primary care (Lapid and Rummans, 2003). Substance abuse in the elderly often goes unrecognized and may directly or indirectly affect the severity of depressive symptoms. Substances most frequently abused by older adults include nicotine, sedative-hypnotics, and alcohol (Wiseman, 2000). Comorbid alcohol abuse and/or dependence increases suicide risk in older adults who are depressed (Lapid and Rummans).

Box 10.2 • Clinical Presentation of Subsyndromal Depression

New medical complaints

Exacerbation of preexisting gastrointestinal symptoms

Arthritic pain

Cardiovascular symptoms

Preoccupation with poor health

Physical limitations

Diminished interest in pleasurable activities

Fatigue

Poor concentration

From Alexopoulos, G. S. (2000). Depression and other mood disorders. *Clinical Geriatrics, 8*(11), 69-82.

Neurologic Disorders

Depression in older adults with neurologic disease is common. It is estimated that depression rates range from 17 to 31 percent in persons with Alzheimer's disease (AD), approximately 50 percent in persons with Parkinson's disease, and about 25 percent in persons with cerebrovascular disorders (primarily strokes) (Lapid and Rummans, 2003). These statistics are particularly sobering for older women. The number of women living with AD at any one time is twice as high as men, and women have a tendency for greater psychiatric involvement (Filley, 1997). About 46,000 more women than men have a stroke every year, and this rate is even higher for racial/ethnic minority women (American Heart Association, 2007); and although the rate of Parkinson's disease is similar between women and men, women live longer with the disease.

Medical Conditions

Diabetes, coronary artery disease, and cancer have been associated with higher rates of depression. Hypothyroidism, autoimmune diseases, connective tissue disorders, and some infections can also cause depressive symptoms. Additionally, many medications have been associated with depression, especially corticosteroids and sedative-hypnotics (Lapid and Rummans, 2003).

Although multiple depression screening scales exist, few have been developed specifically for the geriatric population. Holroyd and Clayton (2002) reported that the Geriatric Depression Scale (available at *www.hartfordign.org/publications/trythis/issue04.pdf*) has good validation but is questionable for use with the moderately to severely cognitively impaired elderly. Because dementia has similar symptoms to depression, discriminating between them may sometimes be difficult. Additionally, the elderly frequently require multiple medications for medical comorbidities, which then increase the risk for drug–drug interactions. These interactions may cause agitation, dementia, and/or depression. Other medical challenges facing the elderly include age-related factors that affect drug accumulation and elimination. Failure to diagnose and treat depression in the elderly is particularly critical because of the high suicide rate.

Treatment Options

Once a medical workup has been completed and no medical cause determined, several treatment options are available depending on the severity of depressive symptoms and if other comorbidities are present.

Nonpharmacologic Interventions

Psychotherapeutic interventions can be beneficial alone or in conjunction with pharmacologic interventions in the treatment of depression in older women. The PCP is able to provide supportive psychotherapy, but when this is insufficient and more intensive therapy is needed, the older woman should be referred to an appropriate mental health provider (Lapid and Rummans, 2003). Cognitive behavioral therapy (CBT) and interpersonal therapy are the two most commonly used psychotherapies, and both have been shown in randomized clinical trials to be as efficacious as medications for cognitively intact older patients with *mild to moderate* depression. A combination of formal psychotherapy and pharmacologic agents is more efficacious on social adjustment for *moderate to severe* depression than either form of treatment alone (Lenze, Dew, Mazumdar, et al., 2002). Other nonpharmacologic interventions with the best evidence of effectiveness in the treatment of depression in older adults include reminiscence therapy, problem-solving therapy, bibliotherapy (for mild to moderate depression), and exercise (Frazer, Christensen, and Griffiths, 2005). There is limited evidence to support the effectiveness of dialectical behavior therapy and light therapy (for people in nursing homes or hospitals) (Frazer et al.).

Pharmacologic Interventions

Four issues must be assessed when pharmacologic interventions are being considered in the treatment of depression in older women: (a) response versus remission, (b) safety, (c) length of short-term treatment, and (d) need for continuation and/or maintenance therapy (Lapid and Rummans, 2003). Based on expert census guidelines, selective serotonin reuptake inhibitors (SSRIs) are the recommended first-line antidepressant (Alexopoulos, Katz, Reynolds, et al., 2001). In choosing a specific SSRI, the guideline experts suggest citalopram (Celexa) or sertraline (Zoloft) as initial first-line agents. These SSRIs have relatively low drug–drug interaction risks, an appropriate half-life that allows once-daily dosing, and well-tolerated side effects. Other antidepressants shown to be effective in geriatric depression include fluoxetine (Prozac), paroxetine (Paxil), venlafaxine (Effexor), and the tricyclic antidepressants nortriptyline and clomipramine (Raj, 2004). In general, it is acceptable to initiate doses at half the usual adult dosage and then titrate slowly for a few weeks to the optimal dose, if tolerated (Lapid and Rummans). Although SSRIs have less cardiovascular and anticholinergic effects than the tricyclic antidepressants, SSRIs have other side effects (e.g., nausea, diarrhea, insomnia, headache, agitation, and anxiety) that may lead the patient to stop taking the medication. Sleep disturbances in older women taking SSRIs was recently reported ($N = 223$) and included poorer sleep

Table 10.1 • Daily Dosages for Various Antidepressants for Older Adults

Antidepressant	Daily Dosage (mg/day) Initial	Daily Dosage (mg/day) Usual Range	Most Common or Potentially Serious Adverse Effect
Selective serotonin reuptake inhibitors			
Citalopram	10	20–40	Gastrointestinal (GI) symptoms, sexual dysfunction
Fluoxetine	10	20–50	GI symptoms, sexual dysfunction, insomnia
Fluvoxamine	50	100–300	GI symptoms, sexual dysfunction
Paroxetine	10	10–40	GI symptoms, sexual dysfunction
Sertraline	25	50–150	GI symptoms, sexual dysfunction
Others			
Trazadone	25	75–300	Sedation
Bupropion	75–100	200–300	GI symptoms, agitation, seizures
Mirtazapine	7.5–15.0	15–45	Sedation, weight changes, pain, bone marrow toxicity
Venlafaxine	50–75	75–225	GI symptoms, hypertension
Tricyclic antidepressants			
Nortriptyline	10–25	50–150	Sedation, cardiac conduction abnormality, anticholinergic reaction, orthostasis
Desipramine	10–25	75–150	Sedation, cardiac conduction abnormality, anticholinergic reaction, orthostasis

From Medical Economics Company, Inc. (2001). *Psychotropic prescribing guide* (4th ed). Montvale, NJ: Author.

efficiency, longer sleep latency, and sleep fragmentation manifested in multiple long-wake episodes (Ensrud, Blackwell, Ancoli-Israel, et al., 2006). Older adults are also at increased risk for developing hyponatremia and the syndrome of inappropriate antidiuretic hormone (SIADH) from SSRIs and venlafaxine (Effexor). Severe SIADH can cause confusion, weakness, and seizures. Consequently, serum sodium levels must be monitored prior to initiating medication and 4 weeks later. An adequate medication trial requires 6 or more weeks of a recommended dosage (Table 10.1).

Although response to antidepressant medications is common, complete remission from depression is less frequent (Lapid and Rammans, 2003). Several psychosocial and clinical factors have been identified as predictors of remission from geriatric depression: adequate social support, better medical health, early and aggressive treatment with antidepressants and/or antipsychotics, and use of electroconvulsive therapy (ECT) when clinically indicated (Bosworth, McQuoid, George, et al., 2002). Treatment of major depression when comorbidities exist (e.g., anxiety, drug dependence, or medical or neurologic disorders) is less clear except for anxiety.

Electroconvulsive Therapy

ECT treatment has been established as being safe and effective for treatment of late-life major depression with an efficacy rate as high as 80 to 90 percent (Greenberg and Kellner, 2005). It has been suggested that ECT should be considered as first-line treatment in older depressed individuals with psychotic depression, for those who cannot tolerate the adverse effects of antidepressant medication, or for those in whom antidepressant medication therapy has failed (Dombrovski and Mulsant, 2007; Greenberg and Kellner). In older patients experiencing unipolar depression with suicide intent, 80.9 percent were relieved of suicidal ideation by the end of ECT treatment (Kellner, Knapp, Petrides, et al., 2006). The most important adverse effect is memory impairment, which is often transient (Lapid and Rummans, 2003). However, it is also important to be aware of the risk for traumatic injury to bones and teeth (Rudorfer, Henry, and Sackeim, 2003). The rate of relapse following ECT ranges from 37.1 percent (mean time to relapse 9.0 ± 7.0 weeks) (Kellner et al.) to 50 percent (mean 6.8 years) including relapse and recurrent depression (van Beusekom, van den Broek, and Birkenhager, 2007). Relapse of depression was similar for patients who received pharmacotherapy (combination of lithium carbonate plus nortriptyline hydrochloride) (31.6 percent) at 6 months.

SUICIDE AND OLDER WOMEN

The most serious consequence of depression is suicide. There were 31,484 completed suicides in the United States in 2003. Of this number, 5,248 (17 percent) were committed by older adults (aged 65 years and older) (Centers for Disease Control and Prevention [CDC], 2006), yet older adults comprised only 12.4 percent of the total population. This is equivalent to a suicide rate of 14.6/100,000, with 14.4 deaths occurring per day (McIntosh, 2006). Females attempt suicide

1.5 times more than males and are more likely to attempt by overdosing on medications compared with men, who use more lethal means (Suicide Prevention Resource Center, 2006). However, 307 (7.9 percent) of older adult women who committed suicide in 2003 used firearms (CDC, 2006). The rate of suicide increases with age, with adults aged 85 years and older having the highest suicide rate. The rate of suicide for women peaks in midlife and remains stable or slightly declines after midlife (Conwell, 2001; Moscicki, 1995).

The assessment and management of suicide ideation and behavior for older adults are especially relevant for PCPs. Several retrospective studies have indicated that >70 percent of older patients who commit suicide visited their PCP within the month of their suicide, and approximately 33 percent visited their PCP within the week of their suicide (Brown, Bruce, Pearson, et al., 2001). In these studies, most of the patients had not been diagnosed with a psychiatric disorder nor had they received or sought mental health services (Brown et al.).

Older suicide attempters often plan for their suicide over a period of time and use methods that are more lethal in comparison to younger adult attempters, who are more impulsive and tend to notify or make warnings before their attempt (Szanto, Gildenger, Mulsant, et al., 2002). Social and functional factors make older adults more isolated and less likely to be rescued after afflicting self-harm than younger adults (Conwell, 2001). Further, older adults who commit suicide are more likely to have major affective disorder compared with younger adults, who are more likely to be diagnosed with schizophrenia, substance use, and/or conduct disorder (Conwell and Brent, 1995).

There are myriad risk factors for suicide in older women, which makes accurate prediction of who will commit suicide difficult. The best predictors of suicidal behavior are a history of a suicide attempt (Brown, Beck, Steer, et al., 2000; Oquendo, Galfalvy, Russo, et al., 2004; Sher, 2004), current suicidal thoughts, and presence of hopelessness that is suggestive of an imminent risk. In fact, hopelessness is consistently found to be a significant predictor of suicidal ideation, the seriousness of suicidal intent, and completed suicide (Szanto, Reynolds, Conway, et al., 1998). Moreover, despite resolution of depression symptoms after treatment, studies report that subjective rates of hopelessness remain high (Szanto et al.) and that hopelessness is a stronger indication of suicidal intent than depression itself (Beck, Kovacks, and Weissman, 1975). Other risk factors include a history of childhood abuse (e.g., physical, emotional, sexual), with the long-terms effects presenting as lifelong depression, poor perception of self-value, hopelessness (negative perception toward the future), and chronic suicidal ideation (Dube, Anda, Felliti et al., 2001; Mann, Waternaux, Haas, et al., 1999; McHolm, MacMillan, and Jamieson, 2003).

Comorbid conditions and social isolation are frequently cited among older adult attempters. The most common psychiatric condition associated with suicide or serious suicide attempts are mood disorders (Szanto et al., 2002). However, personality disorders, alcohol and substance abuse, anxiety disorders, and schizophrenia are also frequently associated with suicidal behavior (Sher, 2004). Other common chronic illnesses associated with suicide are moderate and severe pain, psychoses with agitation, sleep disorders, and bipolar disorder (Juurlink, Herrmann, Szalai, et al., 2004). Juulink, Herrmann, and Szalai found that patients who committed suicide with a firearm and/or by poisoning were more likely to have severe pain. In the same study, patients with three illnesses were found to have a threefold increase in the estimated relative risk of suicide, and patients with five illnesses had about a fivefold increase risk when compared with patients who had no identifiable illness. Lower social interaction pattern, perceived social support, and widowhood are also significantly related to suicidal ideation (Dennis, Baillon, Brugha, et al., 2007; Rowe, Conwell, Schulberg, et al., 2006; Stroebe, Stroebe and Abakoumkin, 2005). The satisfaction with one's relationships and feeling useful to family and friends are significantly associated with a lower likelihood of suicidal ideation and may serve as a protective factor (Rowe et al., 2006).

Buffers to suicide have been identified. Malone, Oquendo, Haas, et al. (2000) found that persons with major depression who had "reasons for living" were less likely to attempt suicide compared with those who had attempted suicide. Other factors noted in those who did not attempt suicide included greater survival and coping beliefs, fear of social disapproval, and moral objections to suicide. Religious affiliation has also been identified as a buffer to suicide. Dervic, Oquendo, Grunebaum, et al. (2004) found that participants in their study who had no religious affiliation reported more lifetime suicide attempts, more suicidal ideation, and were more likely to have first-degree relatives who had committed suicide than religiously affiliated subjects. Hopelessness and depression scores were similar in the religious and nonreligious group, but the two groups differed in regard to perceived reasons for living. This suggests that some positive aspect of religious affiliation overcame the negative effects of depression, stressful life events, feelings of hopelessness, and suicidal ideations (Dervic et al.). It is reasonable to assume that these findings can be extrapolated to older adult women. Older adult women who present in the clinical setting may be experiencing feelings of depression, hopelessness, and not wanting to live. However, those who are without a plan are most often those who are able to state a reason for living. In addition, as the woman enters into and out of the suicidal process, the concept of committing suicide becomes more of an acceptable alternative to living in a state of despair and hopelessness. Once the moral objection is overcome (e.g., suicide is acceptable), then the older adult is more likely to act.

Assessment

Older women who present in the primary care setting with symptoms of depression and anxiety should be assessed for suicide risk. Considerations in the evaluation for suicide risk include (a) presence of suicidal or homicidal ideation, intent, or plans; (b) access to means for suicide and the lethality of those means; (c) presence of psychotic symptoms, command hallucinations, or severe anxiety; (d) presence of alcohol or substance use; (e) history and seriousness of previous attempts; and (f) family history of or recent exposure to suicide (American Psychiatric Association [APA], 2003). Specific questions to ask include: Have you ever felt that life was not worth living? Did you ever wish you could go to sleep and just not wake up? Do you have a suicide plan? Under what conditions would you consider making an attempt? Are there any firearms in the household or workplace? Have you recently purchased a firearm?

Three assessment scales may be useful in developing a line of questioning about suicide; however, they have low predictive values and do not provide reliable estimates of suicide risk. The Scale of Suicide Ideation (Beck, Kovacs, and Weissman, 1979) is a 19-point clinically administered scale. This scale has been widely used in primary care, emergency rooms, rehabilitation programs, and private practices (Brown et al., 2001) and has been used with older adults. Scores above 3 are considered high risk. The Suicide Intent Scale (Beck, Schuyler, and Herman, 1974) assesses the degree of intent, whereas the degree of medical lethality can be measured using the Suicide Lethality Scale (Beck, Beck, and Kovacs, 1975). Both of these scales characterize most recent and most severe past attempt(s). The Beck Hopelessness Scale (Beck, Weissman, Lester, et al., 1974) may also be useful when assessing suicide intent. This scale measures a person's negative expectancies or sense of hopelessness and consists of 20 true/false statements. Scores range from 0 to 20, with higher scores indicating higher levels of hopelessness.

Crisis Management

Crisis management is required in the event that an older woman (or man) expresses active suicide ideation or has a suicide plan. The following approaches for dealing with suicidal patients are based on the recommendations of the Prevention of Suicide in Primary Care Elderly: Collaborative Trial

(PROSPECT) study. PROSPECT is a collaborative, multicenter study that focuses on *primary care*-based interventions to reduce major risk factors for suicide in later life (Brown et al., 2001). Their recommendations include: (a) be very attentive, and take suicidal ideation seriously; (b) remain calm and nonthreatened; (c) give the patient some space and time to vent; (d) stress a team approach to the problem; and (e) be willing to say the word *suicide* (Brown et al.). If the patient is a high risk for suicide, she needs to be informed that a consultation with a psychiatrist will need to be made. The patient should make a verbal consent to the agreement for consultation. If the patient fails to provide consent to see a psychiatrist, the patient is then notified that she cannot be left alone until the psychiatrist is consulted for her own safety. The psychiatrist will develop and suggest the treatment plan, which may consist of voluntary or involuntary hospitalization, intensive outpatient treatment, medication changes, psychotherapy, or any other intervention or further consultation or monitoring as clinically indicated (Brown et al.). If the PCP does not have a consulting psychiatrist, the patient's family must be contacted and the patient taken to the nearest emergency room for further assessment and treatment. If the family is unavailable, then the PCP should contact the local police department or call an ambulance to transport the patient to the hospital. It is important for PCPs to have an understanding of the rules and regulations in the state where they practice regarding their responsibility when they have a suicidal patient and how patients in a crisis situation enter the mental health system (Box 10.3). The APA (2003) has

Box 10.3 • When to Consider Hospitalization for a Suicidal Patient

1. Psychosis is present
2. Significant substance abuse, severe hopelessness, or strong desire to act on ideas
3. Lack of sufficient social support to participate in outpatient treatment
4. Concurrent medical conditions that could make outpatient medication treatment unsafe
5. Patient lacks ability to participate in outpatient care
6. Patient refuses to contract for safety
7. Patient has a definite plan and the means to commit suicide

From Brown, G. K., Bruce, M. L., & Pearson, J. L. (2001). High-risk management guidelines for elderly suicidal patients in primary care setting. *International Journal of Geriatric Psychiatry, 16*, 593–601.

developed guidelines for selecting a treatment setting for patients at risk for suicide or suicidal behavior. These guidelines are available at *www.psychiatryonline.com/pracGuide/pracGuideTopic_14.aspx*.

ANXIETY AND OLDER WOMEN

Older women are more likely to have an anxiety disorder compared with older men based on data from the Epidemiological Catchments Area (ECA) study, one of the largest investigations of the prevalence of mental disorders ever completed. Based on ECA data, older women had rates of 6.8 percent overall for anxiety disorders, with 6.1 percent for phobias, 0.9 percent for obsessive-compulsive disorder (OCD), and 0.2 percent for panic disorder, whereas the rates for men were 3.6 percent overall, with 2.9 percent for phobias, 0.7 percent for OCD, and 0.0 percent for panic disorder (Regier, Boyd, Burke, et al., 1988). In a review of eight random-sample community surveys of anxiety disorders in people aged 60 years and older, agoraphobia and OCD were reported to occur as a primary disorder for the first time in old age for women (Flint, 1994). Although the prevalence of most anxiety disorders is believed to decrease with age (Flint), general anxiety disorder (GAD) remains at a constant prevalence rate throughout life. As a result, GAD is one of the most prevalent anxiety disorders in adults aged 60 years and older (Flint) and is a common illness seen in primary care settings. In addition to GAD, subsyndromal anxiety has been identified in 30 to 60 percent of elderly depressed persons living in the community (Flint and Rifat, 1997). Moreover, anxiety in primary care is a global health concern The 1-month prevalence rate for GAD was 8 percent in a 14-country, World Health Organization–sponsored study conducted in primary care settings (Woodman, Noyes, Black, et al., 1999).

The most frequent and consistent finding regarding late-life anxiety is its high level of comorbidity with major depression (Flint, 2005), with anxiety frequently symptomatic of the depression. A study of 182 depressed subjects aged 60 years and older seen in primary care and psychiatric settings reported a high rate of lifetime (35 percent) and current (23 percent) comorbid anxiety disorders. The most common current comorbid anxiety disorders were panic disorder (9.8 percent), specific phobias (8.8 percent), and social phobia (6.6 percent). Symptoms that met inclusion criteria for GAD, measured separately, were present in 27.5 percent of depressed subjects (Lenze, Mulsant, Shear, et al., 2000). A study conducted in the Netherlands (N = 3,056, aged 55 to 85 years) found that 47.5 percent of those with major depression also met criteria for anxiety disorder, whereas 26.1 percent of those with anxiety disorders also met criteria for major depressive disorder (Beekman, de Beurs, van Balkom, et al., 2000).

The combination of depressive and anxiety disorders can lead to marked functional disability (Mohamed, Osatuke, Aslam, et al., 2006) and poor social functioning (Lenze et al., 2000) and has been associated with a poorer treatment response and a longer time to response compared with either condition alone (Mohamed et al.). Comorbid anxiety has also been associated with higher levels of somatic symptoms and suicidality (Lenze et al.; Sareen, Cox, Afifi, et al., 2005). A recent study investigating the effects of anxiety and depression on cognitive functioning found that anxious older subjects displayed short-term memory impairment, while depressed subjects displayed executive dysfunction (Mantella, Butters, Dew, et al., 2007).

Assessment

Making an appropriate differential diagnosis is critical to the success of any intervention. Although many of the diagnostic strategies are the same for older women as for younger women, there are some characteristics of late-life anxiety that warrant mention. There are several common illnesses in late life that may present with anxiety as part of the clinical presentation. These include cardiovascular diseases, particularly cardiac failure, mitral valve prolapse, and cardiac arrhythmias; respiratory distress, including chronic obstructive pulmonary disease, pulmonary embolus, and sleep apnea; endocrine disorders, especially thyroid and adrenal hyperactivity; neurologic illness; and vitamin B_{12} deficiency. Various drugs commonly cause anxiety or increase preexisting anxiety, such as caffeine, over-the-counter cold preparations, and select antidepressants (monoamine oxidase inhibitors, desipramine, fluoxetine). Lastly, in older adults, anxiety disorders are almost always accompanied by symptoms of depression, and major depressive disorder is almost always accompanied by symptoms of anxiety (Salzman, Roose, and Chatterjee, 2004) (Box 10.4. Refer to Chapter 4 for assessment strategies for specific anxiety disorders).

Treatment Options

As with geriatric depression, treatment options for anxiety include nonpharmacologic and pharmacologic interventions. In terms of nonpharmacologic interventions, CBT is the most frequently studied treatment for GAD (the most common anxiety disorder in older adults). Although CBT is more effective than

Box 10.4 • Potential Differential Diagnoses for Patients with Anxiety Disorders

1. Adjustment disorder secondary to life stressors
2. Anxiety disorder secondary to a medical condition
3. Anxiety symptoms secondary to a medical condition
4. Anxiety secondary to alcohol or substance abuse or dependence
5. Generalized anxiety disorder (GAD)
6. Panic disorder (PD)
7. Social anxiety disorder
8. Specific phobia
9. Posttraumatic stress disorder (PTSD)
10. Obsessive-compulsive disorder (OCD)

From Maddux, R. E., & Rapaport, M. H. (2003). Anxioltyic drugs. In A. Tasman, J. Kay, & J. A. Liberman (Eds.), *Psychiatry therapeutics* (2nd ed., pp. 335–355). West Sussex, England: John Wiley and Sons, Ltd.

a wait-list control condition (list of subjects waiting to obtain treatment), it is not more effective than nondirective therapies and appears to be less efficacious in older adults than younger adults (Flint, 2005).

Pharmacologic interventions include three primary classes of medications: antidepressants, benzodiazepines, and buspirone. Antidepressant medications are the pharmacologic treatment of choice for "pure" anxiety as well as for anxiety comorbid with depression in older adults. SSRIs (e.g., fluoxetine, sertraline, paroxetine, fluvoxamine, citalopram) and new antidepressants (e.g., venlafaxine, mirtazapine, bupropion, nefazodone) are recommended as first-line agents for the treatment of depression and anxiety disorders (Mohammed et al., 2006). Refer to Chapter 4 for additional information on medications.

Benzodiazepines are the second most commonly prescribed medication for anxiety. Older adults are prescribed more benzodiazepines than any other age group (Llorente, Golden, and Silverman, 2000), and older women are more likely to receive prescriptions for benzodiazepines than older men (Blow and Barry, 2002). However, the side effects of benzodiazepines often limit their therapeutic usefulness in this age population. All benzodiazepines can cause sedation, ataxia, falls, hip fractures, function decline, and cognitive impairment (Lantz, 2004) and worsen depressive symptoms (Shader and Songer, 2003).

Table 10.2 • Preferred Benzodiazepines for Use in the Older Adult

Drug	Half-Life	Onset of Action	Geriatric Dose Range
Lorazepam	8–14 hr	1–2 hr	0.5–2.0 mg/day
Alprazolam	10–14 hr	1 hr	0.25–1.00 mg/day
Oxazepam	10–15 hr	1–2 hr	10–0 mg/day
When agent with long half-life preferred:			
Clonazepam	20–50 hr	1–2 hr	0.25–1.00 mg/day

From Lantz, M. S. (2004). Chronic benzodiazepine treatment in the older adult: Therapeutic or problematic? *Clinical Geriatrics, 12*(5), 21–23.

Additionally, drug interactions with benzodiazepines are quite common. When mixed with other sedating compounds (e.g., alcohol, narcotics, antihistamines), the effects are additive. Further, the use of antacids that slow gastric emptying may decrease the rate of absorption from the small intestines, altering both peak and concentration effects (Shader and Songer). If a benzodiazepine must be initiated, pharmacokinetic considerations favor the use of either lorazepam or oxazepam in older adults because of the shorter half-lives (Table 10.2). Discontinuing treatment can be difficult because of dependency and tolerance (Mohamed et al., 2006). Women experience more protracted withdrawal symptoms when undergoing taper of long-term benzodiazepine therapy (Lantz) and will experience both benzodiazepine withdrawal and rebound anxiety if the medications are abruptly discontinued. Dose reductions of 10 to 20 percent per week are recommended in older patients (Lantz). Buspirone also has a more limited role than antidepressants in the treatment of late-life GAD (Flint, 2005).

SUBSTANCE ABUSE AND OLDER WOMEN

Substance abuse and dependence in older adults is less common that in younger adults but is also less apt to be recognized (Lantz, 2005). Diagnosis is often more difficult because older adults are more likely to deny the problem, and impairment in functioning may be attributed to the aging process or health problems rather than drug use/misuse/abuse (Lantz). As noted previously, nicotine, sedative-hypnotics, and alcohol are the substances most commonly abused by older adults (Wiseman, 2000). This section will focus on prescription drug misuse and alcohol.

Prescription Misuse and Abuse

There are no population-based studies on the prevalence of prescription drug misuse and abuse in older adults, and research in this area is scarce. The few observational and retrospective studies that are available offer some insights. A study conducted in 1990 with 50 elderly patients referred for prescription drug abuse reported that diazepam, codeine, meprobamate, and flurazepam were the top four drugs abused. Duration of misuse over 5 years was seen in 92 percent of the patients, with a 60 percent correlation with codependency related to alcoholism and alcohol dependence (Schmader and Moore, 2003). A retrospective case review from the Mayo Clinic inpatient addiction program found 100 older adults admitted between 1974 and 1993 with prescription drug abuse. The majority were women who primarily abused opioids, although many had codependencies on other prescription drugs as well (Schmader and Moore). Women who abuse medications are more likely to be married to an alcoholic or drug abuser, be victims of domestic violence, or suffer from unrecognized psychiatric disorders such as depression and anxiety (Lantz, 2005). It has been suggested that a great deal of problem drug use in older adults may be iatrogenic and only identified after a patient is hospitalized for medication-related disorders (Lantz).

Warning signs of prescription drug abuse include cognitive impairment, delirium, personality change, altered mood, unexpected complaints about chronic pain that do not seem normal, seizures, thinking about withdrawal, tremor, restlessness, agitation, sleep complaints, and withdrawal from family, friends, and normal activities. Medical and functional changes include anorexia, poor eating, malnutrition, frequent falls, functional decline, poor hygiene, and traffic accidents. Signs of drug-related behavior to look for include continuous requests for refills, particularly when the condition for which the prescription was originally made is no longer an issue, complaints about other PCPs who refuse to write prescriptions for preferred drugs, and self-medication (Schmader and Moore, 2003). Older adults who abuse prescription medications are at extremely high risk for suicide due to depression, isolation, and the erratic behavior and impaired judgment that accompanies substance abuse (Lantz, 2005).

Alcohol Dependence and Abuse

It is estimated that between 40 to 50 percent of adults ages 65 years and older drink alcohol (Breslow, Faden, and Smothers, 2003). The ECA study reported that women aged 65 years and older had a 1.5 percent rate of alcohol dependence compared with 14 percent among men (Robins, Helzer, and Przybeck, 1988).

Moreover, an estimated 12 percent of older women regularly drink in excess of recommended guidelines (no more than one drink per day or seven drinks per week) and can be considered at-risk drinkers (Blow, 2000). A study conducted in a clinic setting (e.g., geriatric psychiatry, $N = 140$) reported that over 87.5 percent of subjects diagnosed with benzodiazepine dependence were women, as were 58.3 percent of those with alcohol dependence (Holroyd and Duryee,1997).

Older women experience many physical, social, and psychological factors that make them more vulnerable to at-risk drinking or dependence: loneliness, financial difficulties, isolation, bereavement, retirement, insomnia, pain, depression, anxiety, loss of function, comorbidity, and polypharmacy (Schmader and Moore, 2003). Physiologically, women are at greater risk for alcohol-related illnesses and for swifter progression to those illnesses as they age (Blow, 2000). Age-related changes adversely impact the absorption, metabolism, and distribution of alcohol. A few of these changes include lower levels of alcohol dehydrogenase enzyme, which helps to metabolize alcohol in the stomach, as well as higher body fat and lower body water, which tends to increase blood alcohol levels (Moore, Whiteman, and Ward, 2007). Many of the illnesses common in older women can be worsened by consumption of specific amounts of alcohol: hypertension, diabetes mellitus, upper gastrointestinal conditions, gout, insomnia, depression, and cognitive impairment. Other illnesses, while not necessarily more prevalent in older women, may also be worsened by alcohol use: liver disease, seizures, and breast cancer (Moore et al.). Finally, older women who drink alcohol and take medications (which is >90 percent of older adults) are at risk for a variety of adverse consequences depending on the amount of alcohol and the type of medications consumed (Moore et al.). Thus, it is important for PCPs to know how much alcohol their older women patients are drinking to be able to effectively assess their risks and counsel them about safe use of alcohol and medications (Moore et al.).

Assessment

The goals of screening are to identify at-risk drinkers, problem drinkers, or people with alcohol abuse or dependency disorders and to determine the need for further assessment (Blow and Barry, 2002). Screening may be conducted as part of the physical health services in primary care and updated annually. When assessing for alcohol misuse, it is also important to assess for prescription drug abuse, as there is a high codependency. Many of the screening instruments for at-risk and problem drinking have been developed and validated with younger populations and are not reliable or valid with older women. CAGE, a widely used alcohol screen test, does not have high validity with older adults, in particular older women (Adams, Barry, and Fleming, 1996). (Refer to Chapter 5, Table 5.4, for a summary of screening instruments.) However, two screening instruments have been developed specifically for older adults. The Short Michigan Alcoholism Screening Test-Geriatric Version (SMAST-G), consists of quantity and frequency questions embedded with questions about other health habits. The SMAST-G is available at *www.naatp.org/pdf/secad/05speakers/13MAST-G.pdf.* Moore, Whiteman, and Ward also developed a survey specific for older adults. The Short Alcohol-Related Problems Survey is a 32-item questionnaire that has a reported sensitivity of 89 percent and specificity of 77 percent (Schmader and Moore, 2003). A four-step approach for screening alcohol misuse has been recommended (Box 10.5).

Treatment Options

Substance abuse interventions for older women are similar to those offered to younger adults. These approaches include education, brief structured interventions, cognitive behavioral approaches, group-based approaches, individual counseling, medical/psychiatric approaches, marital and family involvement/family therapy, case management/community linked services and outreach, and formal alcohol treatment (Blow and Barry, 2002). Only a few studies have focused on the effectiveness of substance abuse treatment in older adults, and of these studies, the focus has been on alcohol treatment. These studies found that cognitive behavioral approaches (e.g., teaching older adults skills necessary to rebuild social support networks and using self-management approaches for overcoming depression, grief, and loneliness) were successful in reducing or stopping alcohol use (Blow, Walton, Chermack, et al., 2000). Case management services were found to be helpful for older adults receiving alcoholism treatment and may be the most effective strategy for providing outreach services (Atkinson, 1995). Lastly, screening and brief intervention, 5- to 15-minute sessions of information and advice about the risks of drinking and how to reduce drinking, may be especially useful in minimizing alcohol problems in older women (Blow and Barry).

DEMENTIA AND OLDER WOMEN

The incidence and prevalence of dementia is rapidly expanding as our population of 75 million baby boomers ages. Because cognitive functioning is the key to

Box 10.5 • Four-Step Approach for Screening Substance Misuse and Abuse

Step 1: Ask about alcohol or prescription use.
- How often do you typically drink?
- How much do you have when you have a drink?
- Is it a can of beer, a tall boy, a shot, or a double shot?
- Do you drink more on certain occasions?

Step 2: Assess for alcohol-related problems.
- Why do you drink?
- Does it make you feel good?
- Does it help you sleep?
- Is it just something you do because your friends drink?
- What symptoms do you experience when you drink? Do you think any of the symptoms you experience are related to the interaction between the alcohol and your medications? Between the alcohol and your medical problems?

Step 3: Advise appropriate action.
- Recommend low-risk drinking limits for patients who are not alcohol dependent.
- Ask patients to set specific drinking goals.
- Provide educational material.
- Refer for additional diagnostic evaluation and treatment if there is evidence of dependence.

Step 4: Monitor progress.
- Provide regular follow-up and support.
- If not ready to make a change, try to address the drinking periodically so that patients know you believe it is an issue for them.

From Schmader, K. E., & Moore, A. A. (2003). Misadventures with drugs and alcohol in the older patient: Alcohol use, misuse, and abuse in older persons. *Annals of Long-Term Care, 11*(8), 37-43.

quality of life, the increasing incidence of dementia in the United States and the world is a grave concern, as there is no known prevention or cure. AD is by far the most prevalent of the dementias, with predictions of it affecting 8.5 million Americans by the year 2030. The National Institute on Aging estimated that 4.5 million Americans, or about 5 percent of men and women between the ages of 65 and 74 years, suffered from AD in 2006 (National Institutes of Health,

National Institute on Aging, 2006). For men and women over the age of 85 years, approximately 50 percent may acquire the disease. Women may have an even greater risk for AD than men, regardless of their longer life span (35 percent for women and 20 percent for men) (Potyk, 2005). Despite the high prevalence of dementia with advancing age, it is not inevitable, nor is it a part of, the normal aging process.

With the growing numbers of elderly who seek health care services in primary care settings, PCPs will increasingly be expected to have the expertise to diagnose, treat, and refer patients with AD and other dementias. This is a difficult challenge not only because of the variety of dementias but because of the many medical conditions that may present as dementia in elderly people. As well, diagnostic procedures, treatment, and resources are becoming more complex, which adds to the challenge.

Although many studies have been conducted, more research is needed to determine whether the incidence of AD is greater in women than men and whether there are significant sex differences in cognition and behavioral symptoms. It is also important to determine if there are gender differences in treatment response. Recent research has found that older women who were taking combination hormone therapy had twice the rate of dementia than women who did not take the hormones (Shumaker, Legault, and Rapp, 2003). On the positive side, older women who exercised seemed to have protection against cognitive impairment compared with women who did not exercise (Sumic, Michael, Carlson, et al., 2007).

Types of Dementia

The *Diagnostic and Statistical Manual of Mental Disorders* (*DSM-IV-TR*) lists 12 different types of dementia, including AD (American Psychiatric Association [APA], 2000). The non-AD dementias are reported to encompass approximately 20 to 40 percent of incurable forms of dementia (Boeve, 2006). The non-AD dementias include those due to general medical conditions such as vascular (multiple infarct), HIV, head trauma, substance induced, and multiple etiologies as well as Parkinson, Huntington, Pick's, and Creutzfeldt-Jacob diseases. Less research has been conducted on these dementias; therefore, the clinical and neuropathologic terminology is confusing and still evolving. Reiman (2006), while acknowledging the difficulties inherent in the diagnosis of the non-AD dementias, urges practitioners to become aware of these dementias by being alert to patients who present with atypical symptoms or neuropsychological findings, early age onset, or strong familial patterns.

Etiology of Dementias

Although the dementias share common symptoms, they also have differences based on etiology. The universal common symptom is the development of multiple cognitive deficits including both short- and long-term memory impairments (criterion 1). These cognitive deficits are caused by physiologic effects from a medical condition, a substance, or multiple causes. Besides the memory impairment, the cognitive deficits of dementia include at least one of the following (criterion 2): aphasia (language difficulties), apraxia (deficits in motor function despite normal motor function), agnosia (failure to recognize objects despite intact sensory function), or executive function disturbances (planning, organizing, sequencing, abstracting). The cognitive deficits are pronounced and interfere with social and occupational functioning (APA, 2000).

Typically, the person with dementia will have no awareness of her cognitive deficiencies. She may also be suicidal in the early stages of the disease and, on occasion, violent. Hallucinations (usually visual) and delusions (usually paranoid) are not uncommon. Delirium can occur concurrently with dementia because the person is more vulnerable to side effects from medications, medical conditions, and psychological and environmental stressors. While many theories exist about the exact cause of dementia, the consensus seems to be that there are multiple causes.

An enormous amount of dementia research is being conducted to prevent and reverse this degenerative process. One line of research is focusing on delaying the onset of dementia through disease-modifying therapies. Another focus has been on identifying mild cognitive impairment (MCI), which may precede full-blown dementia. Researchers theorize that early intervention is critical because it may slow and/or prevent the degenerative process. It also gives the patient and family time to plan for the future as the patient continues to deteriorate (Petersen, 2007).

Many risks for dementia have been identified. The two most important risk factors are older age and genetics. Other risk factors include infections, nutritional deficiencies, brain injuries, brain tumors, toxic substances, endocrine disorders, and vascular disorders (APA, 2000).

Many conditions and events can cause dementia or present with similar symptoms. One very important differential diagnosis is between dementia and delirium. While both conditions have cognitive deficits, delirium symptoms tend to fluctuate as opposed to dementia, which has a stable course. The two conditions are not mutually exclusive, as dementia is a significant risk factor for delirium, and it is not uncommon to find delirium superimposed on a preexisting

Table 10.3 • Differences Between Delirium and Dementia

Delirium Characteristics	Dementia Characteristics
Sudden onset (hours to days); fluctuating symptoms through the day	Gradual onset without fluctuation
LOC: varies	LOC: normal
Confused and disoriented	Confused and disoriented
Sleep-wake cycle disruptions	Usually normal
Insight can be present at times	No insight
Memory impairment, especially short term	Memory impairment, especially short term
Mental status varies; improves with recovery	Mental status progressively worse
Evidence of organic cause; not due to primary psychiatric disorder	May be due to a medical condition, chronic substance use, or combinations

dementia. Therefore, it is important to inquire about preexisting cognitive deficits in patients with delirium (Kaufer, 2005). Table 10.3 describes the differences between delirium and dementia.

Some dementias are partially or totally reversible (approximately 10 percent), so it must not be assumed that the person is suffering from an incurable disease without ruling out the possibility of treatable conditions. Anticholinergic medications are a common cause of mental status changes in the elderly, including delirium and vivid visual hallucinations. Antipsychotic medications may also cause mental status changes such as excessive sedation, tremors, and gait problems (Kaufer, 2005). Table 10.4 identifies causes of the reversible dementias and the irreversible dementias.

ALZHEIMER'S DISEASE

The focus of the remainder of this chapter will be on AD, as it is by far the most common dementia and the one most often encountered by the PCP. However, much of what is discussed has application for all the irreversible dementias.

Table 10.4 • Etiologies of Reversible and Irreversible Dementias

Reversible Dementias	Irreversible Dementias
Chronic substance abuse	Alzheimer's disease
Removable tumors	Vascular dementia (multi-infarct)
Subdural hematomas	Parkinson's dementia & similar disorders
Normal pressure hydrocephalus	Pick's disease
Metabolic disorders (including vitamin B_{12} deficiency)	Creutzfeldt-Jacob disease
Hypothyroidism	AIDS dementia
Hypoglycemia	
Depression	
Antipsychotic & anticholinergic medications	
HIV infections	

Assessment

The assessment of AD is challenging because it is a heterogeneous disorder that has multiple clinical presentations. Because there is no confirmatory test, the clinical diagnosis is critical, as it will determine both the prognosis and the management of the disease. Younger patients typically have more reversible causes of dementia, but conversely, they may show a more rapid progression than older patients. Clinical assessments can be supported by magnetic resonance imaging, computed tomography scan, electroencephalogram (EEG), cerebrospinal fluid, and psychometric evaluation, particularly with the younger patient.

Brain changes on autopsy of patients with AD typically show abnormal clumps of material called *amyloid plaques* along with neurofibrillary tangles that contain tau protein. Other brain changes include brain atrophy, widened sulci, and shrinkage of gyri. Usually, the total cerebral cortex is affected while the occipital area is often unaffected (Yaari and Corey-Bloom, 2007).

As a dementia, AD has the two basic symptoms consisting of cognitive deficits (criterion A) and serious impairment due to these deficits (criterion B) (Box 10.6). Unfortunately, a definite diagnosis cannot be made because of the lack of direct pathologic evidence. Therefore, the diagnosis is made after excluding all other possibilities (Table 10.4). The AD subtypes include early onset (before age

Box 10.6 • *DSM-IV-TR* Criteria for Alzheimer's Disease

A. Multiple cognitive deficits including :
   (1) memory impairment
   (2) one or more of the following cognitive disturbances: aphasia, agnosia, and impaired executive functioning
B. These deficits result in significant impairment in functioning as compared to previous level of functioning.
C. The disease has a gradual onset and continuous cognitive decline.
D. The cognitive deficits are not due to other nervous system causes or other Axis 1 disorders.

From the American Psychiatric Association (2000). *Diagnostic and statistical manual of mental disorders* (Revised 4th ed.). Washington, DC: Author.

65 years) and late onset (after age 65 years). The subtypes are further classified according to the presence or absence of behavioral disturbances such as wandering and agitation. As with all dementias, the prevalence of AD increases with age. Progression is gradual, with an average duration of 8 to 10 years from the recognition of symptoms to death. Box 10.6 identifies the *DSM-IV-TR* diagnostic criteria for AD (APA, 2000). The National Institute of Neurological and Communicative Disorders and Stroke and the Alzheimer's Disease and Related Disorders Association have also developed diagnostic criteria for AD. Their criteria are more detailed than that found in the *DSM-IV-TR* and are classified according to levels of diagnostic certainty (McKhann, Drachman, Folstein, et al., 1984).

Some practitioners find the Mini-Mental State Examination helpful in diagnosing dementia, but results alone are not diagnostic (Yaari and Corey-Bloom, 2007). However, no simple tests exist that would be appropriate for screening patients in primary care settings for dementia. Although laboratory tests cannot diagnose or confirm the presence of AD, they are important to rule out differential diagnosis, particularly reversible dementias. The routine recommended lab tests include a complete blood count, chemistry panel, thyroid function tests, and serum vitamin B_{12} levels. Additional laboratory tests, x-rays, EEG, neuroimaging, and other tests are conducted as well.

Frequently, the patient may exhibit MCI but does not qualify for the diagnosis of AD. Ismail (2006) emphasizes that distinguishing between MCI and AD is very challenging, and the difference is quantitative rather than qualitative. As well, patients with MCI have a higher risk for progression to AD than other patients with neuropsychiatric symptoms.

Two other conditions, mixed dementia and Parkinson's disease, should be considered when assessing a patient for AD. Mixed dementia seems to be in the middle of a continuum between AD and vascular dementia. Although similar to AD, mixed dementia presents with a cerebral vascular history and has a faster onset, more fluctuations, uneven cognitive deficits, seizures, and radiographic and neuroimaging changes.

The presence of Parkinson's symptoms does not preclude a diagnosis of AD. Ismail (2006) suggests that when symptoms of AD and Parkinson's coexist, one must consider the possibility of dementia with Lewy bodies. Furthermore, Ismail emphasizes that it is not uncommon to encounter patients with AD who also present with the above conditions and/or other medical conditions as well.

Stages of Alzheimer's Disease

Ismail (2006) describes three stages of AD: mild, moderate, and severe. The stages affect the clinical presentation of the disease regarding activities of daily living (ADLs), behavior, and cognition. The mild stage is characterized by social withdrawal or isolation, less involvement in complex activities, some symptoms of depression, and memory loss. At this time, depression may be difficult to diagnose because of its atypical presentation with symptoms such as anxiety, worry, irritability, and fear.

The moderate stage of AD involves loss of basic ADLs and behavioral symptoms such as paranoia, hallucinations, anxiety, agitation, and aggression. The majority of patients with AD have behavioral disturbances, and these symptoms hasten institutionalization of the patient because of caregiver burnout. The severe stage of AD is marked by medical comorbidities; serious medical conditions; and issues related to safety, placement, and comfort. The most common comorbidities are musculoskeletal; genitourinary; and ear, nose, and throat disorders. Tariot (2006) maintains that one of the principles of patient-focused care for the patient with dementia is that some treatment must be offered at all stages of the illness.

Treatment Options

Pharmacologic Treatment

There is no treatment that directly impacts the *pathophysiologic* processes that cause the various types of dementias and their symptoms. Therefore, the pharmacologic management of dementia must focus on target symptoms. There are several standard antidementia treatments available, and studies have demonstrated that these agents can slow the decline in cognition and daily functioning in patients with AD. However, these agents are being underused (Tariot, 2006). The Food and Drug Administration (FDA) has approved cholinesterase inhibitors (donepezil, galantamine, and rivastigmine) for patients with mild to moderate AD and the N-methyl-D-aspartate (NMDA) receptor memantine for treatment of moderate to severe AD. Recently, donepezil (Aricept) has also been approved for severe AD. Switching cholinesterase inhibitors may improve symptoms, as the profile of these medications varies and patients may respond differently to each. A washout period of 4 days was found to be the most effective procedure to minimize adverse effects (Lyketsos, Colenda, and Beck, 2006).

Because AD is often heterogeneous and treatment may need to be stage specific, combining antidementia medications may result in synergistic effects. Such is the case with adding memantine to existing donepezil, as researchers have reported that the combination preserved or even improved functioning (Lyketsos et al, 2006; Tariot, Farlow, and Grossberg, 2004). Improved cognition was also reported in a study that combined memantine and rivastigmine (Riepe, Adler, and Ibach, 2006).

The most common side effects with cholinesterase inhibitors are gastrointestinal, including nausea and vomiting, diarrhea, and abdominal pain. Less common side effects include bradycardia, fatigue, muscle cramps, and sleep disturbances. Patients with renal disease should receive half-doses of memantine, and other NMDA antagonists should not be used in conjunction with memantine (Tariot, 2006).

Antidementia medications have demonstrated improvement in behavioral symptoms such as hallucinations, delusions, anxiety, irritability agitation, and aggression (Cummings, 2006). When the antidementia medications are ineffective for behavioral symptoms, antipsychotic medications that are cautiously used may have therapeutic value for patients. The main concern in using antipsychotics for AD is the black box warning by the FDA of increased incidence of deaths from cardiac, cardiovascular, and cardiopulmonary complications as well as infections (pneumonia) in elderly patients with dementia-related psychosis (Stone, 2005). Therefore, the risk of agitation and aggression in the patient must be weighed against the risk of increased incidence of cardiac complications and infections. PCPs must thoroughly document the rationale for using the antipsychotic medication, including the consideration of existing cardiac or lung disease, and why the medication is appropriate. The antipsychotic must be started at a low dose and increased slowly while monitoring for adverse effects, particularly

Box 10.7 • Strategies for Prescribing Antipsychotic Medications

1. Evaluate environment and psychosocial possibilities as the basis for the increased agitation and aggression; eliminate or minimize frustrations that may trigger symptoms such as excessive stimulation.
2. Rule out all possible medical conditions as causative (e.g., bladder infection, pain, respiratory infection, electrolyte imbalance).
3. Evaluate all existing medications as causative (e.g., anticholinergic effects).
4. Educate family and obtain informed consent.
5. Justify use of antipsychotic with documentation of psychotic behavior and potential for harm to self and others.
6. Justify use of antipsychotic with documentation on why it is the most appropriate medication.
7. Regularly monitor patient for cardiovascular and other possible medical problems, then document.

cognitive decline, low blood pressure, and parkinsonism (Yaari and Correy-Bloom, 2007). Box 10.7 describes strategies to use when prescribing antipsychotics for patients with dementia.

Benzodiazepines should not be used, as they have a potential for adverse cognitive effects. Buspirone would be the preferred anxiolytic to use (Yaari and Corey-Bloom, 2007).

Other medications that have been used and found to be somewhat effective are the SSRIs for depression and anticonvulsants and mood stabilizers for agitation (Cummings, 2006). Research on vitamins has been inconclusive, although a recent meta-analysis found large doses of vitamin E increased all-cause mortality (Miller, Pastor-Barriuso, Dalal, et al., 2005). No evidence has been found to support the use of anti-inflammatory agents, prednisone, and estrogen for AD (Doody, Stevens, and Beck, 2001). Although much of the pharmacotherapy research has been done with AD, it is believed that the agents identified in Table 10.5 are helpful in the management of other dementias as well because they are targeted to symptoms rather than underlying causes that may often be unknown (Boeve, 2006).

Table 10.5 • Pharmacologic Management of Target Symptoms of Dementia

Target Symptom	Preferred Class of Agents	Other Agents
Cognitive		
Amnesia/forgetfulness	AChEI*, memantine	C/L, DA, PS
Aphasia	DA	
Apraxia	C/L, DA	
Executive function	AChEI*	C/L, DA, memantine
Noncognitive		
Agitation/aggression	AN*, SSRI*	AChEI*, BZD, MS
Anxiety	SSRI*, AN	BZD, AChEI
Apathy	AChEI*, SSRI (with stimulating properties)	PS, S/L, DA
Depression	SSRI*	AN, AChEI
Delusions	AN*, SSRI	AChEI
Disinhibition	AN, SSRI	AChEI, MS
Emotional lability	SSRI*	Dextromethorphan/quinidine*
Hallucinations	AN*, AChEI*, SSRI*	Melatonin
Hyperphagia	AED (topiramate)	AN, AChEI
Hypersomnia	AChEI, SSRI (with stimulating properties)	PS
Insomnia	SSRI (with sedating properties), trazodone, S/H	Melatonin, AN
Parasomnia	Melatonin*, clonazepam	AN

AChEI, acetylcholinesterase inhibitor; AED, antiepileptic drug; AN, atypical neuroleptic; BZD, benzodiazepine; C/L, carbidopa/levodopa; DA, dopamine agonist; MS, mood stabilizer; PS, psychostimulant; S/H, sedative/hypnotic; SSRI, selective serotonin reuptake inhibitor.
*Efficacy has been demonstrated in open-label or randomized clinical trials.
From Boeve, 2006.

General Treatment Strategies

Lyketsos, Colenda, and Beck (2006) identified four principles of dementia care published by the American Association of Geriatric Psychiatry. These four principles are disease treatment, symptom treatment, supportive care for the patient, and supportive care for the family or caregiver. Disease treatment focuses on controlling the factors that lead to progression of the disease. For example, studies have demonstrated that systolic pressure above 140 mm Hg accelerates the progression of dementia, while beta-blockers and diuretics slow the progression

(Lyketsos et al.). Vascular risk can be managed by controlling blood pressure and using low-dose aspirin.

Symptom treatment focuses on the three components of dementia symptoms: cognitive, neuropsychiatric, and functional. While no effective treatment has been discovered for functional symptoms, many pharmacologic and nonpharmacologic treatments are available for cognitive and neuropsychiatric symptoms. PCPs should reevaluate patients every 6 to 12 months once they reach the maximum dose of their medication. The evaluation should include ability to perform ADLs, participation in activities, and neuropsychiatric symptoms. When a lack of response to medication exists, the PCP should consider possibilities of inadequate dose, nonadherence to medication, inadequate length of treatment, and problems with other medications (e.g., anticholinergic effects) (Lyketsos et al., 2006).

There is no designated point at which medications should be discontinued, as studies indicate that patients benefit even with late-stage dementia (Lyketsos et al., 2006). However, once the patient reaches terminal dementia stage, consideration of discontinuing medications will need to be done in conjunction with the family, multidisciplinary staff, and advance directives.

Supportive care for the patient and the family are critical in order to improve quality of life, reduce stress, and maintain the patient in her home as long as possible. Educating the caregiver is critical in improving the care of the patient with dementia. Using a team approach in supporting the caregiver will improve information gathering and ongoing evaluation of both patient and caregiver. Table 10.6 describes the basics of supportive care for the patient and caregiver/family.

CONCLUSION

The majority of older adults cope constructively with life changes associated with later life (e.g., physical limitations, cognitive changes, various losses). However, almost 20 percent do experience specific mental disorders that are not considered part of "normal aging" (DHHS, 1999). Unrecognized and untreated depression, dementias, alcohol and/or drug misuse/abuse, and anxiety can be severely impairing, even fatal. The rate of suicide, which is frequently a consequence of depression, is highest among older adults (especially men) relative to all other age groups. Assessing and diagnosing mental disorders are challenging for a variety of reasons. Many older women present with somatic complaints and experience subsyndromal symptoms; further, mental disorders have high comorbidities with other medical and psychiatric disorders. Pharmacotherapy is effective and available for the treatment of depression, anxiety, and cognitive decline associated with the dementias; however, it is underused, as is combination pharmacotherapy and psychotherapy. More efforts must be directed to educating PCPs in the diagnosis,

Table 10.6 • Supportive Care for Patients and Caregivers/Families

Supportive Care for Patient	Supportive Care for Caregiver/Family
Involve patient in treatment decisions whenever possible (e.g., medications & their effects); also involve in feedback on functioning, cognition, & behavior.	Involve in all treatment decisions to assist with monitoring care & providing feedback; also involve in feedback on functioning, cognition, & behavior. Improving caregiver self-esteem and confidence will improve patient care.
Monitor & maintain a supportive, stimulating physical environment (e.g., music & touch therapy, social contact, pet therapy); reduce noise & glaring lights; use exercise, group games, & singing.	Educate on need for a stable, stimulating, and physical environment; may reduce agitation & aggression, thereby making care easier. Assist caregiver to understand that aggressive behavior & agitation are part of the disease, not a personal attack on them. Look for meaning behind behavior.
Monitor & maintain a safe environment, including locks on doors, cabinets, appliances, & other modifications. Use identification for wandering patients.	Educate on safety. May decrease agitation & aggression, thereby making care easier.
Monitor for any internal physical problems that may create or exacerbate current dementia (e.g., side effects from medications, infection, pain, & electrolytes).	Educate on common internal physical problems (e.g., medication side effects, infections, pain, & electrolytes).
Orientation: Maintain independence as possible. Maintain daily routine: Simplify all requests & communication. Provide clock, calendar, & other orientation aids. Remove physical restraints.	Educate on simplifying environment & providing as much structure as possible.
	Routinely assess for fatigue, depression, & burn-out in caregiver. Assist caregiver to express feelings & frustrations. Encourage use of day care, the Internet, local support groups, & home health services.

treatment, and referral of older women who experience emotional difficulties in late life. While a vast amount of research is being conducted, particularly for drug therapies, the search is still ongoing for more definitive methods to diagnose and treat the different late-life mental disorders.

Resources for Patients

Administration on Aging: *www.aoa.gov/*

Alcoholics Anonymous: *www.alcoholics-anonymous.org/?Media=PlayFlash*

American Association of Retired Persons: *www.aarp.org/*

Area Agency on Aging: *www.n4a.org/*
Call 1-800-677-1116 for local agency

Eldercare Locator: *www.eldercare.org/*

Family Caregiver Alliance: *www.caregiver.org/*

Narcotics Anonymous: *www.na.org/*

National Academy of Elder Law Attorneys, Inc.: *www.naela.org/*

Nursing Homes: *www.medicare.gov/nhcompare*

Substance Abuse and Mental Health Services Administration:
www.samhsa.gov/aging/age_08.aspx

Substance Abuse Treatment Facility Locator: *http://dasis3.samhsa.gov/*

Women for Sobriety, Inc.: *www.womenforsobriety.org/*

References

Adams, W. L., Barry, K. L., & Fleming, M. F. (1996). Screening for problem drinking in older primary care patients. *Journal of the American Medical Association, 276*(24), 1964–1967.

Alexopoulos, G. S. (2000). Depression and other mood disorders. *Clinical Geriatrics, 8*(10), 69–82.

Alexopoulos, G. S. Katz, I., Reynolds, C. F., et al. (2001). *Expert consensus guidelines: Pharmacotherapy of depressive disorders in older patients.* A Postgraduate Medicine Special Report: McGraw-Hill Companies, Inc.

American Heart Association. (2007). *Heart disease and stroke statistics.* Retrieved September 7, 2007, from *www.americanheart.org/downloadable/heart/1166711577754HS_StatsInsideText.pdf.*

American Psychiatric Association (APA). (2000). *Diagnostic and statistical manual of mental disorders* (Revised 4th ed.). Washington, DC: Author.

American Psychiatric Association (APA). (2003). *Practice guideline for the assessment and treatment of patients with suicidal behaviors.* Retrieved June 10, 2007, from *www. Psych.org.*

Atkinson, R. (1995). Treatment programs for aging alcoholics. In T. P. Beresford & E. S. Gomberg (Eds.), *Alcohol and aging* (pp. 186–210). New York: Oxford University Press.

Beck, A. T., Beck, R., & Kovacs, M. (1975). Classification of suicide behaviors: I. Quantifying intent and medical lethality. *American Journal of Psychiatry, 132*(3), 285–287.

Beck, A. T., Kovacs, M., & Weissman, A. (1975). Hopelessness and suicidal behavior. An overview. *Journal of the American Medical Association, 234*(11), 1146–1149.

Beck, A. T., Kovacs M., & Weissman, A. (1979). Assessment of suicidal intention: The scale of suicide ideation. *Journal of Clinical Psychology, 47*, 343–352.

Beck, A. T., Schuyler, D., & Herman, I. (1974). Development of suicidal intent scales. In A. T. Beck, H. L. P. Resnick, & D. J. Lettieri (Eds.), *The prediction of suicide* (pp. 45–56). Bowie, MD: Charles Press.

Beck, A. T., Weissman, A., Lester, D., et al. (1974). The measurement of pessimism: The hopelessness scale. *Journal of Consulting and Clinical Psychology, 42*(6), 861–865.

Beekman, A., de Beurs, E., van Balkom, A., et al. (2000). Anxiety and depression in later life: Co-occurrence and communality of risk factors. *American Journal of Psychiatry, 157*(1), 89–95.

Blow, F. C. (2000). Treatment of older women with alcohol problems: Meeting the challenges for a special population. *Alcoholism: Clinical and Experimental Research, 24*(8), 1257–1266.

Blow, F. C., & Barry, K. (2002). Use and misuse of alcohol among older women. *Alcohol Research and Health, 26*(4), 308–315.

Blow, F. C., Walton, M. A., Chermack, S. T., et al. (2000). Older adult treatment outcome following elder-specific inpatient alcoholism treatment. *Journal of Substance Abuse Treatment, 19*(1), 67–75.

Boeve, B. F. (2006). A review of the non-Alzheimer dementias. *Journal of Clinical Psychiatry, 67*, 1985–2001.

Bosworth, H. B., McQuoid, D. R., George, L. K., et al. (2002). Time-to-remission from geriatric depression. *American Journal of Geriatric Psychiatry, 10*, 551–559.

Breslow, R. A., Faden, V. B., & Smothers, B. (2003). Alcohol consumption by elderly Americans. *Journal Studies on Alcohol, 64*(6), 884–892.

Brown, G. K., Beck, A. T., Steer, R. A., et al. (2000). Risk factors for suicide in psychiatric outpatients: a 20–year prospective study. *Journal of Consulting and Clinical Psychology, 68*, 371–377.

Brown, G. K., Bruce, M. L., Pearson, J. L.; The PROSPECT Study Group. (2001). High-risk management: Guidelines for elderly suicidal patients in primary care settings. *International Journal of Geriatric Psychiatry, 16*, 593–601.

Conwell, Y. (2001). Suicide in late life: A review and recommendations for prevention. *Suicide and Life-Threatening Behavior, 31*(Suppl), 32–47.

Conwell, Y. & Brent, D. (1995). Suicide and aging I: Patterns of psychiatric diagnosis. *International Psychogeriatrics*, 7, 149–164.

Cummings, J. L. (2006). New paradigms in the treatment of Alzheimer's disease. *Journal of Clinical Psychiatry, 67*, 2007–2009.

Dennis, M., Baillon, S., Brugha, T., et al. (2007). The spectrum of suicidal ideation in Great Britain: Comparisons across a 16–74 years age range. *Psychological Medicine, 37*, 795–805.

Dervic, K., Oquendo, M., Grunebaum, M., et al. (2004). Religious affiliation and suicide attempt. *American Journal of Psychiatry, 161*, 2303–2308.

Dombrovski, A., & Mulsant, B. (2007). ECT: The preferred treatment for severe depression in late life. *International Psychogeriatrics, 19(1)*, 10–14.

Doody, R. S., Stevens, J. C., & Beck, C. (2001). Practice parameter: Management of dementia (an evidenced-based review). Report of the Quality Standards Subcommittee of the American Academy of Neurology. *Neurology, 56*, 1154–1166.

Dube, S., Anda, R., Felitti, V., et al. (2001).Childhood abuse, household dysfunction, and the risk of attempted suicide throughout the life span. *Journal of the American Medical Association, 286*(24), 3089–3096.

Ensrud, K. E., Blackwell, T. L., Ancoli-Israel, S., et al. (2006). Use of selective serotonin reuptake inhibitors and sleep disturbances in community-dwelling older women. *Journal of the American Geriatrics Society, 54*(1), 1508–1515.

Filley, C. (1997). Alzheimer's disease in women. *American Journal of Obstetrics and Gynecology, 176*(1), 1–7.

Flint, A. J. (1994). Epidemiology and comorbidity of anxiety in the elderly. *American Journal of Psychiatry, 151*, 640–649.

Flint, A. J. (2005). Generalised anxiety disorder in elderly patients: Epidemiology, diagnosis and treatment options. *Drugs and Aging, 22*(2), 101–114.

Flint, A. J., & Rifat, S. L. (1997). Two-year outcome of elderly patient with anxious depression. *Psychiatry Research, 66*(1), 23–31.

Frazer, C. J., Christensen, H., & Griffiths, K. M. (2005). Systematic review: Effectiveness of treatments for depression in older people. *Medical Journal of Australia, 182*(12), 627–632. Retrieved September 23, 2007, from *www.mja.com.au/public/issues/182_12_200605/fra10160_fm.html.*

Greenberg, R., & Kellner, C. (2005). Electroconvulsive therapy. *American Journal of Geriatric Psychiatry, 13*, 268–281.

Hing, E., Cherry, D. K., & Woodwell, D. A. (2006). National Ambulatory Medical Care Survey: 2004 Summary. Advanced Data from Vital and Health Statistics. 374. U.S. Department of Health and Human Services, Center for Disease Control and Prevention. U.S. Department of Health and Human Services, Health Resources and Services Administration (2005). *Women's Health USA 2005.* Rockville, MD: U.S. Department of Health and Human Services.

Holroyd, S., & Clayton, A. H. (2002). Measuring depression in the elderly: Which scale is best? *Medscape*. Retrieved September 23, 2007, from *www.medscape.com/viewarticle/430554_print.*

Holroyd, S., & Duryee, J. J. (1997). Substance use disorders in geriatric psychiatry outpatient clinics: Prevalence and epidemiologic characteristics. *Journal of Nervous and Mental Disease, 185*(10), 627–632.

Hybels, C. F., & Blazer, D. G. (2003). Epidemiology of late-life mental disorders. *Clinics in Geriatric Medicine, 19*, 663–696.

Ismail, M. S. (2006). New paradigms in the treatment of Alzheimer's disease. *Journal of Clinical Psychiatry, 67*, 2007–2009.

Juurlink, D., Herrmann, N., Szalai, J., et al. (2004). Medical illness and the risk of suicide in the elderly. *Archives of Internal Medicine, 164*, 1179–1184.

Kaufer, D. I. (2005). Parkinson's disease dementia. *Medscape*. Retrieved September 10, 2007, from *www.medscape.com/viewprogram/4035_pnt.*

Kellner, C., Knapp, R., Petrides, G., et al. (2006). Continuation electroconvulsive therapy vs pharmacotherapy for relapse prevention in major depression. *Archives of General Psychiatry, 63*, 1337–1344.

Kockler, M., & Heun, R. (2002). Gender differences of depressive symptoms in depressed and non-depressed elderly persons. *International Journal of Geriatric Psychiatry, 17*(1), 65–72.

Lantz, M. S. (2004). Chronic benzodiazepine treatment in the older adult: Therapeutic or problematic? *Clinical Geriatrics, 12*(5). Retrieved September 19, 2007, from *www.mmhc.com.*

Lantz, M. S. (2005). Prescription drug and alcohol abuse in an older woman. *Clinical Geriatrics, 13*(1). Retrieved September 19, 2007, from *www.mmhc.com.*

Lapid, M. I., & Rummans, T. A. (2003). Evaluation and management of geriatric depression in primary care. *Mayo Clinic Proceedings, 78*, 1423–1429.

Lavretsky, H., Lesser, I. M., Wohl, M. et al. (1999). Managing mood disorders in older patients. *Journal of Gender-Specific Medicine, 2*(4), 40–44.

Lenze, E. J., Dew, M., Mazumdar, S., et al. (2002). Combined pharmacotherapy and psychotherapy as maintenance treatment for late-life depression: Effects on social adjustment. *American Journal of Psychiatry, 159*(3), 466–468.

Lenze, E. J., Mulsant, B. H., Shear, M. K., et al. (2000). Comorbid anxiety disorders in depressed elderly patients. *American Journal of Psychiatry, 157*(5), 722–728.

Llorente, M. D., Golden, A. G., & Silverman, M. A. (2000). Defining patterns of benzodiazepine use in older adults. *Journal of Geriatric Psychiatry and Neurology, 13*(3), 150–160.

Lyketsos, C. G., Colenda, C. C., & Beck, C. (2006). Task Force for the American Association for Geriatric Psychiatry. Position statement of the American Association for Geriatric Psychiatry regarding principles of care for patients with dementia resulting from Alzheimer disease. *American Journal of Geriatric Psychiatry, 14*, 561–562.

Lyness, J. M., Heo, M., Datto, C. J., et al. (2006). Outcomes of minor and subsyndromal depression among elderly patients in primary care settings. *Annals of Internal Medicine, 144*(7), 496–504.

Malone, K., Oquendo, M., Haas., G., et al. (2000). Protective factors against suicidal acts in major depression: Reasons for living. *American Journal of Psychiatry, 157*, 1084–1088.

Mann, J., Waternaux, C., Haas, G., et al. (1999). Toward a clinical model of suicidal behavior in psychiatric patients. *American Journal of Psychiatry, 156*(2), 181–189.

Mantella, R. C., Butters, M. A., Dew, M. A., et al. (2007). Cognitive impairment in late-life generalized anxiety disorder. *American Journal of Geriatric Psychiatry, 15*(8), 673–679.

McHolm, A., MacMillan, H., & Jamieson, E. (2003). The relationship between childhood physical abuse and suicidality among depressed women: Results from a community sample. *American Journal of Psychiatry, 160*(5), 933–938.

McIntosh, J. (2006). Suicide date page: 2003. *American Association of Suicidology*. Retrieved December 30, 2006, from *www.suicidology.org*.

McKhann, G., Drachman, D, Folstein, M., et al. (1984). Clinical diagnosis of Alzheimer's disease: Report of the NINCD-ADRDA work group under the auspices of the Department of Health and Human Services Task Force on Alzheimer's Disease. *Neurology, 34*, 939–944.

Miller, E. R., Pastor-Barriuso, R., Dalal, D., et al. (2005). Meta-analysis: High dosage vitamin E supplement may increase all-cause mortality. *Annals of Internal Medicine, 142*, 37–46.

Mohamed, S., Osatuke, K., Aslam, M., et al. (2006). Escitalopram for comorbid depression and anxiety In elderly patients: A 12–week, open-label, flexible-dose, pilot trial. *American Journal of Geriatric Pharmacotherapy, 4*(3), 201–209.

Moore, A. A., Whiteman, E. J., & Ward, K. T. (2007). Risks of combined alcohol/medication use in older adults. *American Journal of Geriatric Pharmacotherapy, 5*(1), 64–74.

Moscicki, E. K. (1995). Epidemiology of suicide. *International Psychogeriatrics*, 7(2),137–146.

National Institutes of Health, National Institute on Aging. (2006). *Alzheimer's disease fact sheet*. Retrieved September 10, 2007, from *www.nia.nih.gov/Alzheimers/Publications/adfact.htm*.

Oquendo, M., Galfalvy, H., Russo, S., et al. (2004). Prospective study of clinical predictors of suicidal acts after a major depressive episode in patients with major depressive disorder or bipolar disorder. *American Journal of Psychiatry, 161*, 1433–1441.

Petersen, R. C. (2007). Mild cognitive impairment: Current research and clinical implications. *Seminal Neurology*, 27. Retrieved August 29, 2007, from *www.medscape.com/viewarticle/553257_print.*

Potyk, D. (2005). Treatments for Alzheimer disease. *Southern Medical Journal, 98*, 628–635. Retrieved September 10, 2007, from *www.medscape.com/viewarticle/507361_print.*

Raj, A. (2004). Depression in the elderly: Tailoring medical therapy to their special needs. *Postgraduate Medicine, 115*(6). Retrieved September 20, 2007, from *www.postgradmed.com/issues/2004/06_04/raj.shtml.*

Regier, D. A., Boyd, J. H., Burke, J. D., et al. (1988). One-month prevalence of mental disorders in the United States. Based on five Epidemiologic Catchment Area sites. *Archives of General Psychiatry, 45*(11), 977–986.

Reiman, E. M. (2006). The non-Alzheimer dementias. *Journal of Clinical Psychiatry, 67*, 1983–1984.

Riepe, M. W., Adler, G., & Ibach, B. (2006). Adding memantine to rivastigmine therapy in patients with mild-to-moderate Alzheimer's disease: Results of a 12–week, open-label pilot study. *Journal of Clinical Psychiatry, 8*, 258–263.

Robins, L. N., Helzer, J. E., & Przybeck, T. R. (1988). Alcohol disorders in the community: A report from the Epidemiologic Catchment Area. In R. Rose & J. Barret (Eds.), *Alcoholism: Origins and outcome* (pp. 15–29). New York: Raven Press.

Rowe, J., Conwell, Y., Schulberg, H., et al. (2006). Social support and suicidal ideation in older adults using home healthcare services. *American Journal of Geriatric Psychiatry, 14*(7), 758–766.

Rudorfer, M. V., Henry, M. E., & Sackeim, H. A. (2003). Electroconvulsive therapy. In A. Tasman, J. Kay, & J. Lieberman (Eds.), *Psychiatry therapeutics* (2nd ed., pp. 167–203). West Sussex, England: John Wiley and Sons, Ltd.

Salzman, C., Roose, S., & Chatterjee, A. (2004). Treatment of late life depression associated with medical illness. In C. Salzman, *Clinical geriatric psychopharmacology* (4th ed., pp. 335–482). Philadelphia: Lippincott Williams & Wilkins.

Sareen, J., Cox, B. J., Afifi, T. O., et al. (2005). Anxiety disorders and risk for suicidal ideation and suicide attempts. *Archives of General Psychiatry, 62*, 1249–1257.

Schmader, K. E., & Moore, A. A. (2003). Misadventures with drugs and alcohol in the older patient: Alcohol use, misuse, and abuse in older persons. *Annals of Long-Term Care, 11*(8), 37–43.

Schumaker, S. A., Legault, C., & Rapp, S. R. (2003). Estrogen plus progestin and the incidence of dementia and mild cognitive impairment on postmenopausal women. *Journal of the American Medical Association, 289*(20), 2651–2652.

Shader, R. I., & Songer, D. A. (2003). Sedative-Hypnotic agents. In A. Tasman, J. Kay, & J. A. Lieberman (Eds.), *Psychiatry* (2nd ed., pp. 2054–2061). West Sussex, England: John Wiley and Sons, Ltd.

Sher, L. (2004). Preventing suicide. *QJM: An International Journal of Medicine, 97*(10), 677–680.

Stroebe, M., Stroebe, W., & Abakoumkin, G. (2005). The broken heart: Suicidal ideation in bereavement. *American Journal of Psychiatry, 161*(11), 2178–2180.

Steunenberg, B., Beekman, A. T., Deeg, D. J., et al. (2007). Mastery and neuroticism predict recovery of depression in later life. *American Journal of Geriatric Psychiatry, 15*(3), 234–242.

Stone, M. B. (2005). *Mortality and antipsychotic drug use in dementia-related behavioral disorders.* Washington, DC: U.S. Department of Health and Human Services, Food and Drug

Administration, Center for Drug Evaluation and Research, Division of Neuropharmacologic Drug Products.

Suicide Prevention Resource Center. (2006). Suicides, 2000–2004. Retrieved September 17, 2006, from *www.sprc.org/stateinformation/PDF/statedatasheets/sprc_national_data.pdf.*

Sumic, A., Michael,Y. L., Carlson, N. E., et al. (2007). Physical activity and the risk of dementia in oldest old. *Journal of Aging and Health, 19*, 242–259.

Szanto, K., Gildenger, A., Mulsant, B., et al. (2002). Identification of suicidal ideation and prevention of suicidal behaviour in the elderly. *Drugs and Aging, 19*(1), 11–24.

Szanto, K., Reynolds, C. III, Conwell, Y., et al. (1998). High levels of hopelessness persist in geriatric patients with remitted depression and a history of attempted suicide. *Journal of the American Geriatrics Society, 46*(11), 1401–1407.

Tariot, P. N. (2006). Treatment initiation in Alzheimer's disease. *Journal of Clinical Psychiatry, 67*, 2004–2007.

Tariot, P. N., Farlow, M. R., & Grossberg, G. T. (2004). Memantine treatment in patients with moderate to severe Alzheimer disease already receiving donepezil: A randomized controlled trial. *Journal of the American Medical Association, 291*, 317–324.

U.S. Centers for Disease Control and Prevention (CDC), Web-based Injury Statistics Query and Reporting System (WISQARS). Retrieved September 17, 2006, from *www.cdc.gov/ncipc/wisqars/default.htm.*

U.S. Department of Health and Human Services (HDDS). (1999). *Mental health: A report of the surgeon general.* Rockville, MD: U.S. Department of Health and Human Services, Substance Abuse and Mental Health Services Administration, Center for Mental Health Services, National Institutes of Health, National Institutes of Mental Health.

U.S. Department of Health and Human Services (HDDS), Health Resources and Services Administration (2005). *Women's Health USA 2005.* Rockville, MD: U.S. Department of Health and Human Services.

Van Beusekom, B. S., van den Broek, W., & Birkenhager, T. K. (2007). Long-term follow-up after successful electroconvulsive therapy for depression: A 4–to 8–year naturalistic follow-up study. *Journal of ECT, 23*(1), 17–20.

Wiseman, E. J. (2000). Drug and alcohol abuse. In B. J. Sadock & V. A. Sadock (Eds.), *Kaplan & Sadock's comprehensive textbook of psychiatry* (7th ed., Vol. 2, pp. 3081–3085). Philadephia: Lippincott Williams & Wilkins.

Woodman, C. L., Noyes, R., Black, D. W., et al. (1999). A 5–year follow-up study of generalized anxiety disorder and panic disorder. *Journal of Nervous and Mental Diseases, 187*(1), 3–9.

Yaari, R., & Corey-Bloom, J. (2007). Alzheimer's disease. *Seminal Neurology, 27*, 32–41. Retrieved September 10, 2007, from *www.medscape.com/viewarticle/553256_print.*

Jessica Roberts Williams
Marguerite L. Baty
Rosa M. Gonzalez-Guarda
Katherine R. Nash
Jacquelyn C. Campbell

chapter 11

Trauma and Violence

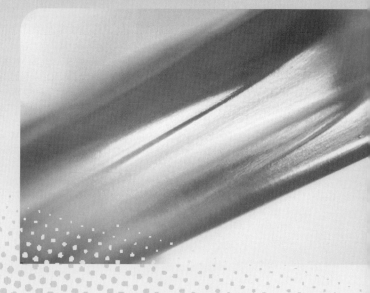

Family violence is a significant public health problem that crosses all demographic and social boundaries. Although both males and females can be victimized by their intimate partners, the vast majority (83 percent) of the victims are females (U.S. Department of Justice, Bureau of Justice Statistics, 2005a). Although this chapter focuses on the female experience of violence, much of the information applies to males as well.

Women who experience violence and trauma are significantly more likely to experience physical and psychological symptoms and seek health care for these ailments compared with nonabused women (Paranjape, Heron, and Kaslow, 2006; Ulrich, Cain, Sugg, et al., 2003). Violence and abuse among women presenting to primary care clinics is common, with lifetime prevalence ranging from approximately 41 to 54 percent (Coker, Smith, and Fadden, 2005; Kramer, Lorenzon, and Mueller, 2004; Wenzel, Monson, and Johnson, 2004) and past year or current prevalence ranging from 5 to 24 percent (Kramer et al.; MacMillan, Wathen, Jamieson, et al., 2006; McCloskey, Lichter, Ganz, et al., 2005; McFarlane, Groff, O'Brien, et al., 2005; Wenzel et al.). Despite these high rates, the majority of women with a history of abuse go undiagnosed, often because of missed opportunities for identification of abuse by providers and disclosure of abuse by clients (Coker, Bethea, Smith, et al., 2002; McCloskey et al.). Identifying women in the primary care setting with current or past history of violence presents the opportunity for treatment, but recognition of these conditions is often challenging and complex.

This chapter begins by examining different forms of abuse and violence, specifically intimate partner violence (IPV), sexual assault, child abuse, and abuse among the elderly and other vulnerable populations. Risk factors for victimization, as well as the physical and psychological outcomes of abuse, are discussed. This chapter also addresses how trauma and violence present in primary care settings and the options available to primary care providers (PCPs) for assessment and treatment. The chapter concludes by discussing legal issues associated with abuse. Additional resources for both clients and providers are presented in the Resources and Client Education section.

ETIOLOGY OF ABUSE

There are several etiologies suggested for IPV, sexual assault, child abuse, and elder/vulnerable adult abuse, but there are none that can definitively identify the cause. Perpetration of abuse has its own etiology, but it is beyond the scope of this chapter to address this particular component of abuse. As for the victims and survivors, the focus has been to examine what may heighten a woman's risk for and what may be protective factors against abuse.

One broad approach that encompasses all forms of abuse is to examine it in the socioecologic context. Factors present at the society, community, family, and individual levels and contribute to higher risks for some individuals and protective factors for others. For instance, on the community level, availability of social services may be mitigated by an individual's awareness of them and ability to access them. Similarly, high neighborhood crime rates can contribute to higher levels of violence among families living in these areas, yet close-knit families appear more resilient to this community context. However, individuals and couples with histories of substance abuse, emotional immaturity, or poor coping skills are highly susceptible to compounding community and societal factors, which in turn play a role in the persistence of violence.

The dynamic process that occurs in abusive relationships and reasons for why women remain in these relationships can be further understood through the theory of the cycle of violence. The "cycle theory of violence" describes violence as involving three cyclical phases (Walker, 1979, 1984). The first of these is the *tension-building phase*. In this phase, there is an escalation of tension that is often characterized by verbal and psychological abuse and minor battering. The woman denies the anger and tries to placate the perpetrator in order to avoid more serious incidents. This phase may last anywhere between days to years until the tension builds up to a breaking point. In the second phase of the cycle of violence, *the acute battering phase*, there is an outbreak of serious battering. This phase may last between 2 and 24 hours. The woman tries to protect herself and her children, feels powerless, and suffers emotional collapse immediately following the acute battering. In the third phase, often called the *honeymoon phase*, there is a period of calm. The perpetrator becomes remorseful and loving and the woman forgives him or her in hopes that the violence will end. This period lasts until tension begins to build up once again, leading the relationship back to the first phase of the cycle of violence. Over time, the honeymoon period occurs less often, and the tension-building and acute phases are more frequent and severe.

Although the causes of abuse and reasons why women remain in abusive relationships still remain somewhat elusive, these models and theories serve as guides in understanding the complexity of the different forms of abuse addressed in this chapter.

INTIMATE PARTNER VIOLENCE

Intimate partner violence is the general term used to describe abuse that exists among current or former boyfriend/girlfriend relationships or spouses. The Centers for Disease Control and Prevention (CDC; 2006a) defines IPV as

Table 11.1 • Intimate Partner Violence by Category

IPV by Category	Definition
Physical violence	The intentional use of physical force with the potential of causing harm (i.e., kicking, slapping, grabbing, throwing, choking, use of weapons, or restraints).
Sexual violence	The use of force to compel a person to participate in any sexual act against his or her will; attempted or completed sexual act involving a person who is unable to understand the nature or condition of the act or communicate unwillingness to participate in the act (i.e., disability, influence of alcohol or drugs, intimidation, or pressure); abusive sexual contact.
Threats of physical and sexual violence	The use of words, gestures, or arms to communicate the intention to cause physical harm.
Psychological/ Emotional violence	Acts, threats of acts, or coercive tactics that cause trauma to the victim (i.e., humiliating, isolating, restricting economic resources).

From Saltzman et al. (2002).

physical, sexual, and/or psychological abuse perpetrated by a current or former intimate partner. As the definition implies, IPV can be manifested in various ways. The specific forms of IPV are often categorized into physical violence, sexual violence, physical and sexual threats, and psychological or emotional violence (Table 11.1). Acts of IPV are often a combination of these specific forms of violence.

IPV is a common cause of physical and psychological injury and illness among women, accounting for a significant proportion of primary care and emergency department visits among this population. Because the immediate and long-term consequences of IPV can be severe, it is essential that PCPs participate in the ongoing assessment and early identification and intervention of IPV.

Epidemiology

Although reported rates of IPV have decreased over recent years, it continues to affect a large proportion of the U.S. population. According to the U.S. Bureau of Justice Statistics (2006a), there were 467,280 nonfatal violence-related crimes committed by a current or former boyfriend/girlfriend or spouse in 2005. However, other studies based on survey data rather than on surveillance systems have indicated that the problem is much more widespread. In a study conducted by the National Institute of Justice and the CDC, researchers reported that nearly 7 million rapes and physical assaults are perpetrated against intimate partners annually (Tjaden and Thoennes, 2000). Because these data are based on the willingness to disclose abuse, it is likely that this is still a gross understatement of the true underlying problem.

Although both males and females can be victimized by their intimate partners, the vast majority (83 percent) of the victims are females (U.S. Department of Justice, Bureau of Justice Statistics, 2005a). In fact, approximately one out of every three women in the United States report being physically or sexually abused by a boyfriend or husband at one point in their lives (The Commonwealth Fund, 1999). IPV occurs at similar rates among both heterosexual and homosexual relationships. However, because males are more often the perpetrators, males in homosexual relationships and females in heterosexual relationships are at greater risk than women in homosexual relationships (Halpern, Young, Waller, et al., 2004; Tjaden and Thoennes, 2000). Consequently, women are also more likely to be killed by a male intimate partner. While 32.7 percent of female murder victims were killed by an intimate partner in 2004, only 3.1 percent of the male homicides were identified as IPV related (U.S. Department of Justice, Bureau of Justice Statistics, 2006b). Women are at greatest risk for homicide when leaving an abusive relationship, when their partner is unemployed, when the perpetrator has access to a gun, or when there has been a previous threat with a gun (Campbell, Webster, Koziol-McLain, et al., 2003).

Risk Factors for Intimate Partner Violence

Although IPV cuts across demographic variables, there are some groups that appear to be at an increased risk including women; adolescents and young adults; ethnic minority groups including blacks, Native American Indians, and Hispanics; and those living below the poverty line (Tjaden and Thoennes, 2000). Pregnancy and new motherhood can also put a woman at increased risk for abuse, as IPV can often begin or worsen during the pregnancy and postpartum periods. Four to 17 percent of pregnant women experience abuse during the gestational period, which is higher than the prevalence of gestational diabetes and pre-eclampsia (Gazmararian, Petersen, Smitz, et al., 2000; Johnson, Haider, Ellis, et al., 2003). Unwanted pregnancies place a woman at three times the risk of physical abuse than a planned pregnancy (Goodwin, Gazmararian, Johnson, et al., 2000).

In addition, a history of child abuse can serve as a risk factor for women, which will be discussed in greater detail later in this chapter. One of the most

Table 11.2 • Risk Factors for the Victimization of Intimate Partner Violence Among Women

Level	Risk Factors
Individual	Young age Ethnic minority groups (black, American Indian/Alaskan Native, Hispanic) Lower education Unemployment Prior history of violence exposure and victimization (child abuse, IPV) Risk behaviors (substance abuse & high-risk sexual behavior)
Relationship	Having a higher education than partner Having a partner who is verbally abusive, jealous, or possessive Couples with disparities in income, education, and job status Male dominance and control in the relationship
Community	Poverty and related factors Low social capital (lack of social support, institutions, prevention programs) Weak sanctions/responses to IPV (i.e., police intervention)
Societal	Traditional gender roles (woman stays at home, female submission)

From the Centers for Disease Control and Prevention (CDC) (2006a).

documented risk factors for IPV is perpetrator substance abuse, which has been consistently linked to the occurrence, recurrence, and severity of IPV as well as intimate partner homicide (Caetano, Field, Ramisetty-Mikler, et al., 2005; Lipsky, Caetano, Field, et al., 2006; Sharps, Campbell, Campbell, et al., 2001; Testa and Leonard, 2001). These and other risk factors are outlined in Table 11.2.

Long- and Short-Term Impact of Intimate Partner Violence

There are a wide range of physical, psychological, social, and economic consequences associated with IPV. Victims of IPV receive repeated physical injuries; are sick more frequently; experience pain (i.e., head, pelvic, back); and tend to have lowered immune status, gynecological disorders, sexually transmitted diseases including HIV/AIDS, pregnancies resulting in intrauterine growth restriction and/or low-birth-weight infants, central nervous system disorders, and other physical consequences that are related to their history of abuse (CDC, 2006b; Champion, Shain, Piper, et al., 2002; Kearney, Munro, Kelly, et al.,

2004). These physical symptoms can intensify along with the recurrence and severity of violence (Campbell, Jones, Dienemann, et al., 2002; Plichta, 2004).

Victims of IPV also suffer from a host of psychological consequences, the most prevalent being depression, posttraumatic stress disorder (PTSD), and anxiety. Studies have indicated that victims of IPV are approximately three to five times more likely to be depressed and experience symptoms of PTSD and twice as likely to be anxious than women who have not been abused (Caetano and Cunradi, 2003; Campbell et al., 2002; Dienemann, Boyle, Baker, et al., 2000; Golding, 1999; Woods, 2000). The mechanisms behind the relationship between IPV victimization and mental health outcomes are not fully understood; however, it is thought that PTSD is not only a consequence of abuse but also a major pathway to negative mental health outcomes of IPV (Dutton, Green, Kaltman, et al., 2006). IPV is also associated with somatization, obsessive compulsiveness, interpersonal sensitivity, paranoia, hostility, sleep and eating disorders, substance abuse, and suicide (Caetano and Cunradi; Champion et al., 2002; Golding; Woods, Wineman, Page, et al., 2005). In fact, it has been documented that more than 20 percent of suicide victims had a fight with an intimate partner immediately before taking their lives (Olson, Huyler, Lynch, et al., 1999). Victims also tend to be isolated from family, friends, and health and social services and have strained relationships with health care providers and employers (Heise and Garcia-Moreno, 2002; Plichta, 2004).

SEXUAL ASSAULT

Rape and sexual assault can have varying and often synonymous meanings. The U.S. Department of Justice (2005b) defines *rape* as forced sexual intercourse that includes both psychological coercion and physical force. Forced sexual intercourse is further defined as vaginal, anal, or oral penetration by the offender and also includes penetration from foreign objects such as a bottle. *Sexual assault* is considered nonconsensual sexual contact outside of penetration, usually fondling. The laws regarding these terms vary from state to state, and the terms are often used interchangeably with varying degrees of severity. This chapter will also use these terms synonymously. Anderson, McClain, and Rivello (2006) have identified three key characteristics to be kept in mind: "force, penetration, and lack of consent" (p. 59).

Sexual assault can occur in all settings and among all demographic groups. As seen with the other forms of abuse presented in this chapter, the mental and physical consequences for a woman who has been raped or sexually assaulted are many.

Epidemiology

According to the National Crime Victimization Survey, there were nearly 200,000 victims of rape and sexual assault in 2005 among individuals 12 years of age or older, equivalent to approximately 1 per 1,000 persons (U.S. Department of Justice, Bureau of Justice Statistics, 2006a). According to this survey, women were far more likely to be victims of sexual assault than men, and victimization was double the rate among the black population than white. Persons between the ages of 16 and 19 years were at the greatest risk for sexual assault. While no difference was noted on the basis of income level, the rate of sexual assault was higher among those who were single (never married or divorced/separated). All regions of the United States reported similar rates of sexual assault, but urban residents showed a substantially higher rate than rural. The majority (73 percent) of female victims are assaulted by someone they know, whereas male victims are typically assaulted by strangers. In fact, 28 percent of female victims are sexually assaulted by an intimate partner (U.S. Department of Justice, Bureau of Justice Statistics, 2006a).

Although the Bureau of Justice Statistics (2006a) reports a significant decline in the incidence of sexual assaults since 1993, the prevalence of sexual assault across the lifetime has not changed (Casey and Nurius, 2006). This is important for PCPs to be aware of when treating clients, as even one incident in a person's life can have long-lasting mental and physical consequences.

Risk Factors

Identifying risk factors for sexual assault is problematic. Rape crosses all nationalities, ages, religions, sexual orientations, and income levels. Recreational drug and alcohol use has been associated with an increased risk of victimization (Champion, Foley, DuRant, et al., 2004). According to Sochting, Fairbrother, and Koch (2004), women who were sexually abused prior to the age of 18 years are at greater risk of being sexually assaulted again as an adult. One possible reason for this finding is that women who have had to deal with abuse in the past may feel more comfortable reporting assault in the future.

Long- and Short-Term Impact of Sexual Assault

Short-term consequences of sexual assault can include genital and nongenital injury, sexually transmitted infections (STIs), and pregnancy. Only about 30 percent of victims of sexual assault suffer injuries, which is consistent with the number of persons who experience injury after consensual intercourse (Anderson et al.,

2006). Injury rates are usually higher with stranger-perpetration assaults (Jones, Wynn, Kroeze, et al., 2004). Only 1 percent of victims suffer injuries severe enough to require hospitalization or surgery (Ledray, 2006).

Experiencing a traumatic event such as sexual assault can have severe consequences on a woman's mental health, manifesting in ways such as physical symptoms, poor general health, substance abuse, and psychological distress. Victims of sexual assault report more intense and frequent health complaints than nonvictims (Conoscenti and McNally, 2006). These women have significantly more gynecologic health problems (Campbell et al., 2002), use health care services more frequently, and report more sick days than nonvictims (Stein, Lang, Laffaye, et al., 2004). Seventy percent of women with substance abuse problems admit to being sexually assaulted (Lincoln, Liebschutz, Chernoff, et al., 2006). Psychological distress is frequently experienced by victims of sexual assault, especially through anxiety, fear, depression, suicidal ideations, and signs of PTSD (Ledray, 2006). As well, the relationship of the assailant to the victim plays a major role in the development of psychological distress; for example, increased PTSD symptoms have been found among women assaulted by relatives and strangers (Ullman, Filipas, Townsend, et al., 2006). Self-blame is a frequent result of sexual victimization and can result in further psychological distress (Ledray; Breitenbecher, 2006).

CHILD ABUSE

A critical element of health history that can impact women's health as adults is whether or not they experienced childhood maltreatment. *Child maltreatment* is an umbrella term that includes physical, sexual, and psychological abuse and neglect of children. Universal definitions of these terms remain elusive. The Federal Child Abuse Prevention and Treatment Act (1998) broadly offers the following definition: "The term 'child abuse and neglect' means, at a minimum, any recent act or failure to act on the part of a parent or caregiver, which results in death, serious physical or emotional harm, sexual abuse or exploitation, or an act or failure to act which presents an imminent risk of serious harm." State laws further define the specific acts that are included under each kind of abuse, which makes child abuse a legal, reportable issue in addition to a health concern (see the Criminal Justice and Legal Systems section for more details). Working definitions of the forms of child abuse are further elucidated in Table 11.3. The primary focus of this chapter with regard to child abuse is the effects of that abuse on an adult female client's well-being.

In their practice setting, PCPs will encounter and care for women who have a history of childhood maltreatment. This is an important element in a

Table 11.3 • Definitions of Child Maltreatment by Type

Child Maltreatment Type	Definition
Neglect	Failure to provide for a child's basic physical, medical, educational, and emotional needs.
Physical abuse	Any nonaccidental physical injury to the child, including but not limited to striking, kicking, burning, or biting the child. Includes any action that results in a physical impairment of the child.
Sexual abuse	Employment, use, persuasion, inducement, enticement, or coercion of any child to engage in or assist in any sexually explicit conduct. Also includes other forms of sexual exploitation of children, statutory rape, molestation, prostitution, and interfamilial incest.
Emotional abuse	Injury to the psychological capacity or emotional stability of the child, including verbal aggression, as evidenced by an observable change in behavior, emotional response, or cognition such as anxiety, depression, withdrawal, or aggressive behavior.

From U.S. Department of Health and Human Services (USDHHS), Children's Bureau (2005).

client's history due to the long-lasting, mental, and physical health effects of child abuse as well as its capacity to put a woman at risk for other forms of abuse in her adult life.

Epidemiology

Several types of child abuse in American society are quite pervasive; therefore, PCPs may have adult clients who experienced abuse as children. Child abuse is all too common, even though the recorded number of substantiated child maltreatment cases has declined in recent years. Among the reported cases, the U.S. Department of Health and Human Services, Administration on Children, Youth and Families (2007) estimates that 899,000 children were substantiated victims of maltreatment in 2005, based on a victim rate of 12.1 per 1,000 children. These statistics show a decrease from the 13.4 per 1,000 children in 1990. In 2005, the majority of substantiated cases of child maltreatment were due to neglect, including medical neglect (62.8 percent). Physical abuse accounted for 16.6 percent of substantiated cases; 9.3 percent were of sexual abuse; 7.1 percent were of psychological abuse;

and 14.3 percent were of "other" forms, including abandonment and threats of harm. It is important to keep in mind that these numbers are likely to be underestimates, as they represent only the substantiated cases that were reported to the Child Protection Services. Many cases go unreported or may not meet legal definitions and therefore are considered to be unsubstantiated. Furthermore, children are often victims of more than one kind of abuse.

Self-reported data on child abuse provide a startling contrast, however. According to the National Survey of Adolescents (Stevens, Ruggiero, Kilpatrick, et al., 2005), 8.2 percent of adolescents between the ages of 12 and 17 years in the United States have been victims of serious sexual assault, 17.8 percent have experienced a serious physical assault, and 10 percent of those have been victimized more than once. Females are more likely than males to have been sexually assaulted (13 percent vs. 3.4 percent), while boys were more likely to experience physical abuse (Stevens et al.). When adults were asked to recall their childhood experiences in the Adverse Childhood Experience study, 21.6 percent reported at least one incident of sexual abuse, 20.6 percent reported physical abuse, and 14.0 percent reported having witnessed domestic violence (Edwards, Holden, Felitti, et al., 2003). While this study captures an aspect of emotional abuse, such experiences as verbal berating or exposing a child to domestic violence slip through the cracks of national reporting mechanisms.

Researchers have reported strong correlations between childhood maltreatment, particularly child sexual abuse, and women's mental health. A national survey reported prevalence rates of child sexual abuse of 21 to 32 percent among adult women over the age of 18 years (Vogeltanz, Wilsnack, Harris, et al., 1999). That percentage increases remarkably among clients in inpatient psychiatric units, where the incidence of adult women who report experiencing sexual abuse as children ranges up to 60 percent (Saleptsi, Bichescu, Rockstroh, et al., 2004; Sansone, Songer, and Miller, 2005; Zanarini, Yong, Fankenburg, et al., 2002). One study, examining adverse childhood experiences among psychiatric inpatients with borderline psychopathology, found that 62.4 percent reported childhood experiences of sexual abuse; of these clients, over 50 percent reported being abused in both childhood and adolescence, on at least a weekly basis, for at least 1 year, and by a parent or other well-known person (Zanarini et al.).

Risk Factors

Child maltreatment does not occur solely within certain demographic groups; therefore, PCPs may find past history of abuse in their adult clients regardless of background. Risk factors can be separated into the realms of the individual, family,

Table 11.4 • Risk Factors for Child Abuse Victimization

Realm	Risk Factors
Community/ Society related	High crime rate Paucity of social services High poverty rate High unemployment rate
Parent/Family related	Single parent Personal history of substance abuse Personal history of mental health problems, including depression Teenage parents and/or emotional immaturity Poor coping skills and/or low self-esteem Lack of preparation for high stress of new infant Domestic violence Personal history of physical or sexual abuse as a child Lack of parenting skills Unwanted pregnancy and/or denial of pregnancy
Child related	Prematurity Low birth weight Handicap

community, and society (Table 11.4), and the presence of some or all of these risks can contribute to acts of child abuse. If a woman reports these risk factors from her childhood, the PCP should be alert to possible past abuse.

Long-Term Impact of Child Abuse

When working with adult female clients in health care settings, PCPs must keep in mind the possible long-term physical and mental health outcomes of child abuse and neglect. Certain factors surrounding the woman's experience of childhood abuse impact her health outcomes: her age and developmental status when the abuse occurred; the type of abuse (physical, sexual, emotional, or neglect); the frequency, severity, and duration of the abuse; and her relationship to the abuser.

Women who experience both sexual and physical abuse as children have greater difficulty forming healthy relationships and are at greater risk for engaging in abusive relationships as adults (Bensley, Van Eenwyk, and Simmons, 2003). Research also suggests that women with a history of child abuse are more likely to engage in health-risk behaviors such as regular smoking, alcohol abuse, and use of other drugs than their nonabused counterparts (Diaz, Simantov, and Rickert, 2002; Fassler, Amodeo, Griffin, et al., 2005). Women who have experienced abuse as children have demonstrated a sevenfold increase in HIV-risk behaviors such as sexual promiscuity and unprotected sex (Bensley et al.). This puts them at an increased risk for unwanted pregnancies in addition to all STIs, including HIV (Senn, Carey, Vanable, et al., 2006). These women have also reported physical symptoms such as chronic pelvic pain, dysmenorrhea, and sexual dysfunction more often than their nonabused counterparts. Complaints of abdominal pain, gastrointestinal problems, and eating disorders are also common among these women (Carter, Bewell, Blackmore, et al., 2006; Nicolaidis, Curry, McFarland, et al., 2004).

These physical symptoms may be the impetus for the woman with a history of child abuse to seek care for her physical problems while ignoring the mental health outcomes of the abuse. The mental health outcomes of child abuse are often manifested by increased risk for major depression, suicide, anxiety disorders, PTSD, and personality disorders. PCPs must keep in mind that the scars of child maltreatment are not limited to the period of time immediately following the event but may persist for a lifetime. Table 11.5 outlines the lifetime consequences most often associated with child abuse.

Table 11.5 • Lifetime Effects of Child Maltreatment in Adolescent and Adult Women

Adolescents	Initiation of smoking Early sexual debut and promiscuity Illicit drug use Adolescent pregnancy Suicide attempts Academic difficulties (10% increase)
Adults	Obesity PTSD (20% increase) Depression (21% increase) Suicide Alcoholism Smoking Illicit drug use Risk for IPV Multiple sex partners (14% increase) Engaging in unprotected sex STIs Unintended pregnancies Fetal death

From Dube et al. (2003); Dube et al. (2001); Paolucci, Genuis & Violato (2001).

ELDER AND VULNERABLE ADULT ABUSE

As PCPs provide care for women in varying life stages, it is important to be knowledgeable of elder and vulnerable adult abuse. *Elder mistreatment* is defined as "(a) intentional actions that cause harm or create a serious risk of harm (whether or not harm is intended) to a vulnerable elder by a caregiver or other person who stands in a trust relationship to the elder or (b) failure by a caregiver to satisfy the elder's basic needs or to protect the elder from harm" (National Research Council [NRC], 2003). Such a term does not include violence by strangers. The term *elder mistreatment* is an umbrella term that encompasses abuse and neglect of a physical, financial, emotional, and psychological nature (Table 11.6). Because self-neglect is frequently encountered and is a common concern among health care professionals, it is also included among the categories of elder mistreatment.

Debate over who constitutes an elder continues. Many authors and researchers place a specific age to this term (i.e., 65 years). However, a specific age does not characterize the essence of this population's vulnerability, which is the key concept in elder mistreatment. An individual must lack the facilities to self-care and/or self-protect to be vulnerable (NRC, 2003). The same concepts of vulnerability noted in elder mistreatment can be applied to a 30-year-old autistic adult who requires a caregiver. To solve this problem, many states have moved away from the term *elder* to the more age-encompassing term *vulnerable adult.*

During the last 15 years, elder and vulnerable adult abuse and neglect has been identified as a national health care concern. As the baby boomer generation ages, the rate is expected to continue to rise significantly. Because of the significant risk placed on this population due to their level of impairment and dependence, PCPs need to carefully evaluate their clients for signs of mistreatment.

Epidemiology

A major concern has arisen around the lack of data to accurately portray incidence and prevalence statistics for elder and vulnerable adult abuse. A recent white paper on the subject identified that lack of common definitions; lack of consistent use of diagnostic codes; and most of all, lack of reporting as reasons for the deficiency of data (Wood, 2006). The most thorough study to date is the National Elder Abuse Incidence Study (National Center on Elder Abuse [NCEA], 1998). They reported that within a 1-year period, nearly half a million elderly individuals (60 years and older) were abused and/or neglected. An additional 50,000 elders suffered self-neglect. However, this number only included reported cases that were then substantiated and did not include those cases originating in

Table 11.6 • Different Categories of Vulnerable Adult Mistreatment

VAM Category	Definition	Examples
Physical abuse	The use of physical force that may result in bodily injury, physical pain, or impairment.	Hitting, grabbing, slapping, or causing bodily injury
Sexual abuse	Nonconsensual sexual contact of any kind with a vulnerable adult.	Exposure, genital touching, penetration
Emotional or psychological abuse	The infliction of anguish, pain, or distress.	Verbal and nonverbal insults humiliation, infantilization, and threats
Neglect	The refusal or failure to fulfill any part of a person's obligations or duties to a vulnerable adult.	Failure to provide basic care, typically with activities of daily living (ADLs)
Abandonment	The desertion of an elderly person by an individual who had physical custody or otherwise had assumed responsibility for providing care for an elder or by a person with physical custody of a vulnerable adult.	Homelessness
Financial or material abuse	The illegal or improper use of an elder's funds, property, or assets.	Theft, misappropriation of funds, and coercion
Self-neglect	The behaviors of a vulnerable adult that threaten his or her own health or safety.	Hoarding

Adapted from National Center on Elder Abuse [NCEA] (1998); Carney, Kahan, & Paris (2003).

facilities (i.e., nursing homes, hospitals). It is estimated that four times as many cases of elder mistreatment were unreported. The overall prevalence rate ranges from 2 to 10 percent for elder abuse (Lachs and Pillemer, 2004).

According to the NCEA study (1998), after controlling for their greater numbers, female elderly have a higher rate of all types of abuse and neglect, except for abandonment. They noted that the oldest elders (80 years and older) accounted for the highest rate abuse in all categories, especially neglect (50 percent of cases). Reported abuse against white elders is consistent with their population size (80 percent) among all categories of mistreatment, but the researchers reported a higher rate of neglect, financial/material abuse, and emotional/ psychological abuse among black elders.

The research surrounding prevalence and incidence rates among vulnerable adults not included in elder mistreatment is even more limited. Current research has been limited to self-reports, relying on the mental capacity of the individuals to be able to participate in a survey or interview. The prevalence rate of self-reported vulnerable adult abuse and neglect ranges from 9.8 to 17.8 percent (Matthais and Benjamin, 2003; McFarlane, Hughes, Nosek, et al., 2001). Persons with disabilities are four to ten times more likely to be abused or neglected (Petersilia, 2001).

Risk Factors

Elder and vulnerable adult abuse and neglect can affect people of all racial, ethnic, and socioeconomic backgrounds. Box 11.1 provides a list of probable and possible evidence-based risk factors for elder abuse and neglect for individuals as well as characteristics of caregivers that may increase their risk of committing elder

Box 11.1 • Risk Factors for Elder Abuse and Neglect

Predictive Factors for Individuals

- Female
- Shared living with caregiver
- Social isolation
- Cognitive impairment
- Spouse of victim
- High level of hostility, passive, or avoidant ways of coping
- Black

Predictive Factors for Caregivers

- Depression, psychiatric hospitalization
- High level of hostility
- Alcohol abuse
- Financial dependency

abuse (NRC, 2003). Lack of sufficient evidence prohibits distinguishing risk between categories of mistreatment. In light of the paucity of research specifically examining risk factors for mistreatment among vulnerable adults, one should infer from Box 11.1 similar predictive factors for this population.

Long- and Short-Term Impact of Elder and Vulnerable Adult Abuse

There are numerous long- and short-term physical and psychological consequences of elder and vulnerable adult abuse and neglect. Physical injury, as a result of physical and sexual abuse and neglect, includes lacerations, abrasions, bruises, fractures, internal organ injury, patterned injury, burns, traumatic alopecia, restraints, and head injuries (Dyer, Connolly, and McFeeley, 2003). Pain and infection are also a major concern. Other medical issues that can arise from abuse and neglect include STIs, untreated chronic diseases, dehydration, malnutrition, decubiti, fecal impaction, and toxic or subtherapeutic medication levels.

The most significant long-term consequence is mortality. A 9 percent survival rate has been established for elderly victims of abuse, neglect, and exploitation (excluding self-neglect) (Lachs, Williams, O'Brien, et al., 1998). Other long-term consequences resulting from all types of maltreatment include depression and PTSD. Psychological abuse can also cause habit, neurotic, and conduct disorders (Kleinschmidt, 1997).

ASSESSMENT AND TREATMENT OF ABUSE AND TRAUMA

Five steps have been identified to assist PCPs in the care of victims of abuse and trauma. These steps can be summarized by the acronym *RADAR* (Massachusetts Medical Society, Committee on Violence, 2004) (Box 11.2).

Routinely Screen for Abuse

Although the clinical value of screening for IPV and other abuses has been widely accepted, the U.S. Preventive Task Force (USPTF) found insufficient evidence to recommend universal screening for IPV (USPTF, 2004). Regardless, hospitals accredited through the Joint Commission are required to incorporate policies and procedures for identifying, treating, and referring IPV victims in their emergency departments and ambulatory settings. Professional organizations for health care providers, such as the American Medical Association (AMA), the American College

Box 11.2 • Steps in Identifying and Treating Abuse

R Routinely screen for abuse.

A Ask direct questions about abuse.

D Document information about suspected or actual abuse in the client's chart.

A Assess the client's safety.

R Review options and refer client to a family violence expert.

From Massachusetts Medical Society, Committee on Violence (2004).

of Obstetricians and Gynecologists (ACOG), the American Academy of Pediatrics (AAP), and the American Nurses Association (ANA), have published guidelines that encourage screening as a way to identify IPV and abuse early and to positively impact health outcomes for their clients (AAP, 1998; ACOG, 2002; AMA, 1992; ANA, 1991). The Family Violence Prevention Fund (1999) has recommended screening of clients in primary care settings at every new encounter, every first visit for a new chief complaint of an established client, every reported new intimate partner relationship, and all regular periodic visits such as regular physicals. Additionally, specialty visits such as prenatal checkups are critical times for screening, given a pregnant woman's increased risk (ACOG, 2002). Screening new mothers and addressing the violence can also help to prevent the intergenerational impact of violence on the children.

PCPs must anticipate working with women who have a history of abuse, given the high prevalence of IPV, child maltreatment, and vulnerable adult abuse and the significant negative physical and mental health outcomes associated with each kind of abuse. Because abuse occurs universally across all demographics, PCPs must have a heightened awareness of clinical indicators of abuse as well as psychological indicators regardless of the client's characteristics.

Practitioners must also be aware that some women may be more reluctant than others to seek help (e.g., going to the emergency room, calling the police) or disclose abuse (Lipsky et al., 2006). Repeatedly screening for abuse in different health care situations (e.g., well-child visits), establishing trust, and providing translation services may be especially important in increasing the likelihood of identifying abuse among victims who are more reluctant to seek help for themselves.

Several simple screening methods have been developed to assist PCPs in identifying abuse. Most of them address IPV, and they have been shown to be as

Box 11.3 • SAFE Questions for Screening of Intimate Partner Violence

Stress/Safety	"Do you feel safe in your relationship?"
Afraid/Abused	"Have you ever been in a relationship where you were threatened, hurt, or afraid?"
Friends/Family	"Are your friends or family aware that you have been hurt? Could you tell them, and would they be able to give you support?"
Emergency Plan	"Do you have a safe place to go and the resources you need in an emergency?"

sensitive as longer questionnaires in detecting violence (Coker, Pope, Smith, et al., 2001; Feldhaus, Koziol-McLain, Amsbury, et al., 1997). A one-question screen has been recommended by the Massachusetts Medical Society Committee on Violence (2004): "At any time, has a partner hit, kicked, or otherwise hurt or threatened you?" Clinicians can adapt the question to the given situation, but asking this question has shown to significantly increase the detection rate of IPV. Other effective screening methods are outlined in Boxes 11.3 and 11.4.

Although women rarely present with a chief complaint of abuse, some may reveal it as part of the history taking or at some point during a visit. If this is the case, the clinician should be aware of her increased risk for the physical and mental health disorders discussed previously, regardless of whether the abuse is current or in the past. Ideally, clinicians would assess for STIs and mental health and substance use disorders at this time.

The physical manifestations of abuse are many and varied. Table 11.7 highlights some of the signs and symptoms that may appear on the physical exam

Box 11.4 • Abuse Assessment Screen for Pregnant Women

1. "Within the last year, have you been hit, slapped, kicked, or otherwise physically hurt by someone?"
2. "Since you've been pregnant, have you been hit, slapped, kicked, or otherwise physically hurt by someone?"
3. "Within the last year, has anyone forced you to have sexual activities?"

Table 11.7 • Signs of Possible Intimate Partner Violence or Other Forms of Abuse on Physical Examination

System Assessed	Findings with Increased Index of Suspicion for IPV
General appearance	Increased anxiety in presence of partner Fatigue Inappropriate or anxious nonverbal behaviors Nonverbal communication suggesting shame about body Flinches or draws away from touch Inappropriately dressed, poor grooming Avoidance of eye contact Flat affect, dissociated
Skin	Bruises, welts, edema, or scars, particularly those in various stages of healing Such marks on breasts, upper arms, abdomen, chest, face, and genitalia Burns inconsistent with history
Head	Subdural hematoma Scalp trauma or clumps of missing hair
Eyes	Periorbital swelling or bruising Subconjunctival hemorrhage
Genital/Urinary	Labial edema, bruising, tenderness, external bleeding
Rectal	Bruising, bleeding, edema, irritation, fissures
Musculoskeletal	Fractures: facial bones, spiral fractures of radius or ulna, ribs Dislocation of the shoulder Limited range of motion of an extremity Old fractures in various stages of healing
Abdomen	Abdominal injuries in pregnant women Intra-abdominal injury Diffuse pain to palpation
Neurologic	Hyperactive reflexes Ear or eye problems secondary to injury Tremors
Mental status examination	Anxiety, fear Depression Suicidal ideation Low self-esteem Memory loss Difficulty concentrating

of an abused woman. A detailed description of the intricacies associated with the physical examination of an abused woman is outside the scope of this chapter. (Refer to Sheridan [2003] for information on this topic).

In addition to the physical manifestations of abuse, many women also experience significant and severe mental health sequelae as a result of family violence, with PTSD, depression, and anxiety being the most common. Many psychiatric illnesses have a genetic component, but according to the multidimensional integrative approach to psychopathology, a genetic predisposition to an illness does not necessarily mean that the illness will manifest itself. Often, an environmental factor serves as a trigger to express the gene(s). Trauma, such as sexual assault or IPV, is cited as one of the most common triggers (Barlow and Durand, 2002). If experiences of violence are found or suspected, the PCP should assess for possible psychological consequences. Chapters 2 and 4 provide a detailed description of the assessment and treatment of the mental health consequences most commonly associated with experiences of family violence.

Ask Direct Questions About Abuse

Therapeutic communication in health care describes a process through which health care providers use a variety of interpersonal communication techniques in order to relate therapeutically with their clients and facilitate the delivery of care. Therapeutic communication may include verbal techniques such as encouragement; seeking clarification and validation; or nonverbal techniques such as eye contact, body movement, and posture. Asking direct questions about abuse is a very important form of therapeutic communication that PCPs can use to identify and determine the extent of the abuse. Examples of direct questions include: Has this happened before? When did it first happen? How were you hurt? Have you needed to go to the emergency room for treatment? Questions should be asked in the PCP's own words and in a nonjudgmental way.

Therapeutic communication with someone who has experienced family violence is often one of the most important interventions a PCP can provide. Women who are victims of family violence are often isolated from others and made to feel that they are to blame or deserve the violence. As a PCP, validation of the client's experiences with violence and acknowledgement that the battering is wrong and that no one deserves to be a victim of violence are important interventions.

Document Information About Suspected or Actual Abuse

Documentation is a critical step in the exam of any form of abuse. It can provide evidence that screening has taken place; it serves as notification for other PCPs who may be caring for the woman that abuse is present in her life; and it may be used in future court proceedings, if necessary. If a woman presents with a chief complaint of abuse or with clear signs of abuse, a thorough history including direct quotes from the client must be taken without correction of grammar or lexicon in those sections of the documentation. If the client is able to name the assailant, detail the surrounding events and location, and describe and quantify the assault (e.g., times she was hit, weapon used, coerced sex involved, etc.); this composes an important part of her history and must be meticulously documented (Sheridan, 2003). In addition to a detailed chief complaint and history of the attack, PCPs should obtain a complete medical history and pertinent social history from the client. The AMA (1992) developed documentation guidelines to assist practitioners when conducting an abuse assessment (Box 11.5).

Box 11.5 • American Medical Association Documentation Guidelines for Abuse

Thorough, well-documented medical records are essential for preventing further abuse. Furthermore, they provide concrete evidence of violence and abuse and may prove to be crucial to the outcome of any legal case. If the medical record and testimony at trial are in conflict, the medical record may be considered more credible. Records should be kept in a precise, professional manner and should include the following:

- Chief complaint and description of the abusive event using the patient's own words whenever possible rather than the physician's assessment. "My husband hit me with a bat" is preferable to "Patient has been abused."
- Complete medical history.
- Relevant social history.
- A detailed description of the injuries, including type, number, size, location, resolution, possible causes, and explanations given. Where applicable, the location and nature of the injuries should be recorded on a body chart or drawing.
- An opinion on whether the injuries were adequately explained.
- Results of all pertinent laboratory and other diagnostic procedures.
- Color photographs and imaging studies, if applicable.
- If the police are called, the name of the investigating officer and any actions taken.

(*Continued*)

Box 11.5 • (Continued)

In addition to complete written records, photographs are particularly valuable as evidence. The physician should ask the patient for permission to take photographs. Imaging studies also may be useful. State laws that apply to the taking of photographs usually apply to x-rays as well.

- When possible, take photographs before medical treatment is given.
- Use color film along with a color standard.
- Photograph from different angles, full body and close-up.
- Hold up a coin, ruler, or other object to illustrate the size of an injury.
- Include the patient's face in at least one picture.
- Take at least two pictures of every major trauma area.
- Mark photographs precisely as soon as possible with the patient's name, location of injury, and names of the photographer and others present.

For medical records to be admissible in court, the doctor should be prepared to testify:

- That the records were made during the "regular course of business" at the time of the examination or interview
- That the records were made in accordance with routinely followed procedures
- That the records have been properly stored and their access limited to professional staff.

From the American Medical Association (AMA) (1992).

Assess the Client's Safety

All forms of family violence can escalate as the relationship continues. As noted previously, women are at greatest risk for homicide when leaving an abusive relationship. Therefore, assessing a client's safety is crucial. The Danger Assessment (Campbell, Webster, Kozid-McLain, et al., 2007) is a 20-item questionnaire that can be used to assess a client's immediate safety within a relationship and risk of lethality or more serious violence in the future (Box 11.6). This instrument asks the woman to respond with yes/no answers to questions identifying the risk factors associated with the incidence of homicide in intimate relationships.

Box 11.6 • Danger Assessment

Several risk factors have been associated with increased risk of homicides (murders) of women and men in violent relationships. We cannot predict what will happen in your case, but we would like you to be aware of the danger of homicide in situations of abuse and for you to see how many of the risk factors apply to your situation.

Using the calendar, please mark the approximate dates during the past year when you were abused by your partner or ex-partner. Write on that date how bad the incident was according to the following scale:

1. Slapping, pushing; no injuries and/or lasting pain
2. Punching, kicking; bruises, cuts, and/or continuing pain
3. "Beating up"; severe contusions, burns, broken bones, miscarriage
4. Threat to use weapon; head injury, internal injury, permanent injury, miscarriage
5. Use of weapon; wounds from weapon

(If **any** of the descriptions for the higher number apply, use the higher number.)

Mark **Yes** or **No** for each of the following.

("He" refers to your husband, partner, ex-husband, ex-partner, or whoever is currently physically hurting you.)

_____ 1. Has the physical violence increased in severity or frequency over the past year?

_____ 2. Does he own a gun?

_____ 3. Have you left him after living together during the past year?

_____ 3a. (If have *never* lived with him, check here: ___)

_____ 4. Is he unemployed?

_____ 5. Has he ever used a weapon against you or threatened you with a lethal weapon?

_____ 5a. (If yes, was the weapon a gun? ____)

_____ 6. Does he threaten to kill you?

_____ 7. Has he avoided being arrested for domestic violence?

_____ 8. Do you have a child that is not his?

(*Continued*)

Box 11.6 • (Continued)

_____ 9. Has he ever forced you to have sex when you did not wish to do so?

_____ 10. Does he ever try to choke you?

_____ 11. Does he use illegal drugs? By drugs, I mean "uppers" or amphetamines, speed, angel dust, cocaine, "crack," street drugs, or mixtures.

_____ 12. Is he an alcoholic or problem drinker?

_____ 13. Does he control most or all of your daily activities? (For instance: Does he tell you who you can be friends with, when you can see your family, how much money you can use, or when you can take the car?) (If he tries, but you do not let him, check here: ____)

_____ 14. Is he violently and constantly jealous of you? (For instance, does he say "If I can't have you, no one can.")

_____ 15. Have you ever been beaten by him while you were pregnant? (If you have never been pregnant by him, check here: ____)

_____ 16. Has he ever threatened or tried to commit suicide?

_____ 17. Does he threaten to harm your children?

_____ 18. Do you believe he is capable of killing you?

_____ 19. Does he follow or spy on you, leave threatening notes or messages on the answering machine, destroy your property, or call you when you don't want him to?

_____ 20. Have you ever threatened or tried to commit suicide?

_____ Total "Yes" Answers

Thank you. Please talk to your nurse, advocate or counselor about what the Danger Assessment means in terms of your situation.

Jacquelyn C. Campbell, PhD, RN, FAAN

When the woman completes the Danger Assessment, she is encouraged to assess her degree of danger within the relationship in conjunction with validation from her PCP. A weighted scoring system for this instrument is available through certification at *www.dangerassessment.org*.

Once a client's degree of safety is determined, the PCP should continue to use therapeutic communication to support the client as she determines her course of action. For numerous reasons, women may decide to stay in the abusive relationship. In these instances, it is important not to convey disappointment or disapproval of this decision but rather to support her in her decision and reiterate that she has options if she decides to leave in the future.

Whether a woman decides to leave or remain in an abusive relationship, it is important that she develop a personalized safety plan to protect herself should her situation become dangerous. The National Coalition Against Domestic Violence (2005) has provided a list of considerations for developing a safety plan (Box 11.7).

Review Options and Refer Client to a Family Violence Expert

Following the above mentioned steps, a PCP should be prepared to review available options and make a referral to a family violence expert or mental health specialist. The most common referrals include those for emergency housing and shelters, legal services, support networks, and counseling services. The ability to make an appropriate referral requires the PCP to be familiar with the resources available in her community. A list of general resources is provided in the Resources for Patients section; many of the organizations listed can provide information about what services are available to victims of family violence in local communities.

CRIMINAL JUSTICE AND LEGAL SYSTEMS

All states recognize acts of family violence as crimes. PCPs who work with survivors of family violence should be knowledgeable of the laws related to family violence. These laws serve to protect victims not only through the prosecution of the abuser but also through mandatory reporting of abuse.

Laws Related to Family Violence

Victims of family violence have several legal options available at both the state and federal levels. Civil and criminal laws exist to protect the victim and hold the offender accountable. Civil laws include civil protection orders at the state level and the Violence Against Women Act at the federal level. Other relevant civil laws include divorce, spousal/child support, child custody, and compensatory

Box 11.7 • Establishing a Safety Plan

If you are still in the relationship:

- Think of a safe place to go if an argument occurs—avoid rooms with no exits (bathroom) or rooms with weapons (kitchen).
- Think about and make a list of safe people to contact.
- Keep change with you at all times.
- Memorize all important numbers.
- Establish a "code word" or "sign" so that family, friends, teachers, or coworkers know when to call for help.
- Think about what you will say to your partner if he or she becomes violent.

If you have left the relationship:

- Change your phone number.
- Screen calls.
- Save and document all contacts, messages, injuries, or other incidents involving the batterer.
- Change locks if the batterer has a key.
- Avoid staying alone.
- Plan how to get away if confronted by an abusive partner.
- If you have to meet your partner, do it in a public place.
- Vary your routine.
- Notify school and work contacts.
- Call a shelter for battered women.

If you leave the relationship or are thinking of leaving, you should take important papers and documents with you to enable you to apply for benefits or take legal action.

Important papers you should take include Social Security cards and birth certificates for you and your children, your marriage license, leases or deeds in your name or both yours and your partner's names, your checkbook, your charge cards, bank statements and charge account statements, insurance policies, proof of income for you and your spouse (pay stubs or W-2s), and any documentation of past incidents of abuse (photos, police reports, medical records, etc.).

From the National Coalition Against Domestic Violence (2005).

and punitive damages for assault and battery. Criminal laws at the state level include arrest and prosecution for crimes such as assault, battery, harassment, child abuse, sexual assault, kidnapping, false imprisonment, stalking, attempted murder, and murder. Federal criminal laws include the Lautenberg Amendment and Violence Against Women Act. Survivors of family violence should be aware of the legal options available to them.

While the justice system in this country has created "legal" definitions for violent crimes, it is important to note that these definitions may not always be fully understood by the general public. Often, an individual may not even realize that she has been the victim of a violent crime such as rape or assault. She may perceive her experience as normal, common behavior, or something that she has brought onto herself. Furthermore, an individual may have experienced some form of abuse, even if there is insufficient proof to meet the legal definition. It is important that PCPs are aware of these differences in definitions, as it can have a great impact on how abuse is diagnosed and treated. The priority for the PCP is to provide a complete assessment, violence screening, safety planning, and referrals and not necessarily focus on an accurate legal definition.

Mandatory Reporting

Every state has specific laws that regulate which types of abuse must be reported to authorities and which people are mandated to report. Because these laws vary from state to state, health care professionals should become familiar with the reporting requirements for the state in which they practice. PCPs can access information specific to their state of practice by searching the state statutes through the Internet or at the local library. A list of websites that provide state specific information related to mandatory reporting can also be found in the Resources for Patients section.

All states have laws mandating health care providers to report suspected child abuse and neglect to appropriate child protective agencies. Acts of child abuse or neglect need not be proven before reporting, only suspected. Child abuse often occurs in situations of IPV, so the children of victims of IPV should be assessed for signs of abuse and neglect, and if suspected, mandatory reporting laws should be followed.

PCPs who work with a primarily adult population may be more likely to encounter disclosures of past child abuse rather than current. While many laws define what constitutes current abuse and neglect, few define how far into the past the mandate to report extends. Most states, however, do require past child abuse to be reported if it is believed that other children may be in danger. If there is still uncertainty as to whether a case is reportable, the child protection services agency should be consulted.

Currently, 42 states also require PCPs to report suspected cases of vulnerable adult abuse or neglect to adult protective services. As with child abuse, these cases do not have to be proven, only suspected.

Unlike child abuse, mandatory reporting of IPV is controversial, with some in favor and others opposed. Most states do have some form of mandated reporting for IPV, particularly if it involves injury resulting from a weapon or other life-threatening situation. Given the differences across states in the mandatory reporting of IPV, it is crucial that PCPs know their state statutes.

If a case requires reporting to authorities, the PCP must fully disclose this obligation to the client and take measures to ensure the individual's safety. In cases of suspected child abuse, the PCP's mandate to report the suspected abuse to the authorities should be disclosed to the parents/guardians unless there is a belief that this would put the child at risk for further abuse. If it is felt that disclosing this to the parents would put the child at greater risk for abuse, then the PCP should not tell the parents but still must report the suspected abuse to the authorities.

RESOURCES AND CLIENT EDUCATION

It is important to provide clients with education and other resources relating to abuse even if a client does not disclose abuse. The Family Violence Prevention Fund (2004) recommends that PCPs offer their clients literature about abuse in exam rooms, waiting areas, and/or bathrooms. Basic information about the commonness of abuse, what constitutes abuse, and the risk factors for abuse are helpful in assisting clients to identify whether they are being victimized or at risk. Any literature (e.g., pamphlets, safety cards, posters) providing information about abuse should include emergency phone numbers/hotlines as well as health and community services in the area. This literature should be developed at an appropriate reading level and language and be culturally appropriate for the client population. Client education materials can be accessed from the websites provided in the Resources for Patients.

CONCLUSION

This chapter has provided a discussion of family violence and the role of the PCP in the identification, treatment, and prevention of family violence and the associated negative health outcomes. Experiences of family violence are common among clients in the primary care setting, and in order to effectively intervene,

PCPs must understand the unique dynamics involved in violence and abuse. This begins with an understanding of the epidemiology, risk factors, and impacts associated with the different forms of family violence.

The focus of the PCP in providing care to victims of abuse and trauma should be on routine screening for abuse, asking direct questions about abuse, documentation of suspected or actual abuse, assessing client safety, reviewing available options, and providing referrals to family violence or mental health experts. Several Internet resources have been provided in this chapter to assist the PCP with these steps. Great progress has been made in the effort to eliminate family violence; however, there is still a long way to go. PCPs are in a unique position to advance these efforts through a continued commitment to providing the best care and advocacy for their clients.

Resources for Patients

General

Family Violence Prevention Fund: *www.endabuse.org/*

National Center for Victims of Crime: *www.ncvc.org/*

National Women's Health Information Center: *http://womenshealth.gov/*

Child Abuse

National Youth Violence Prevention Resource Center: *www.safeyouth.org/*

Intimate Partner Violence

National Center for Injury Prevention and Control (CDC): Intimate Partner Violence
Intimate Partners Violence Prevention: *www.cdc.gov/ncipc/dvp/IPV/default.htm*

National Domestic Violence Hotline:
1-800-799-7233
1-800-787-3224 (TTY)

Nursing Network on Violence Against Women International: *www.nnvawi.org*

WomensLaw.org: *www.womenslaw.org/*
Provides easy-to-understand legal information to women living with or escaping domestic violence

Sexual Assault

National Center for Posttraumatic Stress Disorder, Sexual Assault: *www.ncptsd.va.gov/ncmain/ncdocs/fact_shts/fs_female_sex_assault.html*

National Sexual Assault Hotline:
1-800-656-HOPE

Rape, Abuse, and Incest National Network (RAINN) *www.rainn.org*

Elder and Vulnerable Adult Abuse

Administration on Aging, Department of Health and Human Services: *www.aoa.gov/*

Center for Research on Women with Disabilities (CROWD): *www.bcm.edu/crowd/index.htm*

Clearinghouse on Abuse and Neglect of the Elderly (CANE): *http://db.rdms.udel.edu:8080/CANE/index.jsp*

National Center on Elder Abuse: *http://www.ncea.aoa.gov*

National Disability Rights Network: *www.ndrn.org/*

Mandatory Reporting Laws

Child Abuse: *www.childwelfare.gov/systemwide/laws_policies/state/can/reporting.cfm*

Elder/Vulnerable Adult Abuse: *http://www.ncea.aoa.gov/NCEAroot/Main_Site/Find_Help/APS/Analysis_State_Laws.aspx*

Intimate Partner Violence: *http://endabuse.org/health/mandatoryreporting*

References

American Academy of Pediatrics (AAP). (1998). Policy statement: The role of the pediatrician in recognizing and intervening on the behalf of abused women. *Pediatrics, 101*, 1091–1092.

American College of Obstetricians and Gynecologists (ACOG). (2002). *Guidelines for women's health care* (2nd ed.). Washington, DC: Author.

American Medical Association (AMA). (1992). *Diagnostic and treatment guidelines on domestic violence.* Chicago, IL: Author.

American Nurses Association (ANA). (1991). *Position statement: Physical violence against women.* Washington, DC: Author.

Anderson, S., McClain, N., & Riviello, R. J. (2006). Genital findings of women after consensual and nonconsensual intercourse. *Journal of Forensic Nursing, 2*(2), 59–65.

Barlow, D., & Durand, M. (2002). *Abnormal psychology* (3rd ed.). Belmont, CA: Wadsworth.

Bensley, L., Van Eenwyk, J., & Simmons, K. W. (2003). Childhood family violence history and women's risk for intimate partner violence and poor health. *American Journal of Preventive Medicine, 25*(1), 38–44.

Breitenbecher, K. H. (2006). The relationships among self blame, psychological distress, and sexual victimization. *Journal of Interpersonal Violence, 21*(5), 597–611.

Caetano, R., & Cunradi, C. (2003). Intimate partner violence and depression among whites, blacks and Hispanics. *Annals of Epidemiology, 13*(10), 661–665.

Caetano, R., Field, G.A., Ramisetty-Mikler, S., et al. (2005). The 5-year course of intimate partner violence among white, black and Hispanic couples in the United States. *Journal of Interpersonal Violence, 20*(9), 1039–1057.

Campbell, J. C. (1986). Nursing assessment for risk of homicide with battered women. *Advances in Nursing Science, 8*, 36–51.

Campbell, J. C. (2007). *Assessing dangerousness: Violence by batterers and child abusers.* New York: Springer.

Campbell, J. C., Jones, A. S., Dienemann J., et al. (2002). Intimate partner violence and physical health consequences. *Archives of Internal Medicine, 162*(10), 1157–1163.

Campbell, J. C., Webster, D., Koziol-McLain, J., et al. (2003). Risk factors for femicide in abusive relationships: Results from a multisite case control study. *American Journal of Public Health, 93*(7), 1089–1097.

Carney, M. T., Kahan, F. S., & Paris, B. E. C. (2003). Elder abuse: Every bruise a sign of abuse? *Mount Sinai Journal of Medicine, 70*(2), 69–74.

Carter, J. C., Bewell, C., Blackmore, E., et al. (2006). The impact of childhood sexual abuse in anorexia nervosa. *Child Abuse and Neglect, 30*(3), 257–269.

Casey, E. A., & Nurius, P. S. (2006). Trends in the prevalence and characteristics of sexual violence: A cohort analysis. *Violence and Victims, 21*(5), 629–664.

Centers for Disease Control and Prevention (CDC). (2006a). *Intimate partner violence: Fact sheet.* Retrieved September 4, 2006, from *www.cdc.gov/ncipc/dvp/ipv_factsheet.pdf*

Centers for Disease Control and Prevention (CDC). (2006b). *Sexually transmitted disease treatment guidelines 2006: Sexual assault and STDs.* Retrieved October 8, 2006, from *www.cdc.gov/std/treatment/2006/sexual-assault.htm.*

Champion, H. L., Foley, K. L., DuRant, R. H., et al. (2004). Adolescent sexual victimization, use of alcohol and other substances, and other health risk behaviors. *Journal of Adolescent Health, 35*(4), 321–328.

Champion, J. D., Shain, R. N., Piper, J., et al. (2002). Psychological distress among abused minority women with sexually transmitted diseases. *Journal of the American Academy of Nurse Practitioners, 14*(7), 316–324.

Coker, A. L., Bethea, L., Smith, P. H., et al. (2002). Missed opportunities: Intimate partner violence in family practice settings. *Preventive Medicine, 34*(4), 445–454.

Coker, A. L., Pope, B. O., Smith, P. H., et al. (2001). Assessment of clinical partner violence screening tools. *Journal of the American Medical Women's Association, 56*(1), 19–23.

Coker, A. L., Smith, P. H., & Fadden, M. K. (2005). Intimate partner violence and disabilities among women attending family practice clinics. *Journal of Women's Health, 14*(9), 829–838.

Conoscenti, L. M., & McNally, R. J. (2006). Health complaints in acknowledged and unacknowledged rape victims. *Anxiety Disorders, 20*, 372–379.

Diaz, A., Simantov, E., & Rickert, V. I. (2002). Effect of abuse on health: Results of a national survey. *Archives of Pediatric Adolescent Medicine, 156*(8), 811–817.

Dienemann, J., Boyle, E., Baker, D., et al. (2000). Intimate partner abuse among women diagnosed with depression. *Issues in Mental Health Nursing, 21*(5), 499–513.

Dube, S. R., Felitti, V. J., Dong, M., et al. (2003). Childhood abuse, neglect, and household dysfunction and the risk of illicit drug use: the adverse childhood experiences study. *Pediatrics, 111*(3), 564–572.

Dube, S. R., Anda, R. F., Felitti, V. J., et al. (2001). Childhood abuse, household dysfunction, and the risk of attempted suicide throughout the life span: Findings from the adverse childhood experiences study. *Journal of the American Medical Women's Association, 286*(24), 3089–3096.

Dutton, M. A., Green, B. L., Kaltman, S. I., et al. (2006). Intimate partner violence, PTSD, and adverse health outcomes. *Journal of Interpersonal Violence, 21*(7), 955–968.

Dyer, C. B., Connolly, M. T., & McFeeley, P. (2003). The clinical and medical forensics of elder abuse and neglect. In R. J. Bonnie & R. B. Wallace (Eds.), *Elder mistreatment: Abuse, neglect, and exploitation in an aging America.* Washington, DC: National Academies Press (pp. 339–381).

Edwards, V. J., Holden, G. W., Felitti, V. J., et al. (2003). Relationship between multiple forms of childhood maltreatment and adult mental health in community respondents: Results from the adverse childhood experiences study. *American Journal of Psychiatry, 160*(8), 1453–1460.

Family Violence Prevention Fund. (1999). *Preventing domestic violence: Clinical guidelines on routine screening*. Washington, DC: Author.

Family Violence Prevention Fund. (2004). *The national consensus guidelines on identifying and responding to domestic violence victimization in health care settings* (2nd ed.). Retrieved August 20, 2006, from *www.endabuse.org/programs/healthcare/file/Concensus.pdf.*

Fassler, I. R., Amodeo, M., Griffin, M. L., et al. (2005). Predicting long-term outcomes for women sexually abused in childhood: Contribution of abuse severity vs. family environment. *Child Abuse and Neglect, 29*(3), 269–284.

Federal Child Abuse Prevention and Treatment Act, 42 U.S.C.A. § 5106g (West Supp. 1998).

Feldhaus, K. M., Koziol-McLain, J., Amsbury, H. L., et al. (1997). Accuracy of 3 brief screening questions for detecting partner violence in the emergency department. *Journal of the American Medical Association, 277*(17), 1357–1361.

Gazmararian, J. A., Petersen, R., Spitz, A. M., et al. (2000). Violence and reproductive health: Current knowledge and future research directions. *Maternal and Child Health Journal, 4*(2), 79–84.

Golding, J. M. (1999). Intimate partner violence as a risk factor for mental health disorders: A meta-analysis. *Journal of Family Violence, 14*(2), 99–132.

Goodwin, M. M., Gazmararian, J. A., Johnson, C. H., et al. (2000). Pregnancy intendedness and physical abuse around the time of pregnancy: Findings from the pregnancy risk assessment monitoring system, 1996-1997. *Maternal and Child Health Journal, 4*(2), 85–92.

Halpern, C. T., Young, M. L., Waller, M. W., et al. (2004). Prevalence of partner violence in same-sex romantic and sexual relationships in a national sample of adolescents. *Journal of Adolescent Health, 35*(2), 124–131.

Heise, L., & Garcia-Moreno, C. (2002). Violence by intimate partners. In E. Krug, L. L. Dahlberg, J. A. Mercy, et al. (Eds.). *World report on violence and health* (pp. 87–121). Geneva, Switzerland: World Health Organization.

Johnson, J. K., Haider, F., Ellis, K., et al. (2003). The prevalence of domestic violence in pregnant women. *British Journal of Obstetrics and Gynecology, 110*(3), 272–275.

Jones, J. S., Wynn, B. N., Kroeze, B., et al. (2004). Comparison of sexual assaults by strangers versus known assailants in a community-based population. *American Journal of Emergency Medicine, 22*(6), 454–459.

Kearny, M. H., Munro, B. H., Kelly, U., et al. (2004). Health behaviors as mediators for the effect of partner abuse on infant birth weight. *Nursing Research, 53*(1), 36–45.

Kleinschmidt, K. C. (1997). Elder abuse: A review. *Annals of Emergency Medicine, 30*, 463–472.

Kramer, A., Lorenzon, D., & Mueller, G. (2004). Prevalence of intimate partner violence and health implications for women using emergency departments and primary care clinics. *Women's Health Issues, 14*(1), 19–29.

Lachs, M. S., & Pillemer, K. (2004). Elder abuse. *Lancet, 364*, 1263–1272.

Lachs, M. S., Williams, C. S., O'Brien, S., et al. (1998). The mortality of elder abuse. *Journal of the American Medical Association, 280*(5), 428–432.

Ledray, L. E. (2006). Sexual assault. In V. A. Lynch & J. B. Duval (Eds.), *Forensic nursing* (pp. 279–291). St. Louis, MO: Elsevier-Mosby.

Lincoln, A. L., Liebschutz, J. M., Chernoff, M., et al. (2006). Brief screening for co-occurring disorders among women entering substance abuse treatment. *Substance Abuse Treatment, Prevention, and Policy, 1*(26), 1–9.

Lipsky, S., Caetano, R., Field, C. A., et al. (2006). The role of intimate partner violence, rape and ethnicity in help-seeking behaviors. *Ethnicity and Health, 11*(1), 81–100.

MacMillan, H. L., Wathen, C. N., Jamieson, E., et al. (2006). Approaches to screening for intimate partner violence in health care settings: A randomized trial. *Journal of the American Medical Association, 296*(5), 530–536.

Massachusetts Medical Society, Committee on Violence. (2004). *Partner violence. How to recognize and treat victims of abuse. A guide for physicians and other health care professionals* (4th ed.). Waltham, MA: Author.

Matthias, R. E., & Benjamin, A. E. (2003). Abuse and neglect of clients in agency-based and consumer-directed home care. *Health and Social Work, 28*(3), 174–184.

McCloskey, L. A., Lichter, E., Ganz, M. L., et al. (2005). Intimate partner violence and patient screening across medical specialties. *Academic Emergency Medicine, 12*(8), 712–722.

McFarlane, J., Hughes, R. B., Nosek, M. A., et al. (2001). Abuse Assessment Screen-Disability (AAS-D): Measuring frequency, type, and perpetrator of abuse toward women with physical disabilities. *Journal of Women's Health and Gender-Based Medicine, 10*(9), 861–866.

McFarlane, J. M., Groff, J. Y., O'Brien, J. A., et al. (2005). Prevalence of partner violence against 7,433 African American, white, and Hispanic women receiving care at urban public primary care clinics. *Public Health Nursing, 22*(2), 98–107.

National Center on Elder Abuse (NCEA). (1998). *The national elder abuse incidence study*. Washington, DC: Author.

National Coalition Against Domestic Violence. (2005). *Safety plan*. Retrieved November 9, 2006, from *www.ncadv.org/protectyourself/SafetyPlan_130.html.*

National Research Council (NRC). (2003). *Elder mistreatment: Abuse, neglect, and exploitation in an aging America.* Panel to Review Risk and Prevalence of Elder Abuse and Neglect (R. J. Bonnie & R. B. Wallace, Eds.). Committee on National Statistics and Committee on Law and Justice, Division of Behavioral and Social Sciences and Education. Washington, DC: National Academies Press.

Nicolaidis, C., Curry, M., McFarland, B., et al. (2004). Violence, mental health, and physical symptoms in an academic internal medicine practice. *Journal of General Internal Medicine, 19*, 819–827.

Olson, L., Huyler, F., Lynch, A. W., et al. (1999). Guns, alcohol, and intimate partner violence: The epidemiology of female suicide in New Mexico. *Crisis, 20*(3), 121–126.

Paolucci , E. O., Genuis, M. L., & Violato, C. (2001). Meta-analysis of the published research on the effects of child sexual abuse. *Journal of Psychology, 135*(1), 17–37.

Paranjape, A., Heron, S., & Kaslow, N. (2006). Utilization of services by abused, low-income African American women. *Journal of General Internal Medicine, 21*, 189–192.

Petersilia J. R. (2001). Crime victims with developmental disabilities: A review essay. *Criminal Justice and Behavior, 28*(6), 655–694.

Plitcha, S. B. (2004). Intimate partner violence and physical health consequences: Policy and practice implications. *Journal of Interpersonal Violence, 19*(11), 1296–1323.

Saleptsi, E., Bichescu, D., Rockstroh, B., et al. (2004). Negative and positive childhood experiences across developmental periods in psychiatric patients with different diagnoses—An explorative study. *BMC Psychiatry, 26*(4), 40.

Saltzman , L. E., Fanslow, J. L., McMahon, P. M., et al. (2002). *Intimate partner violence surveillance: uniform definitions and recommended data elements, version 1.0*. Atlanta, GA: Centers for Disease Control and Prevention.

Sansone, R. A., Songer, D. A., & Miller, K. A. (2005). Childhood abuse, mental healthcare utilization, self-harm behavior, and multiple psychiatric diagnoses among inpatients with and without a borderline diagnosis. *Comprehensive Psychiatry, 46*(2), 117–120.

Senn, T. E., Carey, M. P., Vanable, P. A., et al. (2006). Childhood sexual abuse and sexual risk behavior among men and women attending a sexually transmitted disease clinic. *Journal of Consulting and Clinical Psychology, 74*(4), 720–731.

Sharps, P. W., Campbell, J. C., Campbell, D., et al. (2001). The role of alcohol use in intimate partner femicide. *American Journal on Addictions, 10*(2), 122–135.

Sheridan, D. J. (2003). Forensic identification and documentation of patients experiencing intimate partner violence. *Clinics in Family Practice, 5*(1), 113–143.

Sochting, I., Fairbrother, N., & Koch, W. J. (2004). Sexual assault of women: Prevention efforts and risk factors. *Violence Against Women, 10*, 73–93.

Stein, M. B., Lang, A. J., Laffaye, C., et al. (2004). Relationship of sexual assault history to somatic symptoms and health anxiety in women. *General Hospital Psychiatry, 26(*3), 178–183.

Stevens, T. N., Ruggiero, K. J., Kilpatrick, D. G., et al. (2005). Variables differentiating singly and multiply victimized youth: Results from the national survey of adolescents and implications for secondary prevention. *Child Maltreatment, 10*(3), 211–223.

Testa, M., & Leonard, K. E. (2001). The impact of husband physical aggression and alcohol use on marital functioning: Does alcohol "excuse" the violence? *Violence and Victims, 16*(5), 507–516.

The Commonwealth Fund. (1999). *Health concerns across a woman's lifespan: 1998 survey of women's health*. New York: Louis Harris and Associates.

Tjaden, P., & Thoennes, N. (2000). *Full report of the prevalence, incidence, and consequences of violence against women: Finding from the national violence against women survey*. Washington, DC: National Institute of Justice.

Ullman, S. E., Filipas, H. H., Townsend, S. M., et al. (2006). The role of victim-offender relationship in women's sexual assault experiences. *Journal of Interpersonal Violence, 21*(6), 798–819.

Ulrich, Y. C., Cain, K. C., Sugg, N. K., et al. (2003). Medical care utilization patterns in women with diagnosed domestic violence. *American Journal of Preventive Medicine, 24*, 9–15.

U.S. Department of Health and Human Services, Administration on Children, Youth and Families. (2007). *Child maltreatment 2005*. Washington, DC: U.S. Government Printing Office. Retrieved September 03, 2007, from *www.acf.hhs.gov/programs/cb/pubs/cm05/cm05.pdf*.

U.S. Department of Justice, Bureau of Justice Statistics. (2005a). Family violence statistics: Including statistics on strangers and acquaintances. Retrieved July 7, 2006, from *www.ojp.usdoj.gov/bjs/pub/pdf/fvs.pdf*.

U.S. Department of Justice, Bureau of Justice Statistics. (2005b). *Criminal victimization in the United States—Statistical tables index, table index, definitions*. Retrieved October 1, 2006, from *www.ojp.gov/bjs/abstract/cvus/definitions.htm*.

U.S. Department of Justice, Bureau of Justice Statistics. (2006a). *Criminal victimization, 2005*. NCJ Publication no. 214644. Washington, DC: Author.

U.S. Department of Justice, Bureau of Justice Statistics. (2006b). *Homicide trends in the U.S.: Intimate homicide*. Retrieved July 7, 2006, from *www.ojp.usdoj.gov/bjs/homicide/intimates.htm*.

U.S. Preventive Task Force (USPTF). (2004). *Screening for family and intimate partner violence*. Retrieved August 20, 2006, from *www.ahrq.gov/clinic/uspstf/uspsfamv.htm*.

Vogeltanz, N. D., Wilsnack, S. C., Harris, T. R., et al. (1999). Prevalence and risk factors for childhood sexual abuse in women: National survey findings. *Child Abuse and Neglect, 23*(6), 579–592.

Walker, L. E. (1979). *The battered woman*. New York: Harper & Row.

Walker, L. E. (1984). *The battered woman syndrome*. New York: Springer.

Wenzel, J. D., Monson, C. L., & Johnson, S. M. (2004). Domestic violence: Prevalence and detection in a family medicine residency clinic. *Journal of the American Osteopathic Association, 104*(6), 233–239.

Wood, E. (2006). *The availability and utility of interdisciplinary data on elder abuse: A white paper for the National Center on Elder Abuse*. Washington, DC: American Bar Association Commission on Law and Aging.

Woods, S. J. (2000). Prevalence and patterns of post traumatic stress in abused and post abused women. *Issues in Mental Health Nursing, 21*, 309–324.

Woods, S. J., Wineman, M., Page, G. G., et al. (2005). Predicting immune status in women from PTSD and childhood and adult violence. *Advances in Nursing Science, 28*(4), 306–319.

Zanarini, M. C., Yong, L., Fankenburg, F. R., et al. (2002). Severity of reported childhood sexual abuse and its relationship to severity of borderline psychopathology and psychosocial impairment among borderline inpatients. *Journal of Nervous and Mental Disease, 190*(6), 381–387.

Michelle O'Grady
Jody R. Lori

chapter 12

Reproductive Issues

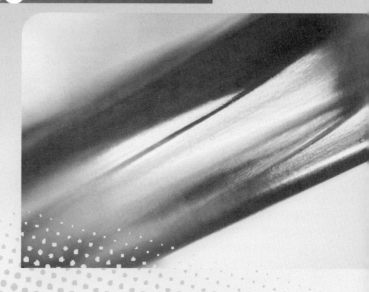

While both men and women experience mental illness, gender does influence its pattern and incidence, as do reproductive status and function. Illnesses associated with transitions in reproductive function are of particular interest to women and society because of quality-of-life considerations as well as their implications for childbearing and parenting.

Progress has been made in understanding gender effects in some major medical illnesses, but the links between mental health, gender, genes, and cellular and reproductive function are unclear and understudied (Blehar, 2003). This gap is critical because women experience a disproportionate burden of some types of mental illness, especially mood and anxiety disorders (Blehar; Steiner, Dunn, and Born 2003). As Steiner, Dunn, et al., (2003) states, "Elucidating the phenomenon of transition-related mental illness is clearly critical to improving women's health" (p. 69). This elucidation requires consideration of race and ethnicity and of physiologic factors such as endocrine function and comorbidity as well as psychosocial issues including lifestyles, habits, stress, and life events (Parry and Newton, 2001).

Mental health is vulnerable in times of biologic or social transition. All women, regardless of childbearing status, experience major biopsychosocial transitions as they age: puberty, reproductive cycles, and menopause; sexual awakening and sexual identity formation; and role formation and relationship changes. As the population of women in developed countries grows (due to improvements in reproductive health care and in differential birth and death ratios) and becomes older, there have been more support for and work being done on elucidating the gendering and mechanisms of mood disorders and other health problems common to women. This work is based on the fairly recent and fundamental recognition that women and men are physiologically, psychologically, and socially different from each other. These differences result in discrepant vulnerabilities to illness. For example, women are twice as likely as men to experience depressive or anxiety disorders (Parry and Newton, 2001; Steiner, Dunn, et al., 2003).

While the attention to female aspects of both mental and general health within the context of transitions has taken some time to develop, knowledge about the neurochemistry underlying many disorders has been increasing rapidly. It is clear that endocrine function and interactions are significantly correlated with mental health (Bell, Donath, Davison, et al., 2006; Feld, Halbreich, and Karkun, 2005; Parry and Newton, 2001; Parry, Sorenson, Meliska, et al., 2003; Payne, 2003; Steiner, 2003) and that normal and abnormal hormonal fluctuations over a woman's life span are associated with and contribute to mood disorders. Since women regularly have significant fluctuations in levels of estrogen and other hormones, the mechanisms of the "tuning" of the synchronicity within the endocrine system are receiving much attention. Disruptions of this synchronicity, or "chronobiological disturbances," are underlying factors across different illnesses (Parry and Newton; Payne; Steiner). Women who have experienced a mental illness during a time of hormonal fluctuation may be more vulnerable to mental illness at another such time (Feld, Halbreich and Karkun, 2006).

This chapter addresses the common and critical problems of premenstrual syndrome (PMS), premenstrual dysphoric disorder (PMDD), postpartum depression (PPD), and infertility as well as problems that may arise during pregnancy and menopause.

PREMENSTRUAL SYNDROME AND PREMENSTRUAL DYSPHORIC DISORDER

PMS and PMDD are related conditions that occur predictably in the luteal phase of the ovulatory cycle (secretory phase of the endometrial cycle), with cessation of symptoms within the first several days of the next cycle. Most women have experienced PMS, with about 30 percent experiencing a moderate form with bothersome symptoms (Parent-Stevens and Burns, 2000; Yonkers, Pearlstein, and Rosenheck, 2003). The most common symptom is irritability, but there is a wide spectrum of symptoms that may be experienced by women in varying degrees (consult an *ICD-10 Manual* for a complete listing of symptoms). The symptoms occur intermittently and vary in intensity for individual women across the cycles and life span. The symptoms of PMDD are much more severe and frequent—to the point of interfering with daily life. Sources vary as to the incidence of PMDD, but it is in the range of 2 to 8 percent (American Psychiatric Association, 2000; Parent-Stevens and Burns; Wihlback, Sundstrom-Poromaa, and Backstrom, 2006). The specific pathophysiology of PMDD is not known. In the late luteal cycle, estrogen and progesterone are at relatively low levels that are inversely related (estrogen is rising as progesterone falls). Current theories are focused on altered signal-response (feedback) loops within the hypothalamic-pituitary-ovarian (HPO) axis that controls cycles. The fluctuating levels of cycle hormones affect the neuroendocrine feedback in affected women such that the serotonergic neurotransmitter system is dysregulated and symptoms occur (Silber and Valadez-Meltzer, 2005; Steiner et al., 2003). This model explains the efficacy of the preferred pharmaceutical treatment, using selective serotonin reuptake inhibitors (SSRIs), which increases serotonin available to brain cells.

Assessment of Premenstrual Dysphoric Disorder

The criteria for the diagnosis of PMDD are set forth in the *Diagnostic and Statistical Manual of Mental Disorders* (*DSM-IV-TR*; APA, 2000): "Five or more of the following symptoms must have been present most of the time during the week prior to a patient's period, remitting within a few days after the onset of the patient's period. At least one of the symptoms must be one of the following:

- Feeling sad
- Hopeless or self-deprecating
- Feeling tense, anxious, or 'on edge'
- Marked lability of mood interspersed with frequent tearfulness
- Persistent irritability, anger, and increased interpersonal conflicts."

Treatment for Premenstrual Dysphoric Disorder

Practitioners may advise pharmacologic, behavioral, and/or nutritional therapies. Women have used many lifestyle adjustments to alleviate PMDD. Aerobic exercise may help and can promote well-being in general (Ling, 2000; Parent-Stevens and Burns, 2000). Dietary approaches have abounded (e.g., decreasing simple sugars), but there is little evidence that any particular food or combination of foods has a predictable effect. Specific nutritional measures may be more effective, including vitamin E, calcium, and/or magnesium supplements and caffeine restriction (Parent-Stevens and Burns). At least one study has found that St. John's wort diminishes PMDD symptoms (Huang and Tsai, 2003) (Table 12.1).

Other nondrug approaches include cognitive behavioral relaxation therapy and aerobic exercise as well as calcium, magnesium, and vitamin B_6 and/or supplementation of L-tryptophan. Some suggest a complex carbohydrate drink (Rapkin, 2003); this may be related to often-mentioned sweet, salty, or chocolate cravings (Steiner et al., 2003). However, there are no nutritional approaches that have been supported with strong evidence.

The most commonly prescribed drug for the treatment of PMDD is an SSRI, usually fluoxetine (Prozac) or sertraline (Zoloft) (APA, 2000; Silber and Valadez-Meltzer, 2005). The dosages will be lower than for depression and are taken just after midcycle (Freeman, Jabara, Sondheimer, et al., 2002; Freeman, Sondheimer, Sammel, et al., 2005; Miner, Brown, McCray, et al., 2002). Some providers have prescribed combined oral contraceptives in an effort to regulate the HPO axis (Rapkin, 2003); the birth control pill "Yaz" is approved for this use (National Women's Health Information Center, 2006) and has been uniquely marketed (Table 12.2).

Table 12.1 • Supplement Treatments for Premenstrual Dysphoric Disorder

Supplement	Dosage	Considerations	Indications
Vitamin E (alpha-tocopherol)	200–1,000 IU/day	Increased bleeding risk with anise, arnica, chamomile, clove, dong quai, fenugreek, feverfew, garlic, ginger, ginkgo, Panax ginseng, licorice.	*Contraindicated* in hypercalcemia, renal calculi, and ventricular fibrillation. *Use cautiously* in patients receiving digitalis glycosides, severe respiratory insufficiency, renal disease, and cardiac disease.
Calcium	1–2 g/day	Encourage patients to maintain a diet adequate in vitamin D.	Possible arrhythmias, constipation
Magnesium	*Women:* 280 up to 400 mg/day; *Pregnant women:* 320 mg/day *Breast-feeding women:* 340–355 mg/day	Caution patient to consult health care professional before taking antacids for more than 2 wk if problem is recurring, if relief is not obtained, or if symptoms of gastric bleeding (black, tarry stools; coffee-ground emesis) occur.	*Contraindicated* in hypermagnesemia, hypocalcemia, anuria, heart block, and active labor or within 2 hr of delivery (unless used for preterm labor). *Use cautiously* in any degree of renal insufficiency.
St. John's wort (*Hypericum perforatum*) *Other names:* Amber, Demon chaser, Goatweed, Hardhay, Klamath weed, Rosin rose, Tipton weed	*Mild depression:* 900 mg/day or 250 mg twice daily of 0.2% hypericin extract *OCD:* 450 mg twice daily of extended-release preparation	Concurrent use with alcohol or other antidepressants (including SSRIs and MAOIs) may increase the risk of adverse CNS reactions. Use with MAOIs and selective serotonin agonists could result in serotonin syndrome.	*Contraindicated* in pregnancy, lactation, or children. *Use cautiously* in history of phototoxicity, history of suicide attempt, severe depression, schizophrenia, or bipolar disorder (can induce hypomania or psychosis).

From Deglin, J. H., & Vallaerand, A. H. (2007).

Table 12.2 • Commonly Prescribed Selective Serotonin Reuptake Inhibitors for Premenstrual Dysphoric Disorder

Drug	Dosage*	Most Common Side Effects	Considerations	Warnings
Fluoxetine (Prozac, Prozac Weekly, Sarafem) *Depression, OCD, PMDD*	20 mg/day to start, up to 80 mg/day *or* Prozac Weekly (90 mg)	Anxiety, drowsiness, headache, insomnia, nervousness, diarrhea, sexual dysfunction, increased sweating, pruritus, tremor	*Pregnancy Category B* 20 mg/day to start, up to 80; 90 mg once/week *or* 20 mg/day starting 14 days prior to expected onset on menses, continued through first full day of menstruation, repeated with each cycle	May cause seizures. D/C/ MAO inhibitors 2 weeks prior to avoid serotonin syndrome. Do not discontinue abruptly.
Sertraline (Zoloft) *Depression, panic disorder, OCD, post-traumatic stress disorder (PTSD), social anxiety disorder, premenstrual dysphoric disorder*	25 mg once daily initially, then 50 mg once daily	Dizziness, drowsiness, fatigue, headache, insomnia, diarrhea, dry mouth, nausea, sexual dysfunction, increased sweating, tremor	*Pregnancy Category B* Risk of serotonergic side effects including serotonin syndrome with St. John's wort and SAMe.	May cause seizures. D/C/ MAO inhibitors 2 weeks prior to avoid serotonin syndrome. Potentially life-threatening: cerebral hemorrhage, cerebral thrombosis, coronary thrombosis, pulmonary embolism.

(Continued)

Table 12.2 • (Continued)

Drug	Dosage*	Most Common Side Effects	Considerations	Warnings
Escitalopram (Lexapro)	10–20 mg/day, through luteal phase or at symptom onset	Usually mild; insomnia, nausea, sleepiness, sexual dysfunction, increased sweating	*Pregnancy Category B* Not advised in 3rd trimester.	See above.
Ethinyl estradiol/ drospirenone (Yaz)	1 po q day	Abdominal cramps, bloating, cholestatic jaundice, gallbladder disease, liver tumors, nausea, vomiting, amenorrhea, breakthrough bleeding, dysmenorrhea, spotting	*Pregnancy Category X* Concomitant use with St. John's wort may decrease contraceptive efficacy and cause breakthrough bleeding and irregular menses.	Contraindicated in pregnancy and lactation or with history of CV disease. Concurrent use with NSAIDs, potassium-sparing diuretics, potassium supplements, ACE inhibitors, angiotensin II receptor antagonists, or heparin may result in hyperkalemia.

*Note that SSRI dosages are smaller than for treatment of depression.
From Deglin, J. H., & Vallaerand, A. H. (2007).

MENOPAUSE

Menopause is a fascinating exemplar of endocrine feedback. It is usually a long process (perimenopause, or the years leading up to final cessation of menses, can last up to 10 years) of progressively diminished response to hypothalamic-pituitary stimulation of the ovaries that begins with diminished fertility related to a decreasing follicular pool resulting in some cycle changes as a result of follicle-stimulating hormone (FSH) stimulating smaller cohorts of follicles. At first, more follicles develop as FSH rises and inhibin B diminishes, therefore promoting even higher FSH. As the levels rise and remaining functional follicles respond, cycle changes occur. Eventually, responsive follicle numbers diminish, inhibin B also diminishes, and cycles become noticeably more irregular and skipped. Luteinizing hormone pulses may also change in frequency and amplitude. FSH continues the valiant struggle for some time, but ultimately, the pool of follicles shrinks. Women often experience heavy or irregular bleeding and hot flushes during perimenopause. When three cycles are missed, the woman is in the later "menopausal transition." When she has passed 1 year without a cycle, she has completed the transition and is postmenopausal (Santoro, 2002). Symptoms often associated with menopause include vasomotor instability such as hot flushes and vaginal/vulvar atrophy.

While vasomotor symptoms occur across cultures, women's psychological responses and experiences vary. One study of Brazilian women indicated that nervousness, hot flushes, and sweating were the most common symptoms experienced and that these symptoms as well as palpitations, dizziness, depression, insomnia, and dyspareunia were associated with poorer quality of life (Conde, Pino-Neto, Santos-Sa, et al., 2006). Australian women were found to have frequent symptoms of forgetfulness, lack of energy, irritability, and weight gain (McVeigh, 2005). They were most negatively impacted by the weight gain and problems with heavy bleeding, poor concentration, leaking of urine, and feeling as though life were not worth living. Mishra, Brown, and Dobson (2003) found that their Australian subjects experienced significant declines over the perimenopause. Swedish women experienced psychological problems as well as hot flushes, vaginal dryness, headache, and muscle-skeletal-joint problems (Li, Wilawan, Samsioe, et al., 2002). Chinese women demonstrated low levels of vasomotor symptoms and anxiety and depression prior to treatment with hormone replacement therapy (HRT) (Haines, Yim, Chung, et al., 2003) (Table 12.3).

Table 12.3 • Menopause Treatment Options

Modalities	Options	Advantages	Disadvantages
Hormone replacement therapy	Conjugated estrogens 0.625 mg/day combined with medroxyprogesterone acetate 2.5 mg/day The FDA recommends that hormone therapy be used at the lowest doses for the shortest duration needed to achieve treatment goals. May consider HRT at the lowest possible dose for a limited time and other options when vasomotor symptoms are the cardinal cause of perimenopausal mental health complaints.	May reduce coronary artery plaque buildup in 50- to 59-year-old women. Relief from vasomotor symptoms including moderate to severe hot flashes, flushing, and symptoms of vulvar and vaginal atrophy. Effective for the prevention of postmenopausal osteoporosis but should only be considered for women at significant risk of osteoporosis who cannot take nonestrogen medications. Effective in diminishing the severity of depression.	Increased risks for invasive breast cancer, heart attacks, strokes, and venous thromboembolism rates, including pulmonary embolism as well as a greater risk of developing probable dementia. The FDA states that HRT should not be taken to prevent heart disease. HRT has also been found to have negative effects on mental well-being.
Complementary and alternative therapies	Black cohosh Red clover Phytoestrogens—most commonly soy products Isoflavone amounts of 40–80 mg/day	Successful in treating vasomotor symptoms. May be helpful in treating severe symptoms. May have a beneficial effect on vasomotor symptoms. Most frequently studied in relation to relief of hot flashes.	Little evidence in the literature to support the use of herbal supplements. Literature is inconclusive.
Cognitive/ mind-body/ social approaches	Education related to menopause and relief measures. Women who learn in groups have been shown to have significant improvements in their symptoms.	Sharing experiences may help women balance their negative perspectives of menopause and ease their symptoms. Able to maintain better dietary adherence & physical activity.	

Mental Health Issues During the Menopause Transition

Because of the cultural differences in the experience of menopause, alternative interventions may be needed, and the questions asked by researchers and primary care providers (PCPs) should reflect these differences. Depression is seen at much higher rates in women seeking care for menopause-related problems than the general perimenopausal population. Women with a previous history of depression are also more vulnerable (Joffe, Soares, Petrillo, et al., 2007; Steiner et al., 2003).

Assessment of the Menopause Transition

Assessment of mental health disorders in the perimenopause period is done similarly to that in the general population and should be informed by the awareness of cultural difference and the potential for increased irritability and risk of depression. The most common psychological symptom for American women in perimenopause is irritability, which may be exacerbated by the discomfort and loss of sleep caused by vasomotor instability. It is critical to determine whether mental distress is related to vasomotor changes or is an independent condition.

Treatment for Menopause

Treatment for menopause varies widely and may include various complementary and alternative medicine (CAM) modalities, specific psychotropics, psychotherapy, and/or daily HRT. The treatment option is based on the woman's history and presenting symptoms. Short-term courses of SSRIs have been effective for combinations of symptoms including depression during the transition to menopause. Joffe, Soares, Petrillo, et al. (2007) found that depression and vasomotor as well as other symptoms significantly improved in women using duloxetine (Cymbalta) for 8 weeks.

Hormone Replacement Therapy

The Women's Health Initiative study has provided significant information since 2001. Emerging findings have altered the management of menopausal symptoms. The primary findings were that (a) postmenopausal women taking conjugated estrogens 0.625 mg/day combined with medroxyprogesterone acetate 2.5 mg/day had increased risks for invasive breast cancer, heart attacks, strokes, and venous thromboembolism rates, including pulmonary embolism as well as greater risk of developing probable dementia; (b) while HRT may reduce coronary artery plaque buildup in 50- to 59-year-old women (Manson, Allison, Rossouw, et al., 2007), the risks of cardiovascular disease in older women still clearly outweigh the benefits; and (c) PCPs should look for alternative modalities to treat menopause-related problems (*http://public.nhlbi.nih.gov/newsroom/home/GetPressRelease.aspx?id= 288*).

Furthermore, the Food and Drug Administration (FDA) states that hormone replacement therapy (HRT) should not be taken to prevent heart disease. These products are approved therapies for relief from moderate to severe hot flashes and symptoms of vulvar and vaginal atrophy. Although hormone therapy is effective for the prevention of postmenopausal osteoporosis, it should only be considered for women at significant risk of osteoporosis who cannot take nonestrogen medications. The FDA recommends that hormone therapy be used at the lowest doses for the shortest duration needed to achieve treatment goals. Postmenopausal women who use or are considering using hormone therapy should discuss the possible benefits and risks to them with their PCP (FDA, 2007).

When considering hormone therapy for the relief of psychological symptoms, there are multiple perspectives and options. HRT does seem to be effective in diminishing the severity of depression (Santoro, 2002; Soares, Almeida, Joffe, et al., 2001; Zarate, Fonesca, Ochoa, et al., 2002) and has other benefits as noted previously. However, it has also been found to have negative effects on mental well-being (Li et al., 2003; McVeigh, 2005; Mishra et al., 2003) and no clear positive effect—and possibly a negative effect—on memory (Rice and Morse, 2003). Given the potential risks of HRT such as those listed previously, women whose primary perimenopausal problem is depression may be treated most specifically and effectively with antidepressants (FDA, 2007; Santoro, 2002).

HRT may best be used for the short-term management of other common perimenopausal problems and for women at risk for osteoporosis. One such problem and indication for HRT is flushing, which is associated with decreased quality of life and mental well-being. Women with flushing in the Heart and Estrogen/Progestin Replacement study (HERS trial) noted improved quality of life with HRT (Hlatky, Boothroyd, Vittinghoff, et al., 2002). Similarly, Newton, Reed, LaCroix, et al. (2006) found that women using estrogen replacement therapy/HRT showed significant improvement in vasomotor symptoms. Practitioners may consider HRT at the lowest possible dose for a limited time and other options when vasomotor symptoms are the cardinal cause of perimenopausal mental health complaints.

Complementary and Alternative Therapies

The CAM modalities used to address the symptoms of menopause are numerous and varied. CAM, as used in this chapter, refers to modalities outside the typical allopathic health care system. Many practitioners utilize one or more modalities with individualized variations and combinations. This breadth of approaches complicates evaluation, often resulting in a confusing and incomplete picture of the effectiveness of most modalities; however, general recommendations may be concluded.

Herbs One of the most promising herbs is black cohosh. Two systematic reviews (Huntley and Ernst, 2003; Kronenberg and Fugh-Berman, 2003) found that black clover was a promising treatment for vasomotor symptoms. Kronenberg and Fugh-Berman as well as Krebs, Ensrud, McDonald, et al. (2004) found no evidence for the efficacy of red clover, although Huntley and Ernst found that it may be effective for severe symptoms.

Phytoestrogens One of the most widely used nutritional categories is phytoestrogens: plant-based extracts of estrogen, most commonly soy. Some women consume soy in dozens of formulations and in variant quantities, primarily to relieve vasomotor symptoms. Extensive reviews of the literature are inconclusive, showing that soy foods may have a beneficial effect on vasomotor symptoms (Kronenberg and Fugh-Berman, 2003), may not have a beneficial effect (Krebs et al., 2004), or may have both (Nedrow, Miller, Walker, et al., 2006). The North American Menopause Society (NAMS) made a cautiously supportive consensus statement about isoflavones and noted that whole food sources are best. Most studies on hot flashes have used isoflavone amounts of 40 to 80 mg/day (NAMS, 2000; Panay, 2007).

Cognitive/Mind-Body/Social Approaches Women who learn about menopause and relief measures may improve their health and perceptions during the menopause transition. Women who learn in groups have been shown to have significant improvements in their symptoms. A cognitive approach that educates women about menopause and provides a venue for sharing experiences may help to women balance their negative perspectives of menopause and ease their symptoms (Rotem, Kushnir, and Levine, et al., 2005). Postmenopausal women who participated in a group dietary intervention program were able to maintain better dietary adherence and better able to sustain their involvement as they improved in mental health and physical activity (Tinker, Perri, Patterson, et al., 2002).

PREGNANCY

Pregnancy is unique in the impact it has across all the dimensions of a woman's life. Even in planned and welcomed pregnancies, stress occurs and women are more vulnerable to maladaptive responses to stress, including mental illness. Some groups may be particularly at risk. For example, lesbian women may have increased stress, less health care, and less social support that their heterosexual peers (Ross, 2005; Trettin, Moses-Kolko, and Wisner, 2006). Another at-risk population is adolescent girls who are simultaneously negotiating very complex transitions (Logsdon and Gennaro, 2005).

Ward and Zamorski (2002) point out that there is little agreement on how pregnancy affects mental illness. Andersson, Sundstrom-Poromaa, Wulff, et al. (2004) found no effect of depression or anxiety on neonatal outcome, and others (Federenko and Wadhwa, 2004; Ross, 2005; Weinstock, 2005) have suggested that preexisting conditions may worsen. Postpartum maternal stress/distress may result in fetal and neonatal problems and disrupted maternal–infant bonding and infant mental health (Federenko and Wadhwa; Ross; Weinstock). This challenge may have increased in the last decade, as more women with chronic mental illness become pregnant (Miller, 1992). This may increase even further as more and more people with chronic mental illness are integrated into community settings. The growing field of infant mental health may help to clarify the impact of maternal mental health on infant and child development. Practitioners should assess for such problems frequently and be prepared to offer appropriate interventions to support the woman, the fetus, and the maternal–infant bond (Spietz and Kelly, 2002).

Depression is the major mental illness associated with pregnancy. In some instances, it may first occur during pregnancy; it also may worsen in pregnant women suffering from depression. The incidence of depression among women of childbearing age is increasing (Sanders, 2006). Practitioners should be aware that depression and anxiety often coexist and that women very often present with anxiety symptoms rather than the classic depressive symptoms (Stocky and Lynch, 2000).

Assessment of Mental Health During Pregnancy

In the initial assessment, most models of prenatal care include broad questions related to mental health issues and support systems. Routine assessment does not usually include tools developed specifically to identify an elevated risk for mental health disorders. This is particularly critical given that providers may not attend to signs of mental distress, either assuming that "happiness" is the expected emotional state in all pregnancies (Morrissey, 2007) or equating mental health symptoms with normal emotional changes of pregnancy (Brown and Solchany, 2004). In women who are already diagnosed with serious mental health problems, Miller (1992) suggests that practitioners minimally assess the woman's adaptation to pregnancy; her perceived and objective competency for

Box 12.1 • Symptoms of Depression

- Depressed mood most of the day, nearly every day
- Markedly diminished interest or pleasure in activities nearly every day
- Weight loss (significant) when not dieting or an increase or decrease in appetite nearly every day
- Insomnia or hypersomnia nearly every day
- Psychomotor agitation or retardation nearly every day and observed by others
- Fatigue nearly every day
- Inappropriate guilt or feeling of worthlessness nearly every day
- Inability to concentrate or indecisiveness nearly every day
- Recurrent thoughts of death, suicidal ideation, suicide attempt, and/or suicide plan

From Lang, Rodgers, et al. (2005).

infant care, bonding, and parenting; and access to care. Lang, Rodgers, and Lebeck, et al. (2006) found the Beck Depression Inventory (BDI) useful in their in-depth survey of 32 pregnant women. Box 12.1 contains the symptoms of depression. A diagnosis of depression should be made if the client has five or more symptoms with depressed mood and/or loss of interest present for a minimum of 2 weeks.

Management of Mental Health Issues During Pregnancy

The current recommendations for medications in pregnancy are in flux, and active debates are ongoing in the literature (Koren, Matsui, Einarson, et al., 2005; Zitner and Bischoff, 2005). Lithium has long been contraindicated in both pregnancy and lactation. Recent reviews have concluded that SSRIs may not be as safe in pregnancy as was formerly believed (Sanders, 2006; Suppaseemanont, 2006). These and other findings have led the FDA to require warnings that the use of selective serotonin norepinephrine reuptake inhibitors (SNRIs) and SSRIs in late pregnancy could result in complications for the newborn. This is in contrast to the previous, though recent, consensus that most SSRIs and tricyclics were safe in pregnancy (Ward and Zamorski, 2002). The National Institute of Mental Health (NIMH) (2002) publishes guidelines on psychotropic medication use for pregnant and postpartum women. Providers and clients should review the patient's previous experiences when unmedicated and weigh the risks and benefits to determine treatment. These recommendations also apply to lactation.

In the United States, women diagnosed with depression have often been treated with medications throughout pregnancy. However, there may be viable alternatives. Andersson et al. (2004) found that neonatal outcomes were *not* worse for Swedish, unmedicated women with preexisting anxiety and/or depression (as diagnosed per the *DSM-IV*). Eberhard-Gran, Eskild, and Opjordsmoen (2005) provide a thorough review of the safety of psychotropic medications in pregnancy and note that in all cases, a multidisciplinary team approach is supported. A team consisting of a nurse, social worker, psychologist, and/or nutritionist will provide a more comprehensive, holistic approach.

Strengthening the social support system has been shown to be an effective tool in promoting maternal mental health, as is providing psychoeducation and psychotherapy (Sanders, 2006; Suppaseemanont, 2006). Physical inactivity (Poudevigne and O'Connor, 2006) and poor nutrition (Bodnar and Wisner, 2005) are related to diminished mood, so prenatal counseling should include encouraging regular physical activity and sound diet to support mental as well as physical health. Specific nutritional recommendations include improving omega-3 fatty acid intake; considering fish oil and folic acid supplements; and correcting any folate, vitamin B_{12}, iron, zinc, and/or selenium deficiencies (Bodnar and Wisner). In all cases, a multidisciplinary approach is advised (D'Afflitti, 2005; Morrissey, 2007; Sanders; Suppaseemanont). PCPs should take particular care to assess and promote maternal–infant attachment (beginning in the antenatal period). Healthy attachment is demonstrated by mothers who are obviously sensitive and responsive to their infants. PCPs can promote attachment by encouraging close attention and proximity to the newborn and teaching the woman about the meaning of the baby's signals (Karl, Beal, O'Hare, et al., 2006).

POSTPARTUM DEPRESSION

Depression following pregnancy (within the first year), or PPD, is a common and serious problem thought to be caused by a combination of hormonal changes and stressors such as sleep deprivation (NIMH, 2000) that occurs in 10 to 15 percent of women and has serious risks for the mother and baby as well as family relationships. Many of these women are not diagnosed and treated, because PCPs may be unable or unwilling to screen, treat, and/or refer them to a mental health provider (Logsdon and Gennaro, 2005). Although clinicians must work within time constraints, Boyd, Le, and Somberg (2005) recommend that PCPs *minimally* assess risk by asking about any history of depression or previous PPD (one of the most important risk factors). PCPs must also understand that cross-cultural differences in response to screening tools and in definitions of PPD exist. Additionally, they recommend that clinicians *universally* screen with tools such as the BPI-II and the Postpartum Depression Screening Scale (PDSS) for highly educated white women and the Edinburgh Postnatal Depression Scale (EPDS) for more diverse populations. The American College of Nurse-Midwives supports universal screening as well as increasing the number of postpartum visits to improve assessment and treatment (American College of Nurse-Midwives, 2002). Screening mothers for PPD at well-child visits may also be an option (Chaudron, Szilagyi, Campbell, et al., 2007). Special care should be taken to assess and support any woman with a history of any mental disorder and, particularly, those women who have stopped or altered their psychotropic medications during the pregnancy and/or lactation (NIMH, 2002).

Treatment for Postpartum Depression

Treatment options for PPD are similar to those for depressed pregnant women. PCPs must be aware of all the medications (including herbs) being used and assess for possible interactions. The safety of the medication for breast-feeding must also be considered since most psychotropic medications are secreted in breast milk. However, these medications are usually at a lower concentration than in the maternal serum and total very small dosages (Loebstein, Lalkin, and Koren, 1997; McCarter-Spaulding, 2005).

Physical activity, healthy diet, avoidance of potentially depressing substances, and adequate sleep as well as medications can ease the symptoms, and an integrated approach will be most effective (Dennis, 2004; Dennis and Stewart, 2004). Peer and/or provider support may be an effective tool to diminish PPD (Ray and Hodnett, 2001). However, cultural differences and variations in the implementation of interventions or how interventions are designed may affect results, as demonstrated in a study by Scottish researchers that showed no significant difference between support- and nonsupport groups (Reid, Glazener, Murray, et al., 2002).

PREGNANCY LOSS

Women who have a pregnancy loss suffer mental distress, whether the loss is spontaneous or induced. Broen, Moum, Bødtker, et al. (2005) found that Norwegian women who had induced abortions exhibited grief, loss, guilt, anger, and anxiety for longer periods than did women with miscarriages (as did New Zealanders; Fergusson, Horwood, and Ridder, 2006). Kero, Högberg, and Lalos (2004) found that while a significant proportion of women did express significant mental distress in the year after induced abortion, almost none experienced long-term distress. Therefore, it is imperative that the PCP be alert to the potential for mental distress following any pregnancy loss.

INFERTILITY

Infertility is defined as a failure to conceive after 12 months of unprotected intercourse. PCPs may often see couples with concerns before the full year elapses. These couples may be simply eager or may have evidence that they are likely to need assistance to conceive. In either case, the couples are likely to have anxiety about the situation. As Hart (2002) notes, infertility is multidimensional and stressful and can cause mental health and relationship problems. In fact, women diagnosed with infertility are more likely to experience psychopathology including anxiety and depression (Lok, Lee, Cheung, et al., 2002; Souter, Hopton, Penney, et al., 2002) than women who are not diagnosed with infertility. Therefore, regular assessment of mental health is indicated along with the initial medical evaluation. Standardized tools such as the Infertility Self-Efficacy scale have been developed for this type of assessment (Cousineau, Green, Corsini, et al., 2006). It is also important to note that women being treated for serious preexisting mental health conditions may have medication side effects, such as hyperprolactinemia, that interfere with conception (Shaw, 2005). Clearly, while PCPs may refer infertile clients to reproductive medicine specialists for advanced assessment and care, initial care should include consideration of mental health (Boivin, 2003; Devine, 2003; Hart, 2002; Himelein and Thatcher, 2006).

Treatment for Infertility

Himelein and Thatcher (2006) concur that treatment as well as assessment of infertile clients (specifically those with polycystic ovarian syndrome) should focus on both physical and psychological function. They advocate a holistic, team model of intervention including nutritionists and mental health professionals. Lacking this ideal approach, providers should be familiar with therapeutic resources in the community. An excellent resource is RESOLVE, a support network established by the National Infertility Association in 1974. The mission of RESOLVE is "to provide timely, compassionate support and information to people who are experiencing infertility and to increase awareness of infertility issues through public education and advocacy" (RESOLVE, 2007).

CONCLUSION

The common and critical mental health issues discussed in this chapter will comprise a significant portion of many PCPs' practices. PCPs must develop the clinical competencies needed to assess and manage common mental health issues. A thorough understanding of vulnerabilities for mental illness during biopsychosocial transitions is imperative for safe comprehensive practice.

Resources for Providers

Association of Women's Health, Obstetric and Neonatal Nurses. (2005). *Journal of Obstetric, Gynecologic, and Neonatal Nursing, 34*(2), 149–286.

Beck Depression Inventory-II (BDI-II): The Beck Depression Inventory (BDI) is copyrighted by the Psychological Corporation and can be ordered at *http://harcourtassessment.com/haiweb/cultures/en-us/productdetail.htm?pid=015-8018-370.*

Publisher: The Psychological Corporation, 555 Academic Court, San Antonio, TX 78204-2498; 2004 review by Paul A. Arbisi (University of Minnesota) and Richard F. Farmer (Idaho State University).

Summary: The BDI-II represents a highly successful revision of an acknowledged standard in the measurement of depressed mood. The revision has improved on the original by updating the items to reflect contemporary diagnostic criteria for depression and utilizing state-of-the-art psychometric techniques to improve the discriminative properties of the instrument. This degree of improvement is no small feat, and the BDI-II deserves to replace the BDI as the single most widely used clinically administered instrument for the assessment of depression.

Postpartum Depression Screening Scale (PDSS):

Publisher: Western Psychological Services, 12031 Wilshire Boulevard, Los Angeles, CA 90025-1251; 2004 review by Paul A. Arbisi, staff clinical psychologist at the Minneapolis VA Medical Center and associate professor at the Department of Psychiatry, University of Minnesota, Minneapolis, MN.

Summary: Although the PDSS is available as a clinical tool and as a screening instrument, several cautions must be emphasized. It is a known fact that self-reporting is vulnerable to underreporting, distortions due to response style bias, inaccurate reporting, defensiveness, and denial. This is true with most self-reporting measures but particularly is true given the mental state of women suffering from PPD. Therefore, test users should proceed with caution when interpreting tests results. Although self-reports have clear limitations, they have some validity related to standardization, economics, and limited training required for administration and administration time. When used with other assessments, the PDSS can be a valuable tool for diagnosing and treating women with PPD.

Source: Spies, R. A., & Plake, B. S. (Eds.). (2005). *The sixteenth mental measurements yearbook*. Lincoln, NE: Buros Institute of Mental Measurements. Hardbound, LC 39-3422, ISBN 0-910674-58-2. $195.00.

Symptom Checklist-90-R (SCL-90-R):

The SCL-90-R instrument from Pearson Assessments helps to evaluate a broad range of psychological problems and symptoms of psychopathology. The instrument is also useful in measuring patient progress or treatment outcomes. The SCL-90-R instrument is used by clinical psychologists, psychiatrists, and professionals in mental health, medical, and educational settings as well as for research purposes. Further information regarding the SCL-90-R is available at *www.pearsonassessments.com/tests/scl90r.htm*.

Resources for Patients

Birth control pill "Yaz": *www.yaz-us.com/home.jsp*.

National Institute of Mental Health: *www.nimh.nih.gov/publicat/medicate.cfm#ptdep12*.

Bibliography

Agency for Healthcare, Research, and Quality, U.S. Preventive Services Task Force. (2002). *Screening for depression*. Retrieved Month Day, Year, from *www.ahrq.gov/clinic/uspstf/uspsdepr.htm*.

American College of Nurse-Midwives. (2002). *Depression in women*. Retrieved July 22, 2007, from http://www.midwife.org/sitefiles/position/depression-in-women-05.pdf.

American College of Obstetricians and Gynecologists. (2003). *Premenstrual syndrome*. Educational Pamphlet AP057. Washington, DC: Author.

American Psychiatric Association (APA). (1996). *Diagnostic and statistical manual of mental disorders: Primary care version* (4th ed.). Washington, DC: Author.

American Psychiatric Association (APA). (2000). The DSM-IV criteria for diagnosing PMDD. *Psychiatric News*. August 10, 2007 (subscriber only page), from *www.psych.org/pnews/00-08-18/pmdd.html*.

American Psychiatric Association (APA). (2000). *Diagnostic and statistical manual of mental -disorders* (Revised 4th ed.). Washington, DC: Author.

Andersson, L., Sundstrom-Poromaa, I., Wulff, M., et al. (2004). Neonatal outcome following maternal antenatal depression and anxiety: A population-based study. *American Journal of Epidemiology, 159*(9), 872–881.

Austin, M. P, & Priest, S. R. (2005). Clinical issues in perinatal mental health: New developments in the detection and treatment of perinatal mood and anxiety disorders. *Acta Psychiatrica Scandinavica, 112*(2), 97–104.

Beeber, L. S., & Canuso, R. (2005). Strengthening social support for the low-income mother: Five critical questions and a guide for intervention. *Journal of Obstetric, Gynecologic, and Neonatal Nursing, 34*(6), 769–776.

Bell, R. J., Donath, S., Davison, S. L., et al. (2006). Endogenous androgen levels and well-being: Differences between premenopausal and postmenopausal women. *Menopause, 13*(1), 65–71.

Bifulco, A., Figueiredo, B., Guedeney, N., et al. (2004). Maternal attachment style and depression associated with childbirth: Preliminary results from a European and US cross-cultural study. *British Journal of Psychiatry, 184,* S31–S37.

Binder, E. F., Schechtman, K. B., Birge, S. J., et al. (2001). Effects of hormone replacement therapy on cognitive performance in elderly women. *Maturitas, 38*(2), 137–146.

Blehar, M. C. (2003). Public health context of women's mental health research. *Psychiatric Clinics of North America, 26*(3), 781–799.

Bodnar, L. M., & Wisner, K. L. (2005). Nutrition and depression: Implications for improving mental health among childbearing-aged women. *Biological Psychiatry, 558*(9), 679–685.

Boivin, J. (2003). A review of psychosocial interventions in infertility. *Social Science and Medicine, 57*(12), 2325–2341.

Boyd, R. C., Le, H. N., & Somberg, R. (2005). Review of screening instruments for postpartum depression. *Archives of Women's Mental Health, 8*(3), 141–153.

Boyd, R. C., Zayas, L. H., & McKee, M. D. (2006). Mother-infant interaction, life events and prenatal and postpartum depressive symptoms among urban minority women in primary care. *Maternal and Child Health Journal, 10*(2), 139–148.

Broen, A. N., Moum, T., Bødtker, A. S., et al. (2005). The course of mental health after miscarriage and induced abortion: A longitudinal, five-year follow-up study. *BMC Medical Information, 3,* 18.

Brown, M. A., & Solchany, J. E. (2004). Two overlooked mood disorders in women: Subsyndromal depression and prenatal depression. *Nursing Clinics of North America, 39*(1), 83–95.

Chaudron, L. H., Szilagyi, P. G., Campbell, A. T., et al. (2007). Legal and ethical considerations: Risks and benefits of postpartum depression screening at well-child visits. *Pediatrics, 119*(1), 123–128.

Conde, D. M., Pinto-Neto, A. M., Santos-Sa, D., et al. (2006). Factors associated with quality of life in a cohort of postmenopausal women. *Gynecological Endocrinology, 22*(8), 441–446.

Condon, J. (2006). What about dad? Psychosocial and mental health issues for new fathers. *Australian Family Physician, 35*(9), 690–692.

Costello, M. F. (2004). Systematic review of the treatment of ovulatory infertility with clomiphene citrate and intrauterine insemination. *Australian and New Zealand Journal of Obstetrics and Gynaecology, 44*(2), 93–102.

Cousineau, T. M., Green, T. C., Corsini, E. A., et al. (2006). Development and validation of the Infertility Self-Efficacy scale. *Fertility and Sterility, 85*(6), 1684–1696.

D'Afflitti, J. G. (2005). A psychiatric clinical nurse specialist as liaison to OB/GYN practice. *Journal of Obstetric, Gynecologic, and Neonatal Nursing, 34*(2), 280–285.

De Berardis, D., Campanella, D., Gambi, F., et al. (2005). Alexithymia and body image disturbances in women with premenstrual dysphoric disorder. *Journal of Psychosomatic Obstetrics* and *Gynecology, 26*(4), 257–264.

Deglin, J. H., & Vallaerand, A. H. (2007). *Davis's drug guide for nurses* (10th ed.). Philadelphia: F.A. Davis Company.

Dening, T., Barapatre, C. (2004). Mental health and the ageing population. *Journal of the British Menopause Society, 10*(2), 49–53, 64. Review.

Dennis, C. L. (2004). Treatment of postpartum depression, part 2: A critical review of nonbiological interventions. *Journal of Clinical Psychiatry, 65*(9), 1252–1265.

Dennis, C. L., & Stewart, D. E. (2004). Treatment of postpartum depression, part 1: A critical review of biological interventions. *Journal of Clinical Psychiatry, 65*(9), 1242–1251.

Devine, K. (2003). Caring for the infertile woman. *American Journal of Maternal Child Nursing MCN, 28*(2), 100–105.

Eberhard-Gran, M., Eskild, A., & Opjordsmoen, S. (2005). Treating mood disorders during pregnancy: Safety considerations. *Drug Safety, 28*(8), 695–706.

Federenko, I. S., & Wadhwa, P. D. (2004). Women's mental health during pregnancy influences fetal and infant developmental and health outcomes. *CNS Spectrums, 9*(3), 198–206.

Feld, J., Halbreich, U., & Karkun, S. (2005). The association of perimenopausal mood disorders with other reproductive-related disorders. *CNS Spectrums, 10*(6), 461–470.

Fergusson, D. M., Horwood, L. J., & Ridder, E. M. (2006). Abortion in young women and subsequent mental health. *Journal of Child Psychology and Psychiatry, 47*(1),16–24.

Freeman, E. W., Jabara, S., Sondheimer, S. J., et al. (2002). Citalopram in PMS patients with prior SSRI treatment failure: A preliminary study. *Journal of Women's Health and Gender-Based Medicine, 11*(5), 459–464.

Freeman, E. W., Sondheimer, S. J., Sammel, M. D., et al. (2005). A preliminary study of luteal phase versus symptom-onset dosing with escitalopram for premenstrual dysphoric disorder. *Journal of Clinical Psychiatry, 66*(6), 769–773.

Haines, C. J., Yim, S. F., Chung, T. K., et al. (2003). A prospective, randomized, placebo-controlled study of the dose effect of oral oestradiol on menopausal symptoms, psychological well being, and quality of life in postmenopausal Chinese women. *Maturitas, 44*(3), 207–214.

Hart, V. A. (2002). Infertility and the role of psychotherapy. *Issues in Mental Health Nursing, 23*(1), 31–41.

Himelein, M. J., & Thatcher, S. S. (2006). Polycystic ovary syndrome and mental health: A review. *Obstetrical and Gynecological Survey, 61*(11), 723–732.

Hlatky, M. A., Boothroyd, D., Vittinghoff, E.; Heart and Estrogen/Progestin Replacement Study (HERS) Research Group. (2002). Quality-of-life and depressive symptoms in postmenopausal women after receiving hormone therapy: Results from the Heart and Estrogen/Progestin Replacement Study (HERS) trial. *Journal of the American Medical Association, 287*(5), 591–597.

Huang, K. L., & Tsai, S. J. (2003). St. John's wort (*Hypericum perforatum*) as a treatment for premenstrual dysphoric disorder: Case report. *International Journal of Psychiatry in Medicine, 33*(3), 295–297.

Huntley, A. L., & Ernst, E. (2003). A systematic review of herbal medicinal products for the treatment of menopausal symptoms. *Menopause, 10*(5), 465–476.

Joffe, H., Soares, C. N., Petrillo, L. F., et al. (2007). Treatment of depression and menopause-related symptoms with the serotonin-norepinephrine reuptake inhibitor duloxetine. *Journal of Clinical Psychiatry, 68*(6), 943–950.

Jose-Miller, A. B., Boyden, J. W., & Frey, K. A. (2007). Infertility. *American Family Physician, 75*(6), 849–856.

Karl, D. J., Beal, J. A., O'Hare, C. M., et al. (2006). Reconceptualizing the nurse's role in the newborn period as an "attacher." *American Journal of Maternal Child Nursing MCN, 31*(4), 257–262.

Kero, A., Högberg, U., & Lalos, A. (2004). Wellbeing and mental growth-long-term effects of legal abortion. *Social Science and Medicine, 58*(12), 2559–2569.

Koren, G., Matsui, D., Einarson, A., et al. (2005). Using antidepressants during pregnancy. *Canadian Medical Association Journal, 173*(10), 1503.

Koundi, K. L., Christodoulakos, G. E., Lambrinoudaki, I. V., et al. (2006). Quality of life and psychological symptoms in Greek postmenopausal women: Association with hormone therapy. *Gynecological Endocrinology, 22*(12), 660–668.

Krebs, E. E., Ensrud, K. E., MacDonald, R., et al. (2004). Phytoestrogens for treatment of menopausal symptoms: A systematic review. *Obstetrics and Gynecology, 104*(4), 824–836.

Kronenberg, F., & Fugh-Berman, A. (2002). Complementary and alternative medicine for menopausal symptoms: A review of randomized, controlled trials. *Annals of Internal Medicine, 137*(10), 805–813.

Lang, A. J., Rodgers, C. S., & Lebeck, M. M. (2006). Associations between maternal childhood maltreatment and psychopathology and aggression during pregnancy and postpartum. *Child Abuse and Neglect: The International Journal, 30*(1), 17–25.

Lang, A. J., Rodgers, C. S., Moyer, R., et al. (2005). Mental health and satisfaction with primary health care in female patients. *Women's Health Issues, 15*(2), 73–79.

Li, C., Wilawan, K., Samsioe, G., et al. (2002). Health profile of middle-aged women: The Women's Health in the Lund Area (WHILA) study. *Human Reproduction, 17*(5), 1379–1385.

Ling, F. W. (2000). Recognizing and treating premenstrual dysphoric disorder in the obstetric, gynecologic, and primary care practices. *Journal of Clinical Psychiatry, 61*(Suppl 12), 9–16.

Loebstein, R., Lalkin A., & Koren G. (1997). Pharmacokinetic changes during pregnancy and their clinical relevance. *Clinical Pharmacokinetics*, 33(5), 328–343.

Logsdon, M.C., & Gennaro, S. (2005). Bioecological model for guiding social support research and interventions with pregnant adolescents. *Mental Health Nursing, 26*(3), 327–339.

Lok, I. H., Lee, D. T., Cheung, L. P., et al. (2002). Psychiatric morbidity amongst infertile Chinese women undergoing treatment with assisted reproductive technology and the impact of treatment failure. *Gynecologic and Obstetric Investigation, 53*(4), 195–199.

Major, B., Cozzarelli, C., Cooper, M. L., et al. (2000). Psychological responses of women after first-trimester abortion. *Archives of General Psychiatry*, 57(8), 777–784.

Makar, R. S., & Toth, T. L. (2002). The evaluation of infertility. *American Journal of Clinical Pathology, 117*(Suppl), S95–S103.

Manson, J. E., Allison, M. A., Rossouw, J. E., et al.; WHI and WHI-CACS Investigators. (2007). Estrogen therapy and coronary-artery calcification. *New England Journal of Medicine, 356*, 2591–2602.

McCarter-Spaulding, D. E. (2005). Medications in pregnancy and lactation. *American Journal of Maternal Child Nursing MCN, 30*(1), 10–17.

McNair, R. P. (2003). Lesbian health inequalities: A cultural minority issue for health professionals. *Medical Journal of Australia, 178*(12), 643–645.

McVeigh, C. (2005). Perimenopause: More than hot flushes and night sweats for some Australian women. *Journal of Obstetric, Gynecologic, and Neonatal Nursing, 34*(1), 21–27.

Miller, L. J. (1992). Comprehensive care of pregnant mentally ill women. *Journal of Mental Health Administration, 19*(2), 170–177.

Miner, C., Brown, E., McCray, S., et al. (2002). Weekly luteal phase dosing with enteric-coated fluoxetine 90 mg in premenstrual dysphoric disorder: A randomized, double-blind, placebo-controlled clinical trial. *Clinical Therapeutics, 24*(3), 417–433.

Mishra, G. D., Brown, W. J., & Dobson, A. J. (2003). Physical and mental health: Changes during menopause transition. *Quality of Life Research, 12*(4), 405–412.

Morrison, J., Carroll, L., Twaddle, S., et al. (2001). Pragmatic randomised controlled trial to evaluate guidelines for the management of infertility across the primary care–secondary care interface. *British Medical Journal, 322*(7297), 1282–1284.

Morrissey, M. V. (2007). Suffer no more in silence: Challenging the myths of women's mental health in childbearing. *Journal of Psychiatric Nursing Research, 12*(2), 1429–1438.

Mravcak, S. A. (2006). Primary care for lesbians and bisexual women. *American Family Physician, 74*(2), 279–286.

Nagata, M., Nagai, S., Sobajima, H., et al. (2000). Maternity blues and attachment to children in mothers of fullterm normal infants. *Acta Psychiatrica Scandinavica, 101*(3), 209–217.

National Institute of Mental Health (NIMH). (2002). *Medications.* A detailed booklet that describes mental disorders and the medications for treating them—Includes a comprehensive list of medications. NIH Publication No. 02-3929. Washington, DC: Author. Retrieved July 21, 2007, from *www.nimh.nih.gov/publicat/medicate.cfm.*

National Institutes of Health. (2005). *NIH state-of-the-science conference statement on management of menopause-related symptoms.* Retrieved April 6, 2007, from *http://consensus.nih.gov/2005/2005MenopausalSymptomsSOS025html.htm.*

National Women's Health Information Center. (2006). *Yaz birth control pill approved for new use.* Washington, DC: Office on Women's Health, U.S. Department of Health and Human Services. Retrieved June 15, 2007, from *www.womenshealth.gov/news/English/535356.htm.*

National Women's Health Information Center. (2007). *Premenstrual syndrome.* Washington, DC: Office of Women's Health, U.S. Department of Health and Human Services. Retrieved July 14, 2007, from *www.womenshealth.gov/faq/pms.htm.*

Nedrow, A., Miller, J., Walker, M., et al. (2006). Complementary and alternative therapies for the management of menopause-related symptoms: A systematic evidence review. *Archives of Internal Medicine, 166*(14), 1453–1465.

Newton, K. M., Reed, S. D., LaCroix, A. Z., et al. (2006). Treatment of vasomotor symptoms of menopause with black cohosh, multibotanicals, soy, hormone therapy, or placebo: A randomized trial. *Annals of Internal Medicine, 145*(12), 869–879.

North American Menopause Society (NAMS). (2000). The role of isoflavones in menopausal health: Consensus opinion of the North American Menopause Society. *Menopause,* 7(4), 215–229.

Nunez, A. E., & Robertson, C. (2003). Multicultural considerations in women's health. *Medical Clinics of North America, 87*(5), 939–954.

Panay, N. (2007). Integrating phytoestrogens with prescription medicines—A conservative clinical approach to vasomotor symptom management. *Maturitas, 57*(1), 90–94.

Parent-Stevens, L., & Burns, E. A. (2000). Menstrual disorders. In M. A. Smith & L. A. Shimp (Eds.), *20 Common problems in women's health care* (pp. 486–502). Chicago, IL: McGraw-Hill.

Parry, B. L., & Newton, R. P. (2001). Chronobiological basis of female-specific mood disorders. *Neuropsychopharmacology, 25*(5 Suppl), S102–S108.

Parry, B. L., Sorenson, D. L., Meliska, C. J., et al. (2003). Hormonal basis of mood and postpartum disorders. *Current Women's Health Reports, 3*(3), 230–235.

Payne, J. L. (2003). The role of estrogen in mood disorders in women. *International Review of Psychiatry, 15*(3), 280–290.

Poudevigne, M. S., & O'Connor, P. J. (2006). A review of physical activity patterns in pregnant women and their relationship to psychological health. *Sports Medicine, 36*(1), 19–38.

Rapkin, A. (2003). A review of treatment of premenstrual syndrome and premenstrual dysphoric disorder. *Psychoneuroendocrinology, 28*(Suppl 3), 39–53.

Ray, K. L., & Hodnett, E. D. (2001). Caregiver support for postpartum depression. *Cochrane Database of Systematic Reviews,* (3), CD000946.

Reid, M., Glazener, C., Murray, G. D., et al. (2002). A two-centred pragmatic randomised controlled trial of two interventions of postnatal support. *BJOG: An International Journal of Obstetrics and Gynaecology, 109*(10), 1164–1170.

RESOLVE: The National Infertility Association. (2007). Retrieved January 23, 2007, from *www.resolve.org/site/PageServer?pagename=abt_home.*

Rice, K., & Morse, C. (2003). Measuring cognition in menopause research: A review of test use. *Climacteric, 6*(1), 2–22.

Ross, L. E. (2005). Perinatal mental health in lesbian mothers: A review of potential risk and protective factors. *Women's Health, 41*(3), 113–128.

Rotem, M., Kushnir, T., Levine, R., et al. (2005). A psycho-educational program for improving women's attitudes and coping with menopause symptoms. *Journal of Obstetric, Gynecologic, and Neonatal Nursing, 34*(2), 233–240.

Sanders, L. B. (2006). Assessing and managing women with depression: A midwifery perspective. *Journal of Midwifery and Women's's Health, 51*(3), 185–192.

Santoro, N. (2002). The menopause transition: An update. *Human Reproduction Update, 8*(2), 155–160.

Shaw, E., Levitt, C., Wong, S., et al. (2006). Systematic review of the literature on postpartum care: Effectiveness of postpartum support to improve maternal parenting, mental health, quality of life, and physical health. *Birth, 33*(3), 210–220.

Shaw, M. (2005). Detecting hyperprolactinaemia in mental health patients. *Nursing Times, 101*(49), 24–26.

Shimp, L. A., Almeida, O. P., Joffe, H., et al. (2001). Efficacy of estradiol for the treatment of depressive disorders in perimenopausal women: A double-blind, randomized, placebo-controlled trial. *Archives of General Psychiatry, 58*(6), 529–534.

Shin, H., Park, Y. J., & Kim, M. J. (2006). Predictors of maternal sensitivity during the early postpartum period. *Journal of Advanced Nursing, 55*(4), 425–434.

Silber, T. J., & Valadez-Meltzer, A. (2005). Premenstrual dysphoric disorder in adolescents: Case reports of treatment with fluoxetine and review of the literature. *Journal of Adolescent Health, 37*(6), 518–525.

Smeenk, J. M., Verhaak, C. M., & Braat, D. D. (2004). Psychological interference in in vitro fertilization treatment. *Fertility and Sterility, 81*(2), 277.

Soares, C. N., Almeida, O. P., Joffe, H., et al. (2001). Efficacy of estradiol for the treatment of depressive disorders in perimenopausal women: A double-blind, randomized, placebo-controlled trial. *Archives of General Psychiatry, 58*(6), 529–534.

Souter, V. L., Hopton, J. L., Penney, G. C., et al. (2002). Survey of psychological health in women with infertility. *Journal of Psychosomatic Obstetrics and Gynecology, 23*(1), 41–49.

Spietz, A., & Kelly, J. (2002). The importance of maternal mental health during pregnancy: Theory, practice, and intervention. *Public Health Nursing, 19*(3), 153–155.

Steiner, M., Dunn, E., & Born, L. (2003). Hormones and mood from menarche to menopause and beyond. *Journal of Affective Disorders, 74*(1), 67–83.

Steiner, M., Macdougall, M., & Brown, E. (2003). The Premenstrual Symptoms Screening Tool (PSST) for clinicians. *Archives of Women's Mental Health, 6*(3), 203–209.

Stocky, A., & Lynch, J. (2000). Acute psychiatric disturbance in pregnancy and the puerperium. *Best Practice and Research Clinical Obstetrics and Gynaecology, 14*(1), 73–87.

Strobino, D. M., Grason, H., & Minkovitz, C. (2002). Charting a course for the future of women's health in the United States: Concepts, findings and recommendations. *Social Science and Medicine, 54*(5), 839–848.

Suppaseemanont, W. (2006). Depression in pregnancy: Drug safety and nursing management. *American Journal of Maternal Child Nursing MCN, 31*(1), 10–15.

Swaab, D., Bao, A., & Lucassen, P. (2005). The stress system in the human brain in depression and neurodegeneration. *Ageing Research Reviews, 4*(2), 141–194.

Taylor, A., Atkins, R., Kumar, R., et al. (2005). A new Mother-to-Infant Bonding Scale: Links with early maternal mood. *Archives of Women's Health, 8*(1), 45–51.

Tinker, L., Perri, M., Patterson, R., et al. (2002). The effects of physical and emotional status on adherence to a low-fat dietary pattern in the Women's Health Initiative. *Journal of the American Dietetic Association, 102*(6), 789–800, 888.

Toth, S. L., Rogosch, F. A., Manly, J. T., et al. (2006). The efficacy of toddler-parent psychotherapy to reorganize attachment in the young offspring of mothers with major depressive disorder: A randomized preventive trial. *Journal of Consulting and Clinical Psychology, 74*(6), 1006–1016.

Trettin, S., Moses-Kolko, E. L., & Wisner, K. L. (2006). Lesbian perinatal depression and the heterosexism that affects knowledge about this minority population. *Archives of Women's Mental Health, 9*(2), 67–73.

U.S. Food and Drug Administration (FDA). (2002). *FDA statement on the results of the Women's Health Initiative*. Retrieved June 10, 2007, from *www.fda.gov/cder/drug/safety/WHI_statement.htm*.

U.S. Food and Drug Administration (FDA). (2005). *Noncontraceptive estrogen drug products for the treatment of vasomotor symptoms and vulvar and vaginal atrophy symptoms—Recommended prescribing information for health care providers and patient labeling*. Retrieved June 10, 2007, from *www.fda.gov/cder/guidance/6932dft.htm*.

U.S. Food and Drug Administration (FDA). (2003; Updated 2007). *Estrogen and estrogen with progestin therapies for postmenopausal women*. Retrieved June 12, 2007, from *www.fda.gov/cder/drug/infopage/estrogens_progestins/default.htm*.

Ward, R. K., & Zamorski, M. A. (2002). Benefits and risks of psychiatric medications during pregnancy. *American Family Physician, 66*(4), 639.

Weinstock, M. (2005). The potential influence of maternal stress hormones on development and mental health of the offspring. *Brain, Behavior, and Immunity, 19*(4), 296–308.

White, A. R. (2003). A review of controlled trials of acupuncture for women's reproductive health care. *Journal of Family Planning and Reproductive Health Care, 29*(4), 233–236.

Wihlback, A. C., Sundstrom-Poromaa, I., & Backstrom, T. (2006). Action by and sensitivity to neuroactive steroids in menstrual cycle related CNS disorders. *Psychopharmacology, 186*(3), 388–401.

Wihlback, A. C., Sundstrom Poromaa, I., Bixo, M., et al. (2004). Influence of menstrual cycle on platelet serotonin uptake site and serotonin 2A receptor binding. *Psychoneuroendocrinology, 29*(6), 757–766.

Williamson, J., White, A., Hart, A., et al. (2002). Randomised controlled trial of reflexology for menopausal symptoms. *British Journal of Obstetrics and Gynecology: An International Journal of Obstetrics and Gynaecology, 109*(9), 1050–1055.

Women's Health Initiative. (2004). *Questions and answers about the WHI Postmenopausal Hormone Therapy trials*. Retrieved May 10, 2007, from *www.nhlbi.nih.gov/whi/whi_faq.htm#q1*.

Yonkers, K. A. (2003). Paroxetine treatment of mood disorders in women: Premenstrual dysphoric disorder and hot flashes. *Psychopharmacology Bulletin, 37*(Suppl 1), 135–147.

Yonkers, K. A., Pearlstein, T., & Rosenheck, R. A. (2003). Premenstrual disorders: Bridging research and clinical reality. *Archives of Women's Mental Health, 6*(4), 287–292.

Zarate, A., Fonseca, E., Ochoa, R., et al. (2002). Low-dose conjugated equine estrogens elevate circulating neurotransmitters and improve the psychological well-being of menopausal women. *Fertility and Sterility, 77*(5), 952–955.

Zitner, D., & Bischoff, A. (2005). Using antidepressants during pregnancy. *Canadian Medical Association Journal, 173*(10), 1205; author reply 1205–1206.

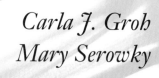

Carla J. Groh
Mary Serowky

chapter 13

Sexuality and Intimacy

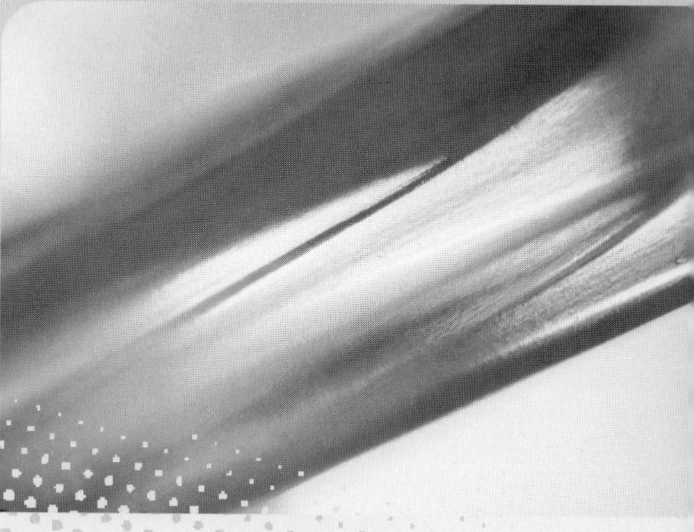

Women's sexual lives have changed dramatically over the last four decades, partly in response to the women's movement of the 1960s and 1970s. Along with the liberalization of women's sexuality came professional and academic interest in the sexual lives of women from multiple points of view: historical, political, cross-cultural, public health, medical, and psychosocial (Tiefer, 2002). From these perspectives emerged a broader understanding that sexual attraction, behavior, and identity are on a continua, ranging from exclusively same gender to exclusively other gender (Garnets and Peplau, 2001). There is increasing awareness that sexual health encompasses not only the physical but also spiritual, emotional, interpersonal, and intellectual aspects of a woman's life, and one of the most important determinants of a woman's sexual satisfaction is the extent of intimacy within that relationship (Byers, 2001). This holds true for heterosexual women and sexual minority women. As women become more comfortable and open about their sexuality, primary care providers (PCPs) will be increasingly asked for advice and recommendations related to their sexual concerns.

The purpose of this chapter is to discuss the various aspects of sexuality that are important in primary care settings. Particular emphasis has been placed on subpopulations of women (e.g., sexual minorities [lesbians, bisexuals, transgender (trans)], women with physical disabilities, women with body-altering surgery) who have traditionally been "invisible" in the literature on sexuality and intimacy.

THEORETICAL FRAMEWORKS OF FEMALE SEXUALITY

Masters and Johnson (1966) were the first to study, describe, and define "normal" sexual functioning. They developed the Human Sexual Response Model (HSRM) to describe the sequence of physiologic changes they observed and measured during sexual activities (masturbation, coitus). They proposed that the sexual response cycle had four stages: excitement, plateau, orgasm, and resolution. Kaplan (1979) collapsed the Masters and Johnson four-stage response cycle into three phases: desire, arousal, and orgasm. This triphasic model of sexual response provided the foundation for the classification system of female sexual dysfunctions (e.g., hypoactive sexual desire disorder, female sexual arousal disorder, and female orgasmic disorder) in the two official diagnostic classification systems: the American Psychiatric Association's *Diagnostic and Statistical Manual of Mental Disorders* (*DSM*) and the *International Classification of Diseases* (*ICD*) from the World Health Organization (WHO).

The *DSM* first included the medical diagnostic system for sexual dysfunctions in 1980, with minor revisions in 1987 and 1994 (Tiefer, Hall, and Tavris, 2002). In the most current edition, the *DSM-IV-TR*, the sexual dysfunction nomenclature is unchanged from the fourth edition and classifies sexual dysfunction into four general categories: sexual desire disorders, sexual arousal disorders, orgasmic disorders, and sexual pain disorder (American Psychiatric Association, 2000). A personal distress criterion is included, meaning that a condition would be considered a disorder only if it creates distress for the woman experiencing the condition. The *ICD-10* (version for 2007) classifies sexual dysfunction similar to the *DSM* in terms of desire, arousal, orgasm, and pain. The *ICD-10* code numbers for sexual problems are found under Mental and Behavioral Disorders.

The medicalization of sexual problems (e.g., *DSM* and *ICD*) and the new diagnosis, "female sexual dysfunction," introduced in 1997 did not go unchallenged. A meeting was convened in 2000 to discuss this emerging situation and to generate a feminist and social science response (Tiefer et al., 2002). The working group identified three major critiques of the *DSM* nomenclature. First, the *DSM* assumes sexual equivalency between men and women. Second, the *DSM* ignores the relational context of sexuality. Third, the *DSM* does not recognize that women's sex needs, satisfactions, and problems are diverse and do not neatly fit into categories of desire, arousal, orgasm, or pain. Thus, the working group developed a "New View of Women's Sexual Problems" and defined women's sexual problems as "discontent or dissatisfaction with any emotional, physical, or relational aspect of sexual experience" (Tiefer et al., p. 229). Within this framework, there is no one normal sexual response or experience. Further, the working group identifies four interrelated aspects of women's sexual lives that could cause sexual discontent or dissatisfaction. These include (a) sociocultural, political, or economic factors; (b) partner and relationship factors; (c) psychological factors; and (d) medical factors (Tiefer et al.). This "New View" offers a woman-centered definition of sexual problems and provides guidance to PCPs in the assessment, diagnosis, and treatment of women's sexual concerns (Box 13.1).

PREVALENCE OF FEMALE SEXUAL PROBLEMS

The most widely cited prevalence rate for sexual dysfunction of women aged 18 to 59 years in the United States is 43 percent (Laumann, Paik, and Rosen, 1999).

Box 13.1 • New View Nomenclature of Causes of Women's Sexual Problems

I. Sexual Problems Due to Sociocultural, Political, or Economic Factors
   A. Ignorance and anxiety due to inadequate sex education, lack of access to health services, or other social constraints:
      1. Lack of vocabulary to describe subjective or physical experience
      2. Lack of information about human sexual biology and life-stage changes
      3. Lack of information about gender roles, sexual expectations, beliefs, and behaviors
      4. Inadequate access to information and services for contraception and abortion, sexually transmitted disease prevention and treatment, sexual trauma, and domestic violence
   B. Sexual avoidance or distress due to perceived inability to meet cultural norms regarding correct or ideal sexuality
      1. Anxiety or shame about one's body, sexual attractiveness, or sexual response
      2. Confusion or shame about sexual orientation or identity, or sexual fantasies
   C. Inhibitions due to conflict between sexual norms of one's culture and the dominant culture
   D. Lack of interest, fatigue, or lack of time due to family and work obligations

II. Sexual Problems Relating to Partner and Relationship
   A. Inhibition, avoidance, or distress arising from betrayal, dislike, or fear of partner; partner's abuse of couple's unequal power; or arising from partner's negative patterns of communication
   B. Discrepancies in desire for sexual activity or in preferences for various sexual activities
   C. Ignorance or inhibition about communicating preferences of initiating, pacing, or shaping sexual activities
   D. Loss of sexual interest and reciprocity as a result of conflicts over commonplace issues such as money, schedules, or relatives or resulting from traumatic experiences
   E. Inhibitions in arousal or spontaneity due to partner's health status or sexual problems

(Continued)

Box 13.1 • (Continued)

III. Sexual Problems Due to Psychological Factors
   A. Sexual aversion, mistrust, or inhibition of sexual pleasure due to (1) past experiences of sexual, physical, or emotional abuse; (2) general personality problems with attachment, rejection, cooperation, or entitlement; and/or (3) depression or anxiety

IV. Sexual Problems Due to Medical Factors
   A. Pain or lack of physical response during sexual activity despite supportive and safe interpersonal situation, adequate sexual knowledge, and positive sexual attitudes. Such problems can arise from (1) local or systemic medical conditions affecting neurologic, neurovascular, circulatory, endocrine, or other systems in body; (2) pregnancy, sexually transmitted diseases, or other sex-related conditions; (3) side effects of drugs, medications, or medical treatments; and (4) iatrogenic conditions.

From Hicks, K. (2005); Tiefer et al. (2002).

However, serious questions revolve around the accuracy of this figure, which was obtained when Laumann, Paik, and Rosen reanalyzed data from the National Health and Social Life survey conducted in 1992. About 1,500 women were asked to answer yes or no to whether they had experienced any of seven problems for 2 months or more during the previous year. If the women answered yes to just one of the seven questions, they were characterized as having sexual dysfunction. These findings are described as exaggerated (Moynihan, 2003) and raise serious concern about when a sexual problem becomes dysfunction and then disease (Balon, Segraves, and Clayton, 2007; Bancroft, Loftus, and Long, 2003).

Laumann, Nicolosi, Glasser, et al. (2005) also attempted to estimate the prevalence and correlates of sexual problems from an international perspective. They interviewed adults aged 40 to 80 years from 29 countries. They reported that lack of interest in sex and the inability to reach orgasm were the most common problems cited by women worldwide, with prevalence ranging from 26 to 43 percent and 18 to 41 percent, respectively. Sexual problems were associated with poor physical and emotional health, negative experiences in sexual relationships, and overall well-being. Based on these data, Laumann, Nicolosi, Glasser, et al.

concluded that sexual difficulties are relatively common among mature women throughout the world.

SEXUAL PROBLEMS ENCOUNTERED IN PRIMARY CARE

The most common sexual problems experienced by women are low sexual desire followed by problems reaching orgasm (Laumann et al., 1999) and problems with lubrication (Ellison, 2001). Community-based studies report that one third of women experience lack of sexual desire (Ellison; Laumann et al.), between 24.0 (Laumann et al.) and 28.5 (Ellison) percent report difficulty reaching orgasm, and 19 percent experience problems with lubrication (Laumann et al.). Other reported sexual problems include male partners' erectile difficulties, lovemaking techniques, and finding a partner (Ellison). While these two studies are informative, both were conducted with white, college-educated women, limiting the generalizability of the findings to other groups of women.

The etiology of sexual problems may be psychosocial or situational (Box 13.2), medical (Box 13.3), substance induced (Box 13.4, page 420), or a combination of these factors. Common sexual problems experienced by older women include decreased libido as a result of decline in estrogen and testosterone and dyspareunia associated with dryness, which is also related to declines in estrogen levels. Sexually transmitted infections (STIs) are also frequently encountered in primary care settings, yet their impact on women's sexual functioning have been inadequately studied. Although there are a large number of studies examining AIDS-related risk and prevention behaviors, this is only one of numerous STIs that cause physical, emotional, and psychological distress for women (Firestein, 2001). Women are affected in acute and chronic ways by the vast array of curable and medically manageable STIs as well as the incurable STIs prevalent in the United States and other countries. STIs have both physical and emotional consequences for women. The physical consequences of an STI are numerous, causing disorders of arousal, orgasm, or pain syndromes (Firestein). The emotional consequences include fear of acquiring another or a different STI, avoidance of intimacy, relationship difficulties, disclosure issues with a new partner (e.g., when, how), and self-rejection. A woman's sexual self-esteem and self-expression may be inhibited, and she may resign herself to a self-imposed life without sexual involvement and pleasure (Firestein).

Box 13.2 • Psychosocial Causes of Female Sexual Problems

Interpersonal Conflicts
- Religious taboos
- Social restrictions
- Sexual identity conflicts
- Guilt

Historical Factors
- Past or current abuse (sexual, verbal, physical)
- Rape
- Sexual inexperience

Interpersonal Conflict
- Relationship conflicts
- Extramarital affairs
- Current physical, verbal, or sexual abuse
- Desires or practices different from partner
- Poor sexual communication

Life Stressors
- Financial
- Family or job problems
- Family illness or death
- Depression

SEXUALITY ISSUES OF SEXUAL MINORITIES

The sexual health of lesbians and bisexual women has been long neglected in health care research and clinical writings (Institute of Medicine [IOM], 1999). The reasons for this neglect vary but include the common misconception that lesbians are a relatively homogenous group of white, middle-class, educated, politically active, or aware women (Solarz, 1999) whose lives revolve around their sexual orientation (Dolan and Davis, 2003). Other reasons are related to

Box 13.3 • Medical Causes of Female Sexual Problems

Cardiovascular
- Hypertension
- Coronary artery disease
- Previous myocardial infarction

Endocrinopathologies
- Diabetes
- Thyroid disorders
- Hyperprolactinemia
- Adrenal disorders

Neurologic Diseases
- Multiple sclerosis
- Peripheral neuropathies
- Stroke

Other Causes
- Autoimmune disorders
- Renal disease (dialysis)
- Bowel disease (colostomy)
- Bladder disease (cystitis)
- Skin disorders (eczema, contact dermatitis)
- Gynecologic malignancies
- Breast cancer

Adapted with permission from Bachmann and Phillips (1998).

the belief that women who have sex with women are less susceptible to contracting STIs or HIV (e.g., lesbian immunity) and therefore do not need regular Papanicolaou (Pap) tests or routine gynecological care (IOM) and that lesbian women have less frequent sex than heterosexual women (also termed *lesbian bed death;* i.e., less sexual activity) (Nichols, 2004). These beliefs and misconceptions may be compounded by a PCP's discomfort and/or lack of knowledge as well as homophobic and heterosexist attitudes related to women's sexual orientation. In addition, lesbians and bisexual women may lack knowledge of their own sexual health risks and are reluctant to disclose their sexual behavior when they seek medical care (Marrazzo and Stine, 2004). Despite these barriers, lesbian women's health issues have received more attention from researchers in recent years (IOM), and there is an increased recognition of the complexity and diversity of their lives. While our knowledge is still incomplete, there is much that we do know that can guide clinical decision making.

One area of particular importance for the PCP is the new paradigm for women's sexual orientation. This paradigm emphasizes the importance of social context and recognizes the multiple pathways that can lead a woman to identify

Box 13.4 • Medications Associated with Female Sexual Problems

Desire	Arousal	Orgasm
Cardiovascular and antihypertensive agents • Antilipid medications • Beta-blockers • Clonidine (Catapres) • Digoxin • Spironolactone (Aldactone) *Hormonal preparations* • Oral contraceptives • Danazol (Danocrine) • GnRH agonists (Lupron, Synarel) *Psychoactive medications* • Antipsychotics • Barbiturates • Benzodiazepines • SSRIs • Lithium • Tricyclic antidepressants *Other* • Histamine H_2 receptor blockers • Indomethacin (Indocin) • Ketoconazole (Nizoral) • Phenytoin sodium (Dilantin)	Anticholingerics Antihistamines Antihypertensives Anorexic drugs *Psychoactive medications* • Benzodiazepines • SSRIs • MAOIs • TCAs	Methyldopa (Aldomet) Amphetamines Antipsychotics Benzodiazepines SSRIs Narcotics Trazodone (Desyrel) TCAs*

*Also associated with painful orgasm.

as lesbian, bisexual, or heterosexual (Garnets and Peplau, 2001). This paradigm suggests that sexual orientation among women is more fluid, more changeable over the life cycle, probably less tied to gender, and therefore more de facto bisexual (Nichols, 2004) compared with the sexual orientation among men. Female sexual development is a potentially continuous, lifelong process in which multiple changes in sexual orientation are possible (Diamond, 1998). It has been reported that the vast majority of lesbians had heterosexual experiences and heterosexual identities prior to self-identifying as lesbian and that almost 50% maintain occasional sexual encounters with men even after "coming out" as gay (Kitzinger and Wilkinson, 1995). The back-and-forth movement between lesbian, bisexual, and heterosexual identities in multiple directions is especially true for younger women (Nichols). Traditionally, Western culture has a need to identify and label what a person is (e.g., heterosexual, lesbian, bisexual, trans), yet some women may not be able to choose one of those options because none represents how they view themselves. Some questions to be asked by PCPs include the following: How does the PCP (and patient) feel about this ambivalence? How is it handled? Can it be discussed? How does it affect the woman's health?

Sexual Health Care for Lesbian and Bisexual Women

The sexual health care for sexual minorities (lesbians, bisexuals, trans) is no different from that of heterosexual women who present for primary care. The IOM (1999) report found that lesbians were not at higher risk for any particular health problem simply because of their sexual orientation, but they often have difficulty accessing appropriate care (e.g., lack of health insurance, low income, hesitancy to disclose their sexual orientation). Working to create a therapeutic provider–patient relationship is critical to overcoming the barriers to appropriate and quality care. Using inclusive language on intake forms (e.g., partner vs. spouse) and displaying posters and patient education materials in the waiting room may increase patient comfort and willingness to disclose (Mravcak, 2006).

Sexually Transmitted Infections

There is no "lesbian immunity" when it comes to contracting an STI. Lesbian women test positive for trichomoniasis, genital herpes, genital human papillomavirus (HPV) (Marrazzo, Coffey, and Bingham, 2005), gonorrhea, chlamydia, and syphilis (Dolan and Davis, 2003). One study ($N = 504$) found that 24 percent of lesbian women and 38 percent of bisexual women reported a lifetime history of an STI (Morrow, 2000), with HPV detected in up to 40 percent of lesbians (Marrazzo, Koutzky, Stein, et al., 1998). Lesbian women also have a high prevalence of bacterial vaginosis, the most common cause of vaginal complaints among U.S. women of reproductive age (Marrazzo, Coffey, et al.). Despite these statistics, routine Pap test screening is performed less frequently among lesbians than national guidelines recommend (Marrazzo, Koutsky, Kiviat, et al., 2001).

Several risk factors have been associated with STI rates in lesbian women: alcohol and other drug use, especially injection drug use (Deren, Estrada, Stark, et al., 1999); unprotected sex with both men and women (Kral, Lorvick, Bluthenthal, et al., 1997); performing oral and digital sex (Dolan and Davis, 2003) on a menstruating partner; as well as other sexual practices (e.g., fisting, insertion of sex toys, oral–anal contact, genital rubbing) (Dolan and Davis). In addition to the potential for STI and HIV transmission between women, many lesbian and bisexual women have had and continue to have sex with men (Dolan and Davis). Studies have found that lesbian and bisexual women underestimate their STI or HIV risk and susceptibility. Many believe that they are invulnerable simply by virtue of being a lesbian (Dolan and Davis; Marrazzo et al., 2005) and because of their abilities to detect, intuit, or sense who among them is infected ("social inoculation") (Dolan and Davis). Further, there is a general lack of knowledge about STIs and safe sex practices (Marrazzo et al.; Stevens and Hall, 2001). Educating lesbians and bisexual women about the risks of STIs and dispelling the misconception that the transmission of STIs between women is negligible will help women make informed decisions about their health and engage in safer sex practices (Box 13.5).

Box 13.5 • Recommended Safer Sex Practices for Women Who Have Sex with Women

Avoid contact with a partner's menstrual blood or with any visible genital lesions.

Cover sex toys that penetrate more than one person's vagina or anus with a new condom for each person; consider using a different toy for each person.

Use a barrier (e.g., latex sheet, dental dam, cut-open condom, plastic wrap) during oral sex.

Use latex or vinyl gloves and lubricant for any manual sex that might cause bleeding.

Adapted with permission from Waitkevicz (2004).

Reproductive Issues

In addition to testing for STIs or HIV, PCPs also need to conduct a comprehensive reproductive health history, regardless if the woman self-identifies as lesbian or bisexual. Marrazzo and Stine (2004) reported that more than 50 percent of the women in their study who self-identified as lesbian had previously used oral contraceptives, 25 percent had been pregnant at least once, and 16 percent had had an abortion ($N = 392$). Further, because of the higher rates of nulliparity among lesbians and bisexual women, the risk of breast and cervical cancers is heightened and the need for screening greater (Marrazzo and Stine).

Risk Factors

In a review of the literature, Hughes and Evans (2003) found that lesbian and bisexual women have greater rates of smoking, alcohol and drug use, higher body mass index, and poorer participation in health-screening programs than heterosexual women. It has been suggested that these high-risk behaviors may in part be due to the stigma of being a sexual minority and leading dual/closeted lives. These issues (e.g., smoking, drug use, obesity, lack of preventive care) can be explored differently if the PCP understands the perspective of lesbian and bisexual women.

Psychological Concerns

Disease is not the only hazard associated with the sexual health of sexual minorities. Other concerns of lesbian and bisexual women include the need for guidance related to the "coming out" process and how disclosure might impact relationships with family, friends, and work colleagues, especially if the woman comes out later in life; the recognition of their emerging sexuality and resulting identity issues; and stigma and sociocultural heterosexism that lead to internalized homophobia. All of these could negatively impact their ability to establish intimate relationships as well as nonsexual friendships.

Sexual Health Care for Transgender Women

The male-to-female trans community is comprised of individuals who were assigned the male gender at birth but who identify and desire to live as women (Israel and Tarver, 1997). Although the exact prevalence is not known, particularly in the United States, international estimates are 1 male-to-female transsexual per 11,900 persons and 1 per 30,400 persons for female-to-male transsexual (Feldman and Bockting, 2003). Trans women are at high risk for being underserved and poorly served by the health care system. Insensitivity and discrimination by health professionals, lack of programs specific to the needs of transgender individuals, and lack of insurance and a PCP (Feinberg, 2001; Lombardi, 2001) all contribute to inadequate health care.

The health of trans women has been described as a health crisis (Feinberg, 2001). This community is high risk for STIs, HIV infection, hepatitis B and C, substance abuse, health concerns related to cross-gender hormone therapy, and the emotional sequelae of discrimination and violence directed toward them. Reported HIV prevalence rates exceed 20 percent and have been shown to be as high as 60 percent among blacks (Lombardi, 2001). High-risk sexual behaviors such as having multiple partners, engaging in sex work, and not using condoms regularly account for the increased prevalence (Feldman and Bockting, 2003). Sharing needles during the injection of hormones (Feldman and Bockting) or drugs (Lombardi) is a contributing factor. It is important for the PCP to ask about transgender-specific interventions that the woman has received (e.g., hormones, surgery), as medically unsupervised use of hormones is common among trans women who have limited access to care (Feldman and Bockting). In addition, PCPs should also inquire about the herbal hormones (e.g., phytoestrogens or androgenlike compounds) sold as dietary supplements (Feldman and Bockting). Trans women on hormones are at higher risk for a number of acute and chronic diseases, including diabetes, cardiovascular disease, thromboembolic events, and liver abnormalities (Feldman and Bockting). All of these factors impact and influence the transgender woman's sexual health and sexuality. For women who have experienced a lifetime struggle for acceptance (Morgan, 2003), the support of a sensitive and informed PCP can make a critical difference in their health outcomes.

SEXUALITY ISSUES OF WOMEN WITH PHYSICAL DISABILITIES

Women with physical disabilities are stereotyped as asexual, without the same desires and needs for sexual and romantic intimacy as able-bodied women (Chance, 2002; Tilley, 1998). However, a national study of women with physical disabilities (N = 475) dispels many of these existing stereotypes, misconceptions, and myths (Nosek, Howland, Rintala, et al., 2001). The major study findings related to sexuality include the following: (a) women with physical disabilities have as much sexual desire as women in general; (b) the vast majority (87 percent) had at least one serious romantic relationship or marriage; (c) more than 75 percent had high self-esteem and a positive body image; (d) slightly less than half (41 percent) reported not having adequate information about how their disability affects their sexual functioning; (e) most reported significantly lower levels of sexual activity, sexual response, and satisfaction with their sex lives; and (f) the level of sexual activity was not significantly related to severity of disability (Nosek et al.). In addition, abuse (emotional, physical, sexual) was identified as a serious problem. Disabled women did not necessarily experience higher rates of abuse when compared with able-bodied women; rather, they experienced abuse for longer periods of time (Nosek et al.). Disabled women were reluctant to leave abusive relationships for fear of losing custody of their children and the lack of options for escaping or resolving the abuse (e.g., access barriers to existing programs).

Since the majority of women with physical disabilities have had at least one serious sexual relationship, it is critical that PCPs perform Pap tests as recommended and screen for STIs. The incidence of STIs is about the same for women with and without disabilities (20 percent), yet disabled women may not be aware of STI symptoms because of mobility and sensory impairments that prevent them from noticing a rash or vaginal discharge or from feeling pain and itching (Nosek et al., 2001). In addition to asking about STIs, it is also important to assess what problems, if any, the woman experiences during sexual activity. The most common problems reported have been weakness, vaginal dryness, lack of balance, hip or knee pain, and spasticity of legs (Nosek et al.). In many cases, relatively minor adjustments can be made in the couple's sexual activity to make intercourse (or alternatives to intercourse) possible or more enjoyable (Chance, 2002). For example, a water-soluble lubricant and stimulation prior to entry can be used for vaginal dryness and the rocking motion of a waterbed may be helpful for those with mobility loss (Chance). Other practical suggestions include changes in coital positioning. If the woman has adductor spasms (legs held tightly together) caused by multiple sclerosis or cerebral palsy, a rear-entry position may be helpful. Rear-entry or side-by-side positions may be more comfortable for women with spinal cord injury (Chance). Sexual aids can also be used in sexual activities. For example, vibrators, special adaptive mitts and handles for vibrators, and dildos can be used with a partner or as an aid to solo masturbation. Another important area where PCPs can offer guidance is to help women with physical disabilities redefine sexuality and the goal of sexual activity for them. Genital intercourse (generally considered the gold standard of sexual activity in our culture) may not be possible with certain disabilities due to pain, decreased genital sensation, and/or impaired mobility. Rethinking and redefining sexual activity to include a broader range of activities that focus on mutual pleasure and intimacy could result in greater sexual satisfaction for women with physical disabilities and their partners.

Another important area for PCPs to assess is whether the disability is lifelong or acquired later in life. A woman with a disability acquired at birth or in childhood develops her sense of self- and sexual esteem within a context of social stereotypes and negative images. She may develop a sense of shame about her sexuality, believe that sexual expression is inappropriate or impossible (Chigier, 1980), struggle with negative body image, and feel inferior as a potential romantic partner (Rousso, 1993). In contrast to a woman disabled from birth or childhood, whose identity was developed incorporating the disability, a newly disabled adult woman has an already existing self-concept that must now be altered (Chance, 2002). The woman's body has changed in profound ways, both in how it functions and in how it appears. The woman must go through a period of adjustment in which she mourns her losses and begins to accept and adjust to the new realities of her life (Chance). PCPs can support and facilitate this oftentimes painful process by addressing the woman's sexual concerns with sensitivity, reassurance, and hopefulness. Researching the more common physical disabilities experienced by women is an important step for PCPs. These include spinal cord injury, polio, muscular dystrophy, cerebral palsy, joint and connective tissue disorders, and skeletal abnormalities (Nosek et al., 2001). Becoming familiar with the basic limitations associated with each disability as well as thinking about how these limitations may or may not affect sexual functioning can help to guide the PCP's questions and comments if a woman indicates an interest in discussing sexual matters (Chance). PCPs are in a position of tremendous influence in helping women with physical disabilities to overcome social and self-perceived obstacles and to enjoy satisfying and meaningful sexual relationships.

SEXUALITY ISSUES OF WOMEN WITH BODY-ALTERING SURGERIES

There is an even greater paucity of research and clinical information regarding sexuality and sexual concerns of women who have experienced body-altering surgeries. The information available has focused on breast cancer surgeries, ostomy surgeries, and limb amputation, with the relationship between breast cancer surgeries and sexuality the most widely studied. This is important, since 182,460 new cases of *invasive* breast cancer are expected to occur among women in the United States during 2008 (American Cancer Society, 2008), and first-line treatment for invasive breast cancer is surgery (e.g., lumpectomy, mastectomy with or without reconstruction). The type of surgery does appear to make a difference in a woman's body image and feelings of attractiveness. Women receiving lumpectomies experienced the most positive outcomes in these two areas, whereas women receiving mastectomy with reconstruction were more likely to feel that breast cancer had a negative impact on their sex lives (Rowland, Desmond, Meyerowitz, et al., 2000; Yurak, Farrar, and Anderson, 2000). Loss of feeling in the reconstructed breast was reported to be sexually troublesome and disappointing (Wilmoth and Ross, 1997). Even though type of surgery does impact a woman's body image and sense of attractiveness, other factors are also predictive of sexual functioning. Women who have positive feelings about the relationship with their partner and perceive their partner to be supportive have less difficulty in the physiologic processes of arousal-lubrication-orgasm and satisfaction (Spree, Hillenberg, Sugrue, et al., 2005). Being older and not receiving adjuvant chemotherapy also resulted in more positive outcomes. A study exploring the quality of life at the end of primary treatment reported that 60 percent of the women were sexually active at the end of their breast cancer treatments. However, younger women and those who had received surgery plus chemotherapy reported more sexual problems (e.g., sexual interest, lubrication, pain during intercourse) than women with surgery only (Ganz, Kwan, Stanton et al., 2004).

Stoma formation surgeries are performed primarily because of cancer (e.g., colon, rectal, bladder, cervix, ovaries) and inflammatory bowel disease (e.g., colitis, ulcerative colitis, Crohn's disease). There are three types of ostomies: colostomy, ileostomy, and urinary diversion. All are considered life-changing events (Turnbull, 2001). In a systematic review of 14 research articles exploring the psychological and social impact of stoma surgery, Brown and Randle (2005) found that (a) many women with colostomies worry about sexual issues, believing that their sexual attractiveness has decreased since having the stoma formed; (b) most women with urostomies reported either decreased or no sexual activity, dyspareunia, and vaginal dryness following surgery; and (c) women who had urinary diversion surgery (e.g., cystectomy) because of incontinence or bladder dysfunction reported increased sexual activity postoperatively. The authors concluded that the reason for the ostomy affected the outcome for women in terms of their sexual function and activity.

Limb amputation and sexuality in women has been the least studied of the body-altering surgeries. Limb amputations can include either upper or lower extremities. Reasons for amputation include traumatic injuries, cancer, infection, and vascular insufficiency or may be secondary to another disease process. For example, more than 60 percent of nontraumatic lower extremity amputations (LEAs) in the United States occur in people with diabetes: 82,000 LEAs were performed on diabetics in 2002 alone (Centers for Disease Control and

Prevention [CDC], 2005a). Although women have traditionally had fewer amputations performed than men, this may change as rates of diabetes continue to increase. One of the first studies that included women with limb amputation (male = 51; women = 25) found that 76 percent of the participants perceived that amputation had a limiting effect on their level of sexual activity. Furthermore, the effects of amputation on sexual activity were the most consistent predictor of depressive symptoms (Williamson and Walters, 1996). Predictors of decreased sexual activity included older age, time since amputation, pain during sexual activity related to the amputation, and self-consciousness in intimate relationships. Being married or having good social support resources contributed to the well-being of the amputees (Williamson and Walters). A more recent study (male = 71; female = 14) reported that although 76 percent of participants did engage in some sexual activities (e.g., intercourse, kissing, caressing), 42 percent experienced some change in their sexual life—in particular, reduced libido (Ide, 2004). A limitation of both studies was that the data were not analyzed separately for women and men; thus, our understanding of the relationship between sexuality and limb amputation in women is neither enhanced nor better informed.

In general, PCPs do not appear to be sufficiently prepared to deal with the sexual issues of women who have experienced a body-altering surgery. While we do know that a woman's reaction to any body-altering surgery is a highly individual issue, there are common issues that can help to guide the PCP. First, women with any body-altering surgery are not only coping with the loss of a body part but are also coping with the impact of the illness related to the surgery (e.g., cancer, traumatic injury, inflammatory process, etc.). Second, women do not typically initiate the conversation related to sexual functioning and sexual concerns—it is up to the PCP to initiate that discussion. Third, the role of supportive partners is a significant contributor to a woman's adjustment to any body-altering surgery; therefore, it is important to include the woman's partner in discussions of sexual concerns and sexual activity when possible. Last, depression is common sequelae of body-altering surgeries and as such can reduce a woman's interest in sexual activity. Therefore, evaluating for depression is an important first step in assessing the contributing factors related to changes in sexual desire.

SEXUALITY ISSUES OF OLDER WOMEN

Sexuality remains an integral aspect of life despite the physical and developmental changes that occur with aging. Promoting the sexual health of older women has increasingly impacted encounters in primary care as a result of the baby boomers turning 60 years of age and their expectations of healthy aging. Confounding factors are the increasing prevalence of chronic illnesses that impact sexual health (e.g., diabetes, vascular disease, dementia, musculoskeletal disease). These diseases do not inherently diminish desire but do create challenges in the expression of such. Maintaining physical fitness (including sexual fitness) may be difficult in the presence of restricted physical mobility and diminished endurance (Vincent, 2002).

Women experiencing perimenopause and menopause are more vulnerable to sexual problems because of the various physical, psychosocial, and disease process changes that happen in this phase of life. Complaints of vaginal dryness and atrophy are amenable to hormone treatment. With improved vaginal lubrication, a male partner engaged in penile–vaginal intercourse may consequently experience a sensation of decreased friction, which contributes to difficulty in maintaining an erection. The partner's own sense of sexual prowess may result in behaviors interpreted as rejection of the woman and a sense of feeling sexually unattractive. Further body changes from the loss of subcutaneous fat, redistribution of fat from inactivity or metabolic disorders, and reduced moisture content of the skin may also changes a woman's perception of self as a desirable woman (Myskow, 2002). The increased incidence of urinary incontinence may result in disagreeable odor and leakage, thus affecting the environment for sexual expression.

Psychosocial and relationship concerns affect arousal and desire. Women in midlife are often juggling multiple roles and responsibilities, perhaps working outside the home, dealing with teenage children, and caring for aging parents. Long-standing relationships with a significant other take on a routine quality, with perhaps less attention given to promoting a sexually exciting environment. In contrast, some women may experience a heightened sexual desire resulting from their loss of reproductive function and the absence of concern for getting pregnant (Myskow, 2002) (Box 13.6).

One must consider that for women, a natural decreased libido may occur without sexual dysfunction. Sex is part of a relationship for women; companionship for older women is often more important than sexual urges. Among women studied, 2 percent report dating to fulfill sexual urges versus 11 percent of men reporting the same. If an interesting partner is encountered for the dating older woman, her libido will likely reawaken (American Association of Retired Persons, 2005).

PCPs should explore with their patients the range of options for innovative sexual expression, such as self-pleasuring, mutual masturbation, sensual massage,

Box 13.6 • Factors Affecting Sexual Expression Among Older Women

Physiologic Factors
- Onset of chronic illness
- Stress incontinence
- Decreased muscle tone and tissue atrophy
- Pain and mobility issues
- Dementia
- Depression
- Substance use disorders

Psychological Factors
- Accepting the negative myths about sexual desire in aging
- Familial expectations
- Cultural and religious attitudes and beliefs
- Loss of partner and spouse
- Satisfaction and quality-of-life issues
- Self-image and body image
- Isolation and withdrawal
- Career, social, and financial concerns

Reproduced with permission from Lenahan, P. M., & Ellwood, A. L. (2004).

and erotic imagery. Having the input of a professional may assist patients to open their thinking to new possibilities. A study examining adaptation to partner loss revealed sensual experiences (such as wearing attractive clothing) were important in the lives of unpartnered women (Vincent, 2002).

The PCP must be prepared to discuss sexual concerns and acknowledge the effects that aging has on sexual expression. PCPs can assist the woman in determining the timing of medications to maximize positive effects on endurance and comfort (e.g., inhalers or oxygen). Communal living situations pose unique challenges in terms of privacy and social norms. PCPs can offer suggestions to patients and families as well as advocate for policy modifications in assisted living or nursing homes. They can help to assure that the patient's right to self-determination is protected, help to modify the environment to ensure privacy for both sexual activity with another person or for self-pleasuring, facilitate conjugal visits with significant others, or promote the use of short-term release passes to allow the patient to return to home.

Assisting couples to maintain a satisfying sex life where one partner has dementia also poses challenges. The PCP can help women manage potential guilt either for wanting one's own sexual needs met (on the part of the well partner) or feeling guilty over rejecting their partner's sexual advances. The PCP may provide anticipatory guidance over changes that may occur during the disease process, such as not recognizing one's partner during or following a sexual encounter or displays of disinhibition. Medications may be indicated to manage depression, and the side effects of selective serotonin reuptake inhibitors (SSRIs) may also help to control hypersexual behavior. Normalizing the discussion of sexuality will help patients and families over embarrassment, which may ensue when discussing private issues (Lenahan and Ellwood, 2004).

Sexual satisfaction for women is often driven by the quality of their relationships with their partners. A common concern for aging males is erectile dysfunction. It has been suggested that the use of tadalafil with the male partner increased the overall sexual satisfaction for the couple. Medical intervention for the male partner can alter the relationship, either in a positive or negative fashion. The PCP must be attentive to the context of the relationship and intervene in a holistic fashion, which may include sexual or couples therapy (Althof, Eid, Talley, et al., 2006; Wylie, 2006).

SEXUALITY ISSUES OF ADOLESCENT GIRLS

The footprints of adult sexuality are laid in childhood and thus the PCP is in a unique position to promote women's health across the life span. Adolescent girls become adult women; in this process, the PCP can assist the teen in developing the foundation of a healthy sexuality. Solid preventative care may prevent disorders in adulthood and promote overall well-being throughout the woman's life. The health care of sexually active teens presents some unique challenges. A hallmark of the developmental phase of adolescence is the search for identity and the breaking away from parental constraints while still being dependent to some extent. Puberty heralds the awakening of sex hormones that produce the secondary sexual characteristics and the capacity for pregnancy. Adolescence is a typical time of risk tasking with little regard to possible consequences (Kirby, Lepore, & Ryan, 2005; National Adolescent Health Information Center, 2007).

Although studies show that the prevalence of sexual activity and pregnancy have generally declined over the past decade, the rates are still substantially high and contribute to the morbidity experienced by teens. During 2005, 46.8 percent of high school students had sexual intercourse, and about two thirds used a condom regularly. Martin, Ruchkin, Carminis, et al. (2005) report that among girls younger than 16 years, early sexual activity is associated with more depressive symptoms, a pessimistic outlook, and poorer academic performance. Although birthrates to teens have declined from 16.1 in 1990 to 10.8 in 2002, the increase in chlamydia is troubling, as is the number of HIV cases. From 2004 to 2005, chlamydia rates in the age group of 15 to 19 years increased from 2,630.7 per 100,000 to 2,761.5 per 100,000. For all age groups, black women are seven times more likely to be affected by this condition. HIV/AIDS cases in the same age group increased from 1,010 in 2001 to 1,213 in 2005 (CDC, 2005b; Eaton, Kahn, Kinchen, et al., 2006; National Adolescent Health Information Center, 2007).

Confidential health care is available for teens without express parental permission or knowledge for concerns of a sexual nature or for mental health/substance use counseling. State laws vary with regard to the location in which this care is delivered. Although teen girls do not usually initiate discussions of sex with their health care providers, they are more likely to have this discussion once they are sexually active (Kaiser Family Foundation, 2001). Difficulty talking about sex extends to their partners as well, particularly negotiating the use of condoms (Kaiser Family Foundation, Hoff, Greene, et al., 2003).

Adolescent girls are less likely to seek health care if they feel that their confidentiality with respect to parental notification will be compromised. Lehrer, Pantell, Tebb, et al. (2007) report several reasons for adolescent girls not seeking health care: being sexually active, not using birth control at last intercourse, prior STIs, alcohol use in the last year, unsatisfactory communication with parents, and depressive symptoms with suicidal ideation or suicide attempts. Although some teens may be concerned about the ability to access and pay for health care, it is the PCP's responsibility to educate them on low-cost, confidential options for care in their communities. Many locales provide services on a sliding fee scale and have laboratory tests subsidized by state-funded programs. These are the exact issues and needs that are so uniquely suited to adolescent health promotion. Confidential teen care is mistakenly cited as contributing to a breakdown in teen–parent communication; however, this is one of the key areas that are addressed in a health encounter: to help teens talk to their parents and seek their support (English, 2007).

Multiple factors account for teens being at high risk for acquiring an STI (Shrier, 2004). Many teens (and adults) hold the assumption that one can tell by visual inspection if a partner is infected with a STI. Adolescent girls have physiologic factors in their cervix and vaginal environment that increase susceptibility to infections such as the persistence of columnar epithelial cells on the ectocervix. Some teens lack the knowledge of safer sex practices and proper genital hygiene. Some are unaware that douching may flush pathogens toward the endocervix as well as alter the normal protective vaginal flora. Many engage in oral and anal sex, not recognizing the inherent risks in each of these practices. In addition, teens with mental health problems (either undiagnosed or untreated) are more likely to have an STI and engage in unprotected intercourse.

Multiple behavioral and social factors impact an adolescent's high-risk sexual behavior, including the concurrent use of mood-altering substances, relationship fluidity, and lack of knowledge regarding healthy communication and negotiation strategies. Teens are less likely to advocate for condom use and notify sexual partners if they are diagnosed with an STI. Some teens do not present for confidential care for STIs or pregnancy because they do not want to risk disclosure of a partner that may be subject to statutory rape law enforcement (Teare, 2002). The PCP needs to be comfortable with and welcoming to teens or needs to have referral resources available for more appropriate settings. Young persons are more likely to discuss private issues when sexual health is a normative discussion in the context of routine physical exams.

ASSESSMENT OF SEXUAL DISORDERS AND THE ROLE OF THE PRIMARY CARE PROVIDER

Patients report that their PCPs infrequently ask them about their sexual health (Feldman and Striepe, 2004; Kingsberg, 2006). One survey reported that American women were queried by their health care providers about their sexual histories and perceptions of health only 14 percent of the time (Pfizer Global Study, 2002). The opportunity to explore a woman's sexual health will likely occur within the context of other health concerns, and it is imperative that PCPs take advantage of these opportunities.

Obtaining a Sexual History

The provider's approach to the patient is critical in establishing an environment of trust and comfort. A few key screening questions can begin to identify patient concerns and difficulties, as it is unlikely that the patient will broach this subject first. When conducting the sexual history, it is always helpful to progress from the least sensitive to the most sensitive questions. Furthermore, PCPs need to be cognizant of their own discomforts with sensitive assessment areas; establish appropriate eye contact; and demonstrate a warm, open, and caring attitude (Box 13.7).

It is important to assess for depression and interpersonal violence as part of the screening process. Women with histories of childhood sexual abuse or adult sexual trauma have higher rates of chronic pelvic pain, headaches, gastrointestinal disorders, fibromyalgia, and other chronic pain conditions (Stein, Lang, Laffaye, et al., 2004). In one study, 20 to 50 percent of primary care patients reported childhood abuse (Springer, 2003). The residual effects of childhood sexual abuse are sobering. Women who were abused in childhood are much more likely to be victims of abuse in adulthood; experience higher rates of posttraumatic stress disorder, depression, and anxiety; and exhibit maladaptive sexual behavior (Brand, 2002). The ability to establish and maintain relationship intimacy is also difficult for many women who were victims of childhood sexual abuse.

PCPs also need to assess the relationship intimacy when a woman presents with a sexual problem or concern (Byers, 2001). Research findings suggest that (a) relationship satisfaction is the most important contributor to sexual satisfaction (Byers); (b) greater relationship satisfaction is associated with fewer sexual problems (Byers and Demmons, 1999); and (c) that women's sexual satisfaction can be increased by improving the quality of the nonsexual aspects of the relationship (Byers, 1999). Furthermore, a woman's ability to self-disclose about specific sexual likes and dislikes also contributes to sexual satisfaction. Therefore, a woman's satisfaction with her partner from both a sexual and nonsexual perspective should be explored during the assessment and diagnosis process.

If screening questions reveal that a concern or problem exists, determine the priority for performing a more thorough sexual history and examination. The provider needs to determine if the sexual difficulty can be addressed at the presenting visit, if a separate visit needs to be scheduled that has sexual concerns as the sole focus of the visit, or if the concern is beyond the scope or expertise of the provider. It is important to help a patient believe that her concerns are legitimate, and if a particular provider is not the best professional to address the issue, then the patient must leave the office with a plan of action. It may be appropriate if the patient is comfortable with the provider for the PCP to begin a sexual history, perform the exam, and order some basic testing with the caveat that if complexities become evident, necessary referrals will be made to provide the best diagnostic and intervention plans. Box 13.8 contains questions that may be asked when a more detailed history is needed.

Box 13.7 • Taking a Sexual History

General Guidelines

- Keep the encounter straightforward.
- Briefly explain the importance of addressing sex as part of holistic care.
- Have the patient clothed during the history.
- Assure a quiet, private room without interruptions.
- Do not introduce sexual questions while performing the physical examination.
- Frame questions and then educate the patient within the context of the woman's current developmental phase.
- Provide examples of common sexual concerns: for example, decreased lubrication associated with menopause or postpartum/lactation. (Be open for discussion.)
- Practice uncomfortable words before using them with a patient.
- Phrase questions to allow for all manner and gender choice for sexual activity. (Do not assume that everyone is heterosexual or that one is gay/lesbian.)

Brief Screening Questions

- Are you currently involved in a sexual relationship?
- If yes, with men, women, or both?
- Do you have any concerns related to your sexual activity?
- Are you satisfied with your level or amount of sexual activity? (If not, explore further.)
- In the past 2 weeks, have you felt down, blue, or tearful?
- In the past 2 weeks, have you lost pleasure in activities that were usually enjoyable?
- When you were growing up, did people in your family hit you so hard that it left you with bruises or marks?
- When you were growing up, did someone try to touch you in a sexual way or make you touch him or her?

From Kingsberg, S. (2006); Thombs, B. D., Bernstein, D. P., Ziegelstein, R. C., et al. (2007).

Box 13.8 • Detailed History of Present Sexual Concern

1. Description/perception of the problem.
2. Duration of the problem. Has the problem been lifelong, or has it occurred after a period of satisfying sexual function?
3. Onset: sudden or gradual?
4. Any precipitating events?
5. Has the problem occurred with all partners?
6. Any problems either in the patient's primary relationship or only in the sexual relationship (if they are not with the same person)?
7. Any current life stressors that may be contributing? How does the patient manage stress?
8. Any underlying guilt, depression, anger?
9. Any history of physical, sexual, or emotional abuse?
10. Does the partner have any sexual or health problems?

From Kingsberg, S. (2006).

Another useful strategy for obtaining a more detailed sexual history is to employ the five Ps: partners, practices, prevention of STIs, past history of STIs, and prevention of pregnancy (Mravcak, 2006). A provider must also consider the possible effects of prescription or over-the-counter medication; therefore, one should add this as a sixth P (Box 13.9). If it becomes apparent that a sexual disorder is likely, additional questioning is necessary to further define the issue.

When a gynecologic exam is indicated, the provider should also evaluate blood pressure, cardiovascular and peripheral vascular status, and neurologic function (particularly sensory competence) in order to rule out common medical conditions affecting sexual function.

Performing a Gynecologic Exam

The procedure inherent in performing a gynecologic exam without modifications for patient comfort is discussed in other sources (Seidel, Ball, Dains, et al., 2003). Performing a vaginal or bimanual exam on a patient suspected of having vaginismus or vulvovestibulitis can be particularly challenging. One approach may be to allow the patient to stand while doing the exam, to enhance her sense

Box 13.9 • Sexual History and Review of Systems: Incorporating the Six Ps

PAST *and Current Medical History, Including Reproductive History*

Attend to the following systems, as they often impact sexual function:

- Endocrine: Diabetes, androgen imbalance, estrogen deficiency, thyroid
- Neurologic: Multiple sclerosis, spinal injuries
- Cardiovascular
- Psychiatric: Medications, depression

Reproductive history

- Menarche and menstrual history
- Pregnancies and losses
- Delivery details including episiotomies
- Infertility
- STIs: Current or previous
- Gynecologic pain
- Surgeries
- Genitourinary

PRESCRIPTION *Medications: Past and Current (Refer to Table 13.2)*

PARTNERS

Are they men, women, or both?

Number of partners in last month, 6 months, lifetime?

How satisfied are you with your/your partner's sexual functioning?

Any changes in your/your partner's sexual desire or frequency of activity?

PRACTICES

Give a brief history of all of your sexual experiences to date, including earliest sexual experience:

Did you agree to all of these experiences?

Other sexual practices—oral, anal, toys

PREVENTION *and* PAST *History of STIs*

Current or past risk factors for HIV/STIs

- Ever tested for HIV, STIs?

(Continued)

Box 13.9 • (Continued)

How do you protect yourself and with which partners?
Number of past partners?

PREVENTION *of Pregnancy*
Trying to get pregnant?
How has contraception fit into your sexual behaviors?
Are you willing to use a contraceptive method at the time of intercourse?
Does your partner actively support your use of a contraceptive?
Are you looking for another method?
How likely is it that you will have more than one sexual partner? (Consider for IUD use.)

From Kingsberg, S. (2006; and Nusbaum, M.R.H., & Hamilton, C. D. (2002).

of control. The lithotomy position can make one feel very vulnerable. Another tactic is to allow the woman to hold a mirror and follow the examination along with the provider. A recent study demonstrated that the use of lithotomy position is not necessary for adequate specimen collection; some women may prefer to place their legs on the end of extended exam table rather than in stirrups. It was reported that their physical discomfort and sense of vulnerability were significantly lower than a control group, and the quality of smears was not compromised (Seehusen, Johnson, Earwood, et al., 2006).

Obtaining Forensic Evidence

One must be aware that if recent or current sexual abuse or assault has occurred, a PCP needs to be attentive to maintaining the integrity of forensic evidence. A rule of thumb is that if the incident happened within the 72 hours prior to the health care visit, a complete forensic exam should be done. Ideally, the woman can be referred to a rape crisis center with a sexual assault nurse examiner available. In the event that this is not possible, there are commercial rape kits available that provide complete explanations of the necessary specimen collection process. The PCP can help the woman to understand the dual purpose of the exam: evidence collection in the event that the patient wishes to press charges and to assess and care for injuries or infections (O'Hanlon and Nikkanen, 2006). If the patient is a minor, it is imperative that child protective services and the police be notified. It is important to be able to question the teen separately from her family members. One must also be able to determine sufficient history to help formulate a plan of care. If the teen has disclosed event details to adult caregivers, these adults should be interviewed separately from the adolescent. Do not confuse the patient or caregivers with excessive questions; allow the police to perform the investigation. The provider should primarily focus on current symptoms, treat the patient's injuries, assess and obtain specimens to test for the presence of STIs, offer emergency contraception, assess immunization status, and provide immune globulin for hepatitis B if immune status cannot be verified (Bernard, Peters, & Makoroff, 2006). The PCP should consider HIV postexposure prophylaxis, provide counseling, and assist in planning for follow-up care.

DIAGNOSIS AND TREATMENT ISSUES RELATED TO SEXUAL DISORDERS IN WOMEN

The primary management of sexual dysfunctions may be beyond the expertise of a PCP who is not working in a specialty area. Establishing an accurate diagnosis is essential, as treatment strategies differ for the various dysfunctions. Management often involves cognitive behavioral therapy, couples therapy, and other modalities that are challenging to institute and maintain in the context of a typical episodic visit day. Referral to sexual therapists or counselors may be indicated in addition to or in lieu of medical management. Nonetheless, if so indicated, medication initiation and management for comorbid conditions are well within the scope of primary care practice. Brief descriptions of the various disorders are included in Table 13.1.

Some general principles should guide the PCP when dealing with sexual disorders. It is important to consider comorbid psychological disorders such as depression, anxiety, and attention deficit disorder. What may appear to be disinterest in sex or difficulty with arousal may in fact be untreated or inadequately managed comorbidities. It is important for all patients to receive counseling and education as it applies to general health promotion. The following strategies specifically address sexual health:

- Educate the patient regarding normal anatomy and expected sexual changes that occur in various developmental phases as a result of hormonal and role changes.
- Assist patients in recognizing that their sexual lives may have taken on a routine and uninteresting nature. PCPs can help them to plan to introduce variety—for example, the use of erotic materials or changing locations for sexual intimacy.

Table 13.1 • Sexual Disorders and Treatments

Disorder	Definition	Treatment	Referral	Differentials
Sexual desire/ Interest	• Diminished feelings of interest • Absent sexual fantasies or thoughts • Lack of interest in sex is beyond what normally occurs with stage of development and length of relationship	• Cognitive behavioral therapy (CBT) • Traditional sex therapy • Estrogen therapy may enhance overall well-being & sleep disturbance • *Under investigation:* Tibolone & bupropion • *With caution:* Androgen therapy	For CBT & other sex therapy	• Menopause • Birth control pill • Depression • *Medications:* SERMS, SSRIs, β blocker, gabapentin, codeine
Arousal • Subjective • Genital • Combined genital & subjective • Persistent	• Absent feelings of arousal • Objective data shows genital vasocongestion & lubrication • Physical response occurs but not recognized/ perceived by client • May experience arousal from nongenital stimulation (e.g., erotic film, pleasuring partner, breast stimulation)	• Vaginal estrogen • *Under investigation:* Phosphodiesterase inhibitors • *With caution:* Androgen therapy • Kegels	Consider referral; rule out medical causes	• Diabetes • Hypothyroidism • MS • Cushing's • Addison's • Atherosclerosis • HTN • Heart disease • Medications above
Orgasmic May be primary or secondary	• Despite self-report of high arousal/excitement, lack of or decreased intensity of orgasm	• Directed masturbation program (see Resources for Patients section) • Relationship therapy	For sexual & couple therapy	*Primary:* Emotional trauma or abuse *Secondary:* Surgery, trauma, hormonal, general medical

	• Any type of stimulation fails to produce orgasm	• Partner education & guidance • Maximize stimulation while minimizing inhibition		
Dyspareunia	• Persistent or recurrent pain with attempted or complete entry into vagina	• Rule out STIs • See vaginismus • Physical exam should attempt to localize source of pain • Recommend position change: Female astride, no deep thrusting	Rule out medical causes	• Vaginal atrophy • Vaginal or cervical infections • PID • Cystitis • Endometriosis • Adnexal mass • Crohn's, UC
Vaginismus/ Vulvar vestibulitis syndrome	• Persistent or recurrent problems with anything entering vagina (finger, penis, object) • Avoidance and involuntary pelvic muscle contraction	• Structural problems must be ruled out • Multidisciplinary • Psychotherapy • CBT • EMG & biofeedback • Vaginal hygiene • Treatment of neuropathic pain: Tricyclics, new AEDs	Yes	• Rape or previous sexual abuse • Ongoing abuse • Gynecologic cancers

From Basson, R., Althor, S., Davis, S., et al. (2004); First Consult.

- Counsel in stress management and scheduled relaxation time.
- Suggest noncoital stimulation such as massage and oral activities.
- Counsel for smoking cessation (smoking affects vascular status).
- Assess for and counsel against alcohol and other drug use.
- Promote increased physical exercise. Activity stimulates increased well-being by acting on the serotonin and other neuroendrocrine hormones.
- Teach sexual hygiene: no douching; cleanse with mild substances without fragrance and deodorant. Specifically address if anal penetration or sex objects are involved to avoid cross-contamination.
- Educate patients in the importance of avoiding high-risk behaviors and multiple partners, which may lead to HIV and other sexually transmitted diseases.
- Assess immunization status for hepatitis A and B and HPV. Order immunizations as indicated.
- Teach women that they need adequate foreplay and lubrication and to avoid contraceptive creams, as they are drying and predispose vaginal tissues to epithelial disruption (nonoxynol-9 spermicidal products are no longer indicated in HIV prevention for this reason).
- Evaluate hypertension or depression medication; if indicated, consider changing to different class that has fewer sexual side effects.
- Encourage women with a history of childhood sexual abuse to learn and read about trauma to better understand what happened to them, and explain some of the aftermath sequelae.
- In addition, women with a history of childhood sexual abuse and/or adult sexual abuse may need individual therapy to deal with the trauma of the abuse. It is important for PCPs to have a list of therapists who are sensitive to abuse and trauma issues and to encourage women to obtain therapy when sexual concerns persist.

Pharmacologic Treatment Options

Some important issues need to be considered if medication intervention is a treatment option. When prescribing estrogen, the PCP needs to bear in mind the patient's risk profile (i.e., risk for venous thrombosis, unopposed estrogen in presence of uterus, risk for breast cancer). Before prescribing androgens, carefully ascertain that there is an absence of other psychological or physical factors affecting interest or arousal. Androgens are contraindicated in those with polycystic ovarian syndrome or any preexisting seborrhea, acne, alopecia, or hirsute conditions. If a trial of testosterone is attempted, the need for careful monitoring of lipid and glucose profiles is indicated as well as testosterone and sex hormone–binding globulin levels. There is no established norm for testosterone levels in women, nor is there any clinical correlation with symptoms (Feldman and Striepe, 2004). The typical side effects of testosterone supplementation must be assessed, particularly skin and hair distribution changes. The transdermal drug delivery method may minimize adverse effects. There has not been enough investigation into the use of phosphodiesterase inhibitors in women, although this class of drugs may hold some promise. The mechanism of action is to increase smooth muscle relaxation and enhance vascular congestion. The results of double-blind, placebo-controlled trials are mixed, although sildenafil may improve local sensation for some select groups such as those with spinal cord injury or multiple sclerosis. The drug has not demonstrated any improvements in overall desire or sexual enjoyment. Sildenafil may also have a place in ameliorating the side effects of SSRI-induced sexual arousal disorders. Generally, more study of this class of drugs is necessary. Any prescribing of these agents would be considered off-label.

Dehydroepiandrosterone (DHEA), a weak androgen precursor of estrogen and testosterone, has been examined for the treatment of low libido. DHEA is used by some as a dietary supplement. At this writing, no deleterious effects have been discovered. The dose studied was 300 mg, which is higher that that usually recommended (15–25 mg). This study demonstrated increased libido and sexual satisfaction in postmenopausal women.

Medications in Clinical Trials

Tibolone, a synthetic steroid with estrogenic, androgenic, and progestagenic properties, has been used in Europe for the last two decades (Basson, Althor, Davis, et al., 2004; Modelska and Cummings, 2002). One study of tibolone reported a significant improvement in vaginal blood flow, lubrication, subjective desire, and arousability; however, the measures of frequency of intercourse and other sexual activity showed no change compared with women receiving a placebo. Physiologic responses show an increase in free testosterone and lower sex hormone–binding globulins, but this effect may not correlate clinically with improved sexual function. Despite some promising effects, tibilone is not currently available in the United States.

Phentolamine, a nonspecific alpha-adrenergic blocker, shows some promise with male erectile dysfunction, as it promotes vascular smooth muscle relaxation. A pilot study in women showed enhanced blood flow and improved subjective arousal; however, no randomized controlled trials of this medication have been completed in the United States (First Consult, 2006). The same cautions apply as with all nonspecific alpha blockers and their effect on orthostatic changes in blood pressure. Prostaglandin E_1 (marketed as MUSE, an intraurethral application for males) is under study as an intravaginal medication. Apomorphine, a short-acting dopamine agonist used in Parkinson's disease, may have some promise, as it has shown some effects in medicating sexual desire and arousal in men (First Consult).

CONCLUSION

Sexual problems are common in the lives of many women both in the United States and around the world, yet these problems are frequently overlooked by PCPs. There are many reasons why this occurs: time constraints of a busy practice, lack of knowledge, difficulty broaching such personal areas, and lack of disclosure by women. However, when problems in the sexual and relationships aspects of a woman's life go unaddressed, psychological and physical health is potentially compromised. There has been a renewed interested in research focusing on women's sexuality. The findings have expanded our understanding of the etiologies and treatments for primary and secondary sexual dysfunctions, and PCPs can now offer women multiple intervention options that focus on restoring sexual functioning and satisfaction. All women have unique needs and desires in the areas of sexuality and intimacy. Individual treatment plans should be formulated in collaboration with the woman (and her partner if possible), with special emphasis placed on the emotional, spiritual, relational, and cultural elements that impact the woman's life.

Resources for Patients

Books on Sexuality

Bass, E., Davis, L. (2002). *The courage to heal: A guide for women survivors of child sexual abuse* (3rd ed.). New York: Harper & Row.

Boston Women's Health Book Collective. (2005). *Our bodies, our selves: A new edition for a new era.* New York: Touchstone.

Boston Women's Health Book Collective. (2006). *Our bodies, our selves: Menopause.* New York: Touchstone.

Daniluk, J. (2003). *Women's sexuality across the life span: Challenging myths, creating meaning.* New York: Guilford Press.

Kerner, I. (2004). *She comes first: The thinking man's guide to pleasuring a woman.* New York: HarperCollins.

Kliger, L., & Nedelman, D. (2006). *Still sexy after all these years? The 9 unspoken truths about women's desire beyond 50.* New York: Perigee/Penguin.

Lev, A. (2004). *Transgender emergence: Therapeutic guidelines for working with gender-variant people and their families.* New York: Haworth Press.

Sexuality Information and Education Websites

American Medical Association, Guidelines for Adolescent Preventive Services: *www.ama-assn.org/ama/pub/category/1980.html*
A tool for risk assessment

Bisexual Resource Center: *www.biresource.org*
Devoted to the subject of bisexuality

Gay and Lesbian Medical Association: *www.glma.org*
Resources for health care providers and researchers, including guidelines for clinicians on how to create a welcoming environment for lesbian, gay, bisexual, and transgender patients; articles and research papers; and links to other websites

Our Bodies, Ourselves: *www.ourbodiesourselves.org*
Supported by the Boston Women's Health Book Collective; Spanish language translations for most information available

Project Respect: *www.yesmeansyes.com*
Prevention program for youth ages 14 to 19 years that aims to stop sexual violence, particularly acquaintance assault, and gives youths tools to communicate their sexual limits and have safe, healthy relationships

SexualHealth.com: *www.sexualhealth.com*
Devoted to sexuality issues for people with disabilities

Sexuality Information and Education Council of the United States: *www.siecus.org*
Comprehensive sexuality education books and pamphlets (including Spanish versions), downloadable and free information sheets by various topics, and bibliographies of articles arranged by various topics

References

Althof, S. E., Eid, J. F., Talley, D. R., et al. (2006). Through the eyes of women: The partners' perspective on tadalafil. *Urology, 68*(3), 631–635.

American Association of Retired Persons. (2005). *Sexuality at midlife and beyond.* Retrieved October 29, 2007, from *http://assets.aarp.org/rgcenter/general/2004_sexuality.pdf.*

American Cancer Society. *Cancer facts and figures 2007.* Atlanta, GA. Retrieved on August 24, 2007, from *www.cancer.org/docroot/home/index.asp.*

American Psychiatric Association. (2000). *Diagnostic and statistical manual of mental disorders* (Revised 4th ed.). Washington, DC: Author.

Bachmann, G. A., Phillips, N. A. (1998). Sexual dysfunction. In: J. F. Steege, D. A. Metzger, B. S. Levy (Eds.), *Chronic pelvic pain: an integrated approach*. Philadelphia: Saunders, 77–90.

Balon, R., Segraves, R. T., & Clayton, A. (2007). Issues for DSM-V: Sexual dysfunction, disorder, or variation along normal distribution: Toward rethinking DSM criteria of sexual dysfunction. *American Journal of Psychiatry, 164*(2), 198–200.

Bancroft, J., Loftus, J., & Long, J. S. (2003). Distress about sex: A national survey of women in heterosexual relationships. *Archives of Sexual Behavior, 32*, 193–208.

Basson, R., Althor, S., Davis, S., et al. (2004). Summary of the recommendations on sexual dysfunctions in women. *Journal of Sexual Medicine, 1*, 24–34.

Bernard, D., Peters, M., & Makoroff, K. (2006). The evaluation of suspected pediatric sexual abuse. *Clinical Pediatric Emergency Medicine*, 7, 161–169.

Brand, B. (2002). Trauma and violence. In S. G. Kornstein & A. H. Clayton (Eds.), *Women's mental health: A comprehensive textbook*. New York: Guilford Press.

Brown, H., & Randle, J. (2005). Living with a stoma: A review of the literature. *Journal of Clinical Nursing, 14*, 74–81.

Byers, E. S. (1999). The interpersonal exchange model of sexual satisfaction: Implications for sex therapy with couples. *Canadian Journal of Counseling, 33*, 95–111.

Byers, E. S. (2001). Evidence for the importance of relationship satisfaction for women's sexual functioning. In E. Kaschak & L. Tiefer (Eds.), *A new view of women's sexual problems*. New York: Haworth Press, Inc.

Byers, E. S., & Demmons, S. (1999). Sexual satisfaction and sexual self-disclosure within dating relationships. *Journal of Sex Research, 36*, 180–189.

Centers for Disease Control and Prevention (CDC). (2005a). National diabetes fact sheet, United States, 2005. Retrieved August 24, 2007, from *http://cdc.gov/diabetes/pubs/pdf/ndfs_2005.pdf.*

Centers for Disease Control and Prevention (CDC). (2005b). *STD surveillance 2005, national profile, chlamydia*. Retrieved October 29, 2007, from *http://www.cdc.gov/std/stats05/chlamydia.htm.*

Chance, R. (2002). To love and be loved: Sexuality and people with physical disabilities. *Journal of Psychology and Theology, 30*(3), 195–208.

Chigier, E. (1980). Sexuality of physically disabled people. *Clinics in Obstetrics and Gynecology*, 7(2), 325–343.

Deren, S., Estrada, A., Stark, M., et al. (1999). Sexual orientation and HIV risk behaviors in a national sample of injection drug users and crack smokers. *Drugs and Society, 9*, 97–108.

Diamond, L. M. (1998). Development of sexual orientation among adolescent and young women. *Developmental Psychology, 34*, 1085–1095.

Dolan, K. A., & Davis, P. W. (2003). Nuances and shifts in lesbian women's constructions of STI and HIV vulnerability. *Social Science and Medicine, 57*, 25–38.

Eaton, D. E., Kahn, L., Kinchen, S., et al. (2006). Youth risk behavior surveillance-United States, 2005. *Morbidity and Mortality Weekly Report, 55*, 1–22.

Ellison, C. R. (2001). A research inquiry into some American women's sexual concerns and problems. In E. Kaschak & L. Tiefer (Eds.), *A new view of women's sexual problems.* New York: Haworth Press, Inc.

English, A. (2007). More evidence supports the need to protect confidentiality in adolescent health care. *Journal of Adolescent Health, 40,* 199–200.

Feinberg, L. (2001). Trans health crisis: For us it's life or death. *American Journal of Public Health, 91*(6), 897–900.

Feldman, J., & Striepe, M. (2004). Women's sexual health. *Clinics in Family Practice, 6,* 839–861.

Firestein, B. A. (2001). Beyond STD prevention: Implications of the new view of women's sexual problems. In E. Kaschak & L. Tiefer (Eds.), *A new view of women's sexual problems.* New York: Haworth Press, Inc.

First Consult. (2006). *Medical topics, sexual dysfunction in women.* Retrieved June 2, 2007, from *www.firstconsult.com/fc_home/members/?urn=com/firstconsult/1/101/1016356.*

Ganz, P. A., Kwan, L., Stanton, A. L., et al. (2004). Quality of life at the end of primary treatment of breast cancer: First results from the moving beyond cancer randomized trial. *Journal of the National Cancer Institute, 96*(5), 376–387.

Garnets, L. D., & Peplau, L. A. (2001). A new paradigm for women's sexual orientation: Implications for therapy. In E. Kaschak & L. Tiefer (Eds.), *A new view of women's sexual problems.* New York: Haworth Press, Inc.

Hicks, K. (2005). The "new view" approach to women's sexual problems. *Medscape CME/CE* . Release date November 7, 2005, through November 7, 2006.

Hughes, C., & Evans, A. (2003). Health needs of women who have sex with women. *British Medical Journal, 327,* 939–940. Retrieved July 23, 2007, from *www.bmj.com.*

Ide, M. (2004). Sexuality in persons with limb amputation: A meaningful discussion of re-integration. *Disability and Rehabilitation, 26*(14/15), 939–943.

Institute of Medicine (IOM). (1999). *Lesbian health: Current assessment and directions for the future.* Washington, DC: National Academy Press.

Israel, G. E., & Tarver, D. E. (1997). *Transgender care: Recommended guidelines, practical information and personal accounts.* Philadelphia: Temple University Press.

Kaiser Family Foundation. (2001). *Sexual health care and survey: SexSmarts.* Retrieved July 11, 2007, from *www.kff.org/youthhivstds/3113-index.cfm.*

Kaiser Family Foundation, Hoff, T., Greene, L., et al. (2003). *National survey of adolescents and young adults: Sexual health knowledge, attitudes, and experiences.* Retrieved July 11, 2007, from *www.kff.org/youthhivstds/3218-index.cfm.*

Kaplan, H. S. (1979). Hypoactive sexual desire disorder. *Journal of Sex and Marital Therapy, 3,* 3–9.

Kingsberg, S. (2006). Taking a sexual history. *Obstetrics and Gynecology Clinics of North America, 33,* 535–547.

Kirby, D., Lepore, G., & Ryan, J. (2005). *Executive summary: Sexual risk and protective factors.* Retrieved July 10, 2007, from *www.teenpregnancy.org.*

Kitzinger, C., & Wilkinson, S. (1995). Transitions from heterosexuality to lesbianism: The discursive production of lesbian identities. *Developmental Psychology, 31*(1), 95–104.

Kral, A. H., Lorvick, J., Bluthenthal, R. N., et al. (1997). HIV risk profile of drug-using women who have sex with women in 19 United States cities. *Journal of Acquired Immune Deficiency Syndromes and Human Retrovirology, 16*, 211–217.

Laumann, E. O., Paik, A., & Rosen, R. C. (1999). Sexual dysfunction in the United States: Prevalence and predictors. *Journal of the American Medical Association, 281*, 537–544.

Laumann, F., Nicolosi, A., Glasser, D. B., et al. (2005). Sexual problems among women and men aged 40-80 year: Prevalence and correlated identified in the global study of sexual attitudes and behaviors. *International Journal of Impotence Research, 17*(1), 39–57.

Lehrer, J. A., Pantell, R., Tebb, K., et al. (2007). Foregone health care among U.S. adolescents: Associations between risk characteristics and confidentiality concern. *Journal of Adolescent Health, 40*, 218–226.

Lenahan, P. M., & Ellwood, A. L. (2004). Sexual health and aging. *Clinics in Family Practice, 6*, 917–939.

Lombardi, E. (2001). Enhancing transgender health care. *American Journal of Public Health, 91*(6), 869–872.

Marrazzo, J. M., Coffey, P., & Bingham, A. (2005). Sexual practices, risk perception and knowledge of sexually transmitted disease risk among lesbian and bisexual women. *Perspectives on Sexual and Reproductive Health, 37*(1), 6–12.

Marrazzo, J. M., Koutsky, L. A., Kiviat, N. B., et al. (2001). Papanicolaou test screening and prevalence of genital human papillomavirus among women who have sex with women. *American Journal of Public Health, 91*, 947–952.

Marrazzo, J. M., Koutsky, L. A., Stine, K. L., et al. (1998). Genital human papillomavirus infection in women who have sex with women. *Journal of Infectious Diseases, 178*, 1604–1609.

Marrazzo, J. M., & Stine, K. (2004). Reproductive health history of lesbians: Implications for care. *American Journal of Obstetrics and Gynecology, 190*, 1298–1304.

Martin, A., Ruchkin, V., Caminis, A., et al. (2005). Early to bed: A study of adaptation among sexually active urban adolescent girls younger than sixteen. *Journal of the American Academy of Child and Adolescent Psychiatry, 44*, 358–367.

Masters, W., & Johnson, V. (1966). *Human sexual response*. Boston: Little, Brown and Company.

Modelska, K., & Cummings, S. (2002). Tibolone for postmenopausal women: Systematic review of randomized trials. *Journal of Clinical Endocrinology and Metabolism, 87*, 16–23.

Morgan, S. W. (2003). Transgender life experiences and expressions: A narrative inquiry into identity recognition and development, bodily experiences, relationships with others, and health care experiences. Dissertation (unpublished).

Morrow, K. M. (2000). Sexual risk in lesbians and bisexual women. *Journal of the Gay and Lesbian Medical Association, 4*(4), 159–165.

Moynihan, R. (2003). The making of a disease: Female sexual dysfunction. *British Medical Journal, 326*, 45–47.

Mravcak, S. A. (2006). Primary care for lesbians and bisexual women. *American Family Physician, 74*(2), 279–286.

Myskow, L. (2002). Perimenopausal issues in sexuality. *Sexual and Relationship Therapy, 17*, 253–260.

National Adolescent Health Information Center. (2007). *2007 fact sheet on reproductive health: Adolescents and young adults*. Retrieved July 10, 2007, from *http://nahic.ucsf.edu/*.

Nichols, M. (2004). Lesbian sexuality/female sexuality: Rethinking "lesbian bed death." *Sexual and Relationship Therapy, 19*(4), 363–371.

Nosek, M. A., Howland, C., Rintala, D. H., et al. (2001). National study of women with physical disabilities: Final report. *Sexuality and Disability, 19*(1), 5–39.

Nusbaum, M .R. H., & Hamilton, C. D. (2002). The proactive sexual health history. *American Family Physician, 66*, 1705–1712.

O'Hanlon, K. M., & Nikkanen, H. E. (2006). Sexual assault. *First Consult*. Retrieved June 2, 2007, from *www.firstconsult.com/fc_home/members/?urn=com.firstconsult/1/101/1017269*.

Pfizer Global Study of Sexual Attitudes and Behaviors. (2002). *Selected results from the Pfizer Global Study of Sexual Attitudes and Behaviors*. Retrieved July 7, 2007, from *www.pfizerglobalstudy.com/study/study-results.asp*.

Rousso, H. (1993). Special considerations in counseling clients with cerebral palsy. *Sexuality and Disability, 11*(1), 99–108.

Rowland, J. H., Desmond, K. A., Meyerowitz, B. E., et al. (2000). Role of breast reconstructive surgery in physical and emotional outcomes among breast cancer survivors. *Journal of the National Cancer Institute, 92*(17), 1422–1429.

Seehusen, D. A., Johnson, D. R., Earwood, J. S., et al. (2006). Improving women's experience during speculum examinations at routine gynaecological visits: randomised clinical trial. *British Medical Journal, 333*, 171–173. Retrieved August, 4, 2007, from *www.bmj.com/cgi/content/full/333/7560/171*.

Seidel, H. M., Ball, J. W., Dains, J. E., et al. (2003). *Mosby's guide to physical examination* (5th ed.). Philadelphia: Mosby.

Shrier, L. A. (2004). Sexually transmitted disease in adolescents: Biologic, cognitive, psychologic, behavioral, and social issues. *Adolescent Medicine Clinics, 15*. Retrieved June 2, 2007, from *http://www.popline.org/docs/1704/305894.html*.

Solarz, A. (1999). *Lesbian health: Current assessment and directions for the future*. Washington, DC: National Academies Press.

Spree, J. J., Hillenberg, B., Sugrue, D. P., et al. (2005). Study of sexual functioning determinants in breast cancer survivors. *Breast Journal, 11*(6), 440–447.

Springer, K. W. (2003). The long-term health outcomes of childhood abuse. An overview and a call to action. *Journal of General Internal Medicine, 18*, 864–870.

Stein, M. B., Lang, A. J., Laffaye, B. A., et al. (2004). Relationship of sexual assault history to somatic symptoms and health anxiety in women. *General Hospital Psychiatry, 26*, 178–183.

Stevens, P. E., & Hall, J. M. (2001). Sexuality and safer sex: The issues for lesbians and bisexual women. *Journal of Obstetric, Gynecologic, and Neonatal Nursing, 30*(1), 439–447.

Teare, C. (2002). Nursing practice and statutory rape. Effects of reporting and enforcement on access to care for adolescents. *Nursing Clinics of North America, 37*, 393–404.

Thombs, B. D., Bernstein, D. P., Ziegelstein, R. C., et al. (2007). A brief two-item screener for detecting a history of physical or sexual abuse in childhood. *General Hospital Psychiatry, 29*, 8–13.

Tiefer, L. (2002). Beyond the medical model of women's sexual problems: A campaign to resist the promotion of "female sexual dysfunction." *Sexual and Relationship Therapy, 17*(2), 127–135.

Tiefer, L., Hall, M., & Tavris, C. (2002). Beyond dysfunction: A new view of women's sexual problems. *Journal of Sex and Marital Therapy, 28(s)*, 225–232.

Tilley, C. M. (1998). Health care for women with physical disabilities: Literature review and theory. *Sexuality and Disability, 16*(2), 87–102.

Turnbull, G. B. (2001). Sexual counseling: The forgotten aspect of ostomy rehabilitation. *Journal of Sex Education and Therapy, 26*(3), 189–195.

Vincent, C. (2002). Health challenges for older women: Some implications for sexual health. *Sexual and Relationship Therapy, 17*, 241–252.

Waitkevicz, H. J. (2004). Lesbian health in primary care. Part 2: Sexual health care and counseling for women who have sex with women. *Women's Health in Primary Care*, 7, 231.

Williamson, G. M., & Walters, A. S. (1996). Perceived impact of limb amputation on sexual activity: A study of adult amputees. *Journal of Sex Research, 33*(3), 221–230.

Wilmoth, C. C., & Ross, J. A. (1997). Women's perception: Breast cancer treatment and sexuality. *Cancer Practice, 5*(6), 353–359.

Wylie, K. R. (2006). Optimising clinical interventions for sexual difficulties within a relationship. *Journal of Men's Health and Gender, 3*(4), 350–355.

Yurak, D., Farrar, W., & Anderson, B. L. (2000). Breast cancer surgery: Comparing surgical group and determining Individual differences in postoperative sexuality and body change stress. *Journal of Counseling and Clinical Psychology, 68*(4), 697–709.

Catherine Judd

chapter 14

Sleep Disorders

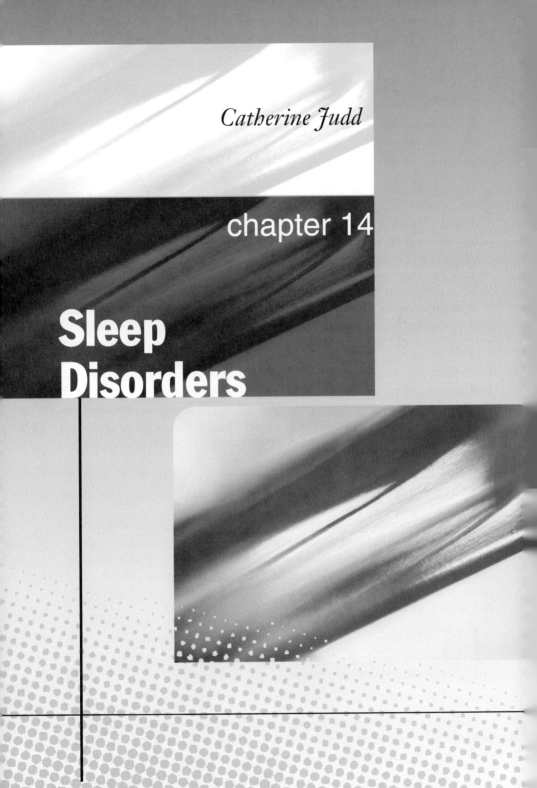

Approximately 40 million people experience sleep problems each year, with women experiencing more problems than men. These sleep disturbances are among the most common complaints reported to health care providers. In addition, approximately 20 percent of women complain of excessive daytime sleepiness, fatigue, or both (Theorell-Haglow, Lindberg, and Janson, 2006).

Sleep disorders also impact mental health (Collier, Skitt, and Cutts, 2003). In women who note sleep disturbance as a prominent symptom complaint, there is an increased prevalence of a number of psychiatric disorders, including anxiety and depression (Roth, 2001; Voderholzer, Al-Shajlawi, Weske, et al., 2003). Screening must take place for psychiatric disorders in the search for the etiology of sleep disturbances because psychotic disorders, mood disorders, anxiety and panic disorders, posttraumatic stress disorder (PTSD), substance abuse, and alcoholism are prominent symptoms in these disorders. Sleep disorders are associated with medical illnesses as well, including neurologic disorders such as Parkinson's disease, seizure disorder, diseases involving the airways, gastroesophageal reflux, peptic ulcer disease, and fibromyalgia.

The prevalence of sleep disorders and insomnia has serious economic consequences as well. According to the National Commission on Sleep Disorders, direct costs of sleep disorders have been estimated at $16 billion and the indirect costs at $150 billion per year (Walsh, 2006). Although the risks of inadequate sleep have been well documented along with data regarding the effect of insufficient sleep on mental and overall health, the amount of time women spend sleeping has decreased by 20 percent over the past 100 years.

The *International Classification of Sleep Disorders: Diagnostic and Coding Manual* provides a detailed list of sleep disorders divided into four categories: dysomnias, parasomnias, sleep disorders associated with medical-psychiatric disorders, and proposed sleep disorders (Diagnostic Steering Committee, 1990). In more recent years, a classification based on the following four categories of sleep disorders has been developed:

1. Disorders of initiating and maintaining sleep (insomnia)
2. Disorders of excessive sleepiness (narcolepsy)
3. Circadian rhythm disturbance
4. Parasomnias (e.g., sleepwalking, night terrors, enuresis)

This chapter covers the most commonly encountered sleep disorders in primary care, including insomnia, sleep movement disorders, narcolepsy, and sleep apnea. Women experience insomnia more often than men (63 percent vs.

54 percent), with complaints of disturbed sleep more prevalent among women across the entire life span with increasing incidence with age (Mauri, 1990; Moline, Brock, and Zack, 2004; Morgenthaler, Kramer, Alessi, et al., 2007).

Health care providers frequently have limited training and experience in treating sleep complaints, and many of them might have misconceptions regarding the risks and benefits of prescribing sedative hypnotic medication. Recognition and appropriate treatment of insomnia are implicit in promoting overall health, mental health, wellness, and quality of life. Clinicians must take a detailed history, conduct a physical examination, and use sleep questionnaires along with polysomnography to make an accurate diagnosis and develop an appropriate treatment plan for the various sleep disorders.

Most patients do not seek treatment for insomnia, resigning themselves to poor sleep and blaming the problems on stress, aging, or illness. Insomnia all too often goes undiagnosed and untreated. In a survey by the National Sleep Foundation (2006), an overwhelming majority (69 percent) of patients acknowledged never discussing their sleep problems with their health care providers, and only 26 percent discussed their insomnia in the context of a visit for another problem. Only 5 percent visited a health care provider specifically for a sleep-related complaint even though three times that number consider insomnia a serious problem (Roth and Ancoli-Isreal, 1999).

DEFINITION OF INSOMNIA

Historically, insomnia has been defined as a symptom rather than a disorder. More recently, with evidence-based diagnostic criteria for insomnia, expert consensus, and an increasing convergence of research data, insomnia is now considered a disorder that may present with specific sleep-related symptoms. Insomnia causes disruption of important nocturnal (sleep) and diurnal (daytime impairment) rhythms and involves "predisposing," "precipitating," and "perpetuating" variables (Fig. 14.1).

The *Diagnostic and Statistical Manual of Mental Disorders* (*DSM-IV-TR*) defines insomnia as difficulty falling asleep (initial insomnia), awakening in the middle of the night and eventually falling back to sleep but with difficulty (middle insomnia), early morning awakening or awakening too early (terminal insomnia), or the perception of insufficient or poor quality sleep, despite an adequate opportunity to sleep resulting in consequences for next-day functioning and impairment in social, occupational, personal, or other important life areas (American Psychiatric Association, 2000). Previously, the definition included the

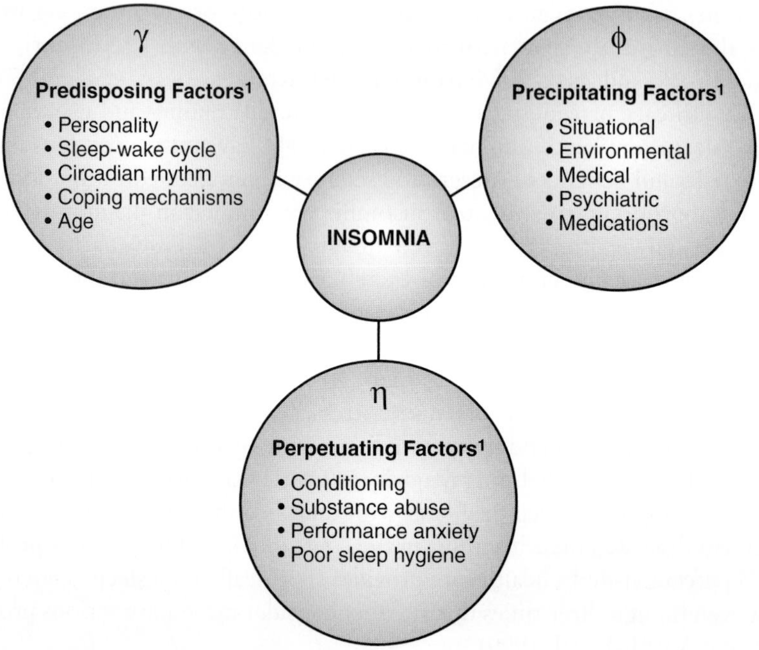

Figure 14.1. Factors in the genesis and progression of insomnia. [Hauri, P. J. (1998); Spielman, A. J., Caruso, L. S., & Glovinsky, P. B. (1987).]

idea of "nonrestorative" sleep; however, because of the limited data regarding "nonrestorative" sleep, the term was replaced by the phrase "waking too early" (National Institutes of Health, 2005).

Transient, Short-Term, and Chronic Insomnia

Insomnia may be classified as being transient, short term, or chronic. *Transient insomnia* lasts only a few days and occurs in response to acute situational stresses or changes in the patient's environment. It may also be a response to a situational stress, such as anxiety regarding anticipated events like starting a new job, moving, marriage, or the birth of child. Additionally, acute medical illness, abrupt changes in normal circadian rhythms due to changes in daily schedule, jet lag, or shift work may cause transient insomnia. Insomnia may also be pharmacologically induced by such substances as caffeine, nicotine, and alcohol as well as by prescription medicine. Most common symptoms of transient insomnia are difficulty falling asleep (initial insomnia) and middle insomnia with early morning awakening. Transient insomnia lasting for more than a few days may cause significant impairment in daytime functioning as well as excessive daytime sleepiness.

Short-term insomnia has a duration of up to 3 weeks and is frequently precipitated by situational stress or environmental changes. It may also be pharmacologically induced. Stresses may include events such as bereavement, emotional trauma, hospitalization, or chronic pain as well as major life events such as marriage, divorce, moving or a change in living situation, or prolonged stress in the family or work environment. A careful history will usually point to the etiology, which may be other than situational or environmental factors. Patients with short-term insomnia may be effectively treated with education regarding good sleep hygiene and short-term use of an appropriate sedative hypnotic. Psychotherapy may be useful in patients who are dealing with loss, trauma, or severe stress. Insomnia that persists for longer than 3 weeks is considered chronic.

Chronic insomnia can be a consequence of physical or emotional illness, such as cardiovascular insufficiency, hyperthyroidism, chronic obstructive pulmonary disease, asthma, Parkinson's disease, and a number of psychiatric disorders, including depression, panic disorder, PTSD, or adjustment disorder. Use of illicit drugs or alcohol can also exacerbate insomnia and cause disturbances in normal sleep. Use of prescription medications may also contribute to chronic insomnia (Box 14.1).

INSOMNIA IN WOMEN

By far, the most common sleep complaint in primary care is insomnia, and women complain of insomnia more often than do men (Morgenthaler et al., 2007). It is estimated that approximately one third of the population in the United States is affected. Population surveys estimate a 1-year prevalence rate in adults of 30 to 45 percent, with approximately 37 percent of Americans reporting they experience daytime sleepiness affecting daytime functioning at least a few days every month (Drake, Roehrs, Richardson, et al., 2002). Women report more insomnia a few nights per week than do men (63percent vs. 54 percent) and more frequent complaints of daytime sleepiness (Morgenthaler et al., 2007). Among individuals who report insomnia, 17 percent rate it as a serious problem.

Most patients do not seek treatment for insomnia, resigning themselves to poor sleep and blaming the problems on stress, aging, or illness. Therefore, insomnia is a symptom that all too often goes undiagnosed and untreated. In a survey by the National Sleep Foundation (2006), an overwhelming majority

Box 14. 1 • Agents That May Contribute to Insomnia

Prescription Medications	*Over-the-Counter Substances*
• Anticholinergics	• Alcohol
• Antidepressants	• Caffeine (including diet pills)
• Antihypertensives	• Nicotine
• Antineoplastic agents	• Various herbs and supplements
• Bronchodilators	
• CNS stimulants	
• Corticosteroids	
• Decongestants	
• Diuretics	
• Histamine-2 blockers	
• Smoking cessation aids	

CNS, central nervous system.
From Becker, P. M., et al. (1993).; Pingdahl, E. N., et al. (2004).

(69 percent) acknowledged never discussing their sleep problems with their health care providers, and only 26 percent discussed their insomnia in the context of a visit for another problem. Only 5 percent visited a health care provider specifically for a sleep-related complaint even though three times that number consider insomnia a serious problem (Roth and Ancoli-Isreal, 1999).

Women, however, are more likely than men to report insomnia. Complaints of disturbed sleep are more prevalent among women across the entire life span, with increasing incidence with age (Mauri, 1990; Moline et al., 2004). Complex hormonal cycles influence in large part the increased prevalence of insomnia in women. The role of hormonal changes as they are related to menstruation (Owen and Matthews, 1998), the decrease in sleep quality during menopause (Manber and Armitage, 1999; Mindell and Jacobson, 2000), and disrupted sleep during pregnancy (Bjoeklund, Bengtssom, Lissner, et al., 2002) have been studied and may be a contributing factor. These hormonal variations may further account for the differences in prevalence and patterns of disrupted sleep between younger women and older women associated with the onset of menses and menopause.

Insomnia and Hormonal Changes

Female sex hormones involved in the reproductive cycle across a woman's life span that fluctuate and change during menarche, pregnancy, lactation, and the perimenopause period have a significant impact on sleep. Premenstrual insomnia and premenstrual hypersomnia (excessive sleeping) are included in the *International Classification of Sleep Disorders* within the category of menstrual-associated sleep disorder. Sleep quality is decreased in women with premenstrual dysphoric disorder, with worsening of anxiety and mood symptoms. These symptoms may be relieved by administering selective serotonin reuptake inhibitors (SSRIs) during the luteal phase of the menstrual cycle (Luisi and Pawasauskas, 2003).

Changes in sleep architecture have been shown to occur during pregnancy (Santiago, Nolledo, Kinzler, et al., 2001). There are increases and subsequent decreases in total sleep time during the first and third trimesters, respectively. There is also an increase in middle insomnia and lengthening of wake time after sleep onset in addition to an overall decrease in sleep quality. The physiologic changes that accompany fluctuations in steroid and hypothalamic-pituitary-adrenal axis–related hormones during pregnancy and following parturition include disruption of normal circadian rhythms and the sleep–wake cycle. These changes are most likely consequences of changes in prolactin, cortisol, thermoregulation, pulmonary function, body mass, and sex steroid hormones (Santiago Nolledo, Kinzler, et al. 2001).

Women also experience a decrease in quality of sleep during menopause, although there is a lack of agreement regarding the relationship of hot flashes to sleep quality. In older women, disruption in sleep may be related to vasomotor disturbance in addition to mood disorders.

Insomnia and Psychiatric Disorders

There is a higher correlation with life events and sleep disruption in women than in men as well as a higher prevalence of underlying depression and anxiety (Piccinelli and Wilkinson, 2000). Insomnia occurs with high frequency in patients with major depressive disorder. It is estimated that approximately 65 percent of outpatients and 90 percent of inpatients with major depression meet criteria for insomnia (McCall, Reboussin, and Cohen, 2000; Nowell and Buysse, 2001). Conversely, patients with primary insomnia have nearly four times the relative risk of developing major depressive disorder as compared with the general population. Furthermore, patients with a history of insomnia have a relative risk of developing an anxiety disorder double that of the general population (Breslau, Roth, Rosenthal, et al., 1996).

Insomnia and Depression

There are marked sex differences in sleep architecture on polysomnography, which shows that women have more delta (slow-wave sleep and rapid eye movement [REM]) sleep than men. Studies of sleep architecture and sleep patterns using electroencephalography in depressed patients have described a number of characteristics, including decreased REM latency, decreased slow-wave sleep, and an increase in early awakening. Positron emission tomography and functional magnetic resonance imaging have shown a relationship between insomnia and depression. Primary insomnia has demonstrated increased activity in the reticular activating system, basal forebrain and hypothalamus, thalamus, and the ventromedial frontal cortex (Nofzinger, Nichols, Meltzer, et al.,1999). Patients with primary insomnia demonstrate hypoactivity in the thalamocortical circuit involving the prefrontal cortex during sleep and wakefulness. Depressed patients exhibit hyperactivity in limbic and paralimbic structures, such as the amygdala, in addition to hypofunctioning in the prefrontal cortex associated with both REM and alterations in slow-wave sleep (Ho, Gillin, Buchsbaum, et al., 1996). These important studies point to an overall hyperarousal in subcortical regions and hypoactivity in the prefrontal cortex both in depressed patients and in patients with insomnia, which suggests at least a partial explanation for their comorbidity. One study further suggested a shared neurobiology between depression and insomnia by demonstrating a polymorphism in the monoamine oxidase-A gene, which is associated with both insomnia and depression in depressed patients (Du, Bakish, Ravindran, et al., 2004).

Insomnia and Age

Epidemiologic data have demonstrated a higher prevalence of insomnia in older persons, with older women reporting insomnia more often than older men, when compared with younger individuals. In a survey completed by the National Institute on Aging with more than 9,000 patients age 65 years or older, 28 percent reported difficulties initiating sleep and 42 percent reported symptoms of both difficulties in sleep initiation and maintenance (Foley, Monjan, Brown, et al., 1995). While the need for sleep may not decrease with age, the ability to sleep and the distribution of sleep during the day and night can change dramatically. Elderly individuals frequently experience longer periods of nighttime wakefulness with an increase in daytime fatigue, napping, and daytime sleepiness. Although this may appear to be a typical pattern of sleep for elderly individuals, it is not considered normal.

Other factors may contribute to insomnia in aging individuals, including depression, chronic pain, and anxiety, along with medications that may disrupt normal sleep patterns. Physical symptoms frequently affect sleep (e.g., the need to void during the night may result in nocturia and frequent awakenings), and changes in lifestyle such as retirement may result in opportunities to nap during the day resulting in fragmentation of nocturnal sleep. Additional stressors may include sharply reduced income, significant losses of family and friends due to illness and death, and concern over personal health problems. Elderly persons may live in crime-ridden areas and be at risk for robbery and victimization, creating an atmosphere of anxiety, apprehension, and helplessness. Other stresses can include leaving familiar surroundings to live in a senior citizen residence or nursing home.

Assessment of Insomnia

Insomnia requires a differential diagnosis based on a careful history and thorough evaluation. Evaluation of insomnia should include an assessment of the impact of the insomnia on daytime functioning. When assessing the patient's sleep habits, it is important to acknowledge individual differences.

A careful patient assessment and history is a prerequisite to identifying the underlining cause of a sleep disorder. The first step should be to obtain a thorough sleep history, which can help to quantify the duration of the problem and determine whether the disorder is transient, short term, or chronic. Patients should be asked about the frequency of episodes as well as the extent to which their daytime functioning is impaired. Evaluation should determine what time the patient usually goes to bed and awakens as well as what, if anything, is used as a sleep aid. Remember that while most adults require approximately 8 hours of sleep to feel rested and restored the next day, some can perform quite well with less (whereas others need more).

The primary care provider (PCP) should be sure to obtain information regarding the use of over-the-counter (OTC) medications, alcohol, illicit drugs, caffeine, and nicotine. Interviewing the bed partner regarding snoring, movements, and any other unusual sleep behaviors can provide useful information. Having the patient keep a sleep diary containing the time she went to bed, the time she thinks she went to sleep, periods of wakefulness, quality of sleep, and effect on functioning the following day can also be helpful.

Treatment Options

Physiologic, psychological, and behavioral factors may, alone or in combination, contribute to and perpetuate insomnia. Treatment for insomnia must address multiple etiologic variables and should be targeted with an integrated approach that is appropriate and most effective, whether the cause is a medical, psychiatric, or circadian rhythm disturbance. The goals of treatment are to resolve the underlying problem, prevent progression, and improve quality of life.

Medication

The ideal pharmacologic agent for insomnia induces and maintains sleep, has no adverse affect on sleep architecture, causes no impairment on next-day functioning or memory, and has no rebound insomnia or addiction potential. Several classes of medications are available for the treatment of insomnia, with distinct class differences in half-life, next-day functioning, side effects, affect on sleep architecture, and safety profile. It is important for clinicians to be aware of these differences when prescribing sedative hypnotics.

Sedative hypnotics are not intended for long-term use, and only one, ramelteon (Rozerem), has Food and Drug Admistration (FDA) approval for such usage. Use of OTC agents, sedating antidepressants such as trazodone (Desyrel), doxepin (Adapin), and amitriptyline (Elavil) as well as nonhypnotic benzodiazepines may actually worsen insomnia as a result of rebound insomnia, withdrawal effects, and next-day drowsiness. They may also cause cognitive impairment, accidents, and falls (Becker, 2005). Long-term use of older sedative hypnotics may perpetuate sleep problems in addition to masking an underlying disorder. Patients should use medication for two or three nights, abstain for several nights, and then repeat the process while implementing sleep-hygiene practices and learning behavioral techniques.

Benzodiazepines. Benzodiazepines have traditionally been used to help patients sleep; however, given alternative new compounds, this class of medication should be avoided. There are important considerations regarding the onset of action, duration of action, and presence of active metabolites. Patients who rely on short-acting benzodiazepines as a sleep aid are at risk for rebound insomnia and have a higher risk for anterograde amnesia when compared with agents with a longer half-life. Longer-acting agents can affect next-day performance and leave patients with a "hung over" or "drugged" feeling the following day. Benzodiazepines interfere with normal sleep architecture with effects on stage 3 and 4 sleep as well as REM sleep. This class of compounds is contraindicated in elderly

Table 14.1 • Nonbenzodiazepine Sedative Hypnotic Medications Available in the United States

Drug Name	Indication	Approximate Half-Life	Dose Formulations
Eszopiclone	"Insomnia . . . decreased sleep latency and improved sleep maintenance."	6 hr	1-, 2-, and 3-mg tablets
Zaleplon	"Short-term treatment of insomnia . . . decrease the time to sleep onset."	1 hr	5- & 10-mg tablets
Zolpidem	"Short-term treatment of insomnia . . . decrease sleep latency and increase duration of sleep."	2.5 hr	5- & 10-mg tablets
Zolpidem CR	"Insomnia characterized by difficulties with sleep onset and/or sleep maintenance."	2.8 hr	6.25- & 12.5-mg tablets
Ramelteon	"Insomnia characterized by difficulty with sleep onset."	1.0–2.6 hr	8-mg tablets

Package information available at *www.accessdata.fda.gov*.

patients who may need to get up in the middle of the night to void and may be at risk for falls and injury. Patients should also be cautioned not to use alcohol while taking benzodiazepines due to the additive central nervous system (CNS) depressant effects. Benzodiazepines should not be administered without ruling out sleep apnea because of the risk of further CNS depression of respiratory drive.

Benzodiazepine-Receptor Agonists. Benzodiazepine-receptor agonists are a relatively new class of compounds and alternative to benzodiazepines (Table 14.1). The first of these agents to be released in the United States was zolpidem (Ambien). Zolpidem is a selective agonist of the type 1 $GABA_A$ alpha subunit (BZ1) with a rapid onset of action and short half-life. It is effective for initial insomnia (i.e., difficulty falling asleep). Zolpidem has a short half-life and is less effective for problems with sleep maintenance. Selectively binding to the omega-1 $GABA_A$ receptor, it does not have the residual side effects of benzodiazepines, impairment in next-day cognitive functioning, and effects on memory. It is nonaddictive, and tolerance does not develop. Patients using zolpidem for up to

30 days did not experience rebound insomnia on abrupt discontinuation. Zolpidem has also been demonstrated to preserve normal sleep architecture; has few drug–drug interactions; and demonstrates significant improvement in sleep latency, number of awakenings, and total sleep time (Perlis, McCall, Krystal, et al., 2004). Zolpidem CR has a fast and slow dissolving layer, producing a biphasic absorption profile. The ability to attain higher plasma levels later during sleep translates into reduced time to get back to sleep after awakening 4 to 5 hours following the first administration.

Zaleplon (Sonata) with specificity for the BZ1 receptor, has the shortest half-life of the currently available sedative hypnotics and is used for sleep induction, with minimal next-day side effects and residual sedation (Verster, Volkerts, Schreuder, et al., 2002). It can be used in the middle of the night for sleep initiation if there are at least 4 hours remaining for sleep. Doses of 20 mg increase sleep duration and reduce the number of awakenings, and as with zolpidem, there does not appear to be any alteration in sleep architecture (Walsh, Vogel, Scharf, et al., 2000).

Eszopiclone (Lunesta) has a half-life of 5 to 6 hours, and it too binds to the 1 $GABA_A$ alpha subunits. It is approved by the FDA for treatment of sleep onset and sleep maintenance insomnia and has been studied in long-term, randomized, double-blind, placebo-controlled trials. Patients with chronic primary insomnia showed significant reduction of time to sleep onset and decreased number of awakenings, with improvement in sleep quality, daytime alertness, sense of well-being, and daytime functioning, with no evidence of significant tolerance or residual next-day sedation. The most common side effect is unpleasant aftertaste (Zammit, Gillin, McNabb, et al., 2003).

Ramelteon (Rozerem), approved by the FDA in 2005, is an MT_1 melatonin receptor agonist. It is unique in that its site of action is at the MT_1 and MT_2 receptors located on the suprachiasmatic nucleus, suggesting its potential effect on circadian regulation. It has neglible affinity for other binding sites, including benzodiazepine, dopamine, and opiate receptors (Jochelson, Scharf, and Roth, 2004).

Antidepressants. Antidepressants are often used with patients who have insomnia because sleep disturbance is one of the cardinal symptoms of depression. It would follow that a sedating antidepressant can serve a dual purpose in the early stages of treatment. As a rule, the depression should be treated aggressively, with insomnia viewed as one of the symptoms that will improve as the depression remits. However, a resolution of sleep complaints early in treatment for depression is not a predictor of antidepressant response. There is some evidence that SSRIs are especially effective in the treatment of women with depression and insomnia (Krystal, 2004), but some of the tricyclic antidepressants (TCAs) and SSRIs (i.e., fluoxetine) may exacerbate insomnia or underlying conditions such as periodic limb movement or restless legs syndrome (RLS). Other sedating non-SSRI antidepressants such as amitriptyline (Elavil), trazodone (Desyrel), doxepin (Adapin, Sinequan), and mirtazapine (Remeron) can be used alone or in combination with an SSRI to treat comorbid depression and insomnia; however, patients may experience residual daytime sedation. TCAs are potentially lethal in overdose and must be used with extreme caution, particularly in depressed patients at risk for suicide.

Antipsychotics. Antipsychotic medications such as quetiapine (Seroquel) have sedative effects for patients who are psychotic and have sleep disturbance but are not approved for and should not be used to treat insomnia. Antihistamines (i.e., diphenhydramine [Benadryl]) are sedating as well. Sedation is a prominent side effect of diphenhydramine but does not treat insomnia directly. Nonetheless, it is the active ingredient included in a number of OTC sleep-inducing preparations. L-Dopa has been found to be successful when used in low doses for patients with periodic limb movements by suppressing muscle activity, which is the cause of nocturnal awakenings. However, caution must be exercised to avoid a drug-induced psychosis or movement disorder.

Alternative Medications. Melatonin is a neuropeptide produced by the pineal gland with several neuromodulating and neuroregulatory functions that affect sleep and mood. Exposure to darkness stimulates nerve pathways from the retina to the suprachiasmatic nucleus, which in turn signals release of melatonin. With the rise in melatonin levels, alertness is decreased and there is a propensity for sleep. Melatonin is sold without a prescription under the provisions of the U.S. Dietary and Supplement Health and Education Act of 1994. Melatonin is produced without regulation by the FDA. Accuracy regarding the quantity of active compound, concentration, and bioequality of doses is not standardized. Exogenously administered melatonin causes melatonin levels in blood to rise to much higher levels than are naturally produced in the body. Systematic controlled trials regarding therapeutic dose, long-term effects, and toxicity are lacking. Doses of 3 mg to 6 mg at bedtime are commonly used by shift workers and individuals with insomnia related to jet lag.

Experimental work with melatonin has proven successful in treating circadian rhythm disturbances in blind persons, where it acts as a biologic substrate for the internal circadian oscillator. In animal studies, melatonin can cause hypertension and infertility. It is contraindicated in persons with cardiac disease, hypertension, cerebrovascular disease, renal disease, and sleep apnea (National Sleep Foundation, 2007).

Table 14.2 • Psychological and Behavioral Strategies

Strategy	Goal
Sleep hygiene	Develop and practice habits that promote and are conducive to sleep.
Stimulus control	Reinforce bedroom and bed as a cue and stimulus for sleep.
Sleep restriction	Restrict time in bed to improve sleep consolidation.
Relaxation training and visual imagery	Decrease tension and anxiety.
Cognitive behavioral therapy (CBT)	Reframe thoughts and beliefs that interfere with sleep.
Psychotherapy	Address psychological issues and interpersonal issues related to insomnia.

Behavioral Interventions

Treatment approaches for insomnia vary. Appreciating the fact that insomnia may be a sign of underlying problems is of utmost importance when a patient complains of difficulty sleeping and excessive daytime sleepiness. Insomnia may be improved with behavioral interventions or environmental changes. Some interventions produce more immediate results for some patients than others. It is important to remember that successful intervention and treatment depend on the patient's willingness and acceptance of alternative treatment approaches (Table 14.2).

Sleep Hygiene. Sleep hygiene is designed to promote conditions favorable to sleep and addresses environmental conditions conducive to sleep. Patient education is directed toward the need for a regular sleep–wake schedule, a regular schedule of exercise, a moderate bedroom temperature free from excessive noise, and a warm beverage or light snack at bedtime, although patients should be advised to avoid caffeine and alcohol because both disrupt sleep. It is also important for the PCP to emphasize the importance of using the bed only for sleep (and sex) and to suggest patients resolve emotional conflicts and disagreements before retiring (Box 14.2).

Stimulus Control. For many individuals, the bed is used for activities other than sleep and sex. The bed becomes a place for watching TV, eating, doing homework, balancing the checkbook, and talking on the telephone. These activities

Box 14.2 • General Sleep Hygiene Measures

Get up at the same time each day, including weekends. Avoid daytime naps, except shift workers.

Avoid caffeine intake 4–6 hours before bedtime. Decrease daytime consumption.

Avoid smoking near bedtime or when waking in the middle of the night, because nicotine is a stimulant.

Avoid alcohol. Do not use alcohol to induce sleep onset.

Avoid heavy meals close to bedtime, since they may interfere with sleep. A light snack or warm beverage may be sleep inducing.

Avoid vigorous exercise within 3–4 hours of bedtime. Exercise regularly earlier in the day.

Minimize noise and light. Keep room cool.

Keep the clock out of sight.

result in the bed no longer being a stimulus cue for sleep, and the activities should be conducted in another room.

Sleep Restriction. Sleep restriction can be helpful for patients who lie in bed worrying about not being able to fall asleep. The goal of sleep restriction is to reduce the amount of time spent in bed to time sleeping, thereby improving sleep efficiency. Sleep restriction reduces the time awake in bed that may perpetuate insomnia. It combines sleep deprivation with deconditioning to increase sleep consolidation. Initially, patients may experience an increase in daytime sleepiness.

The first step is to determine how many hours are spent in bed and how many hours are spent sleeping. If 7 hours are spent in bed, 5 hours are spent asleep, and 2 hours are spent awake, sleep efficiency is 71.5 percent. Therefore, retiring to bed should be delayed by 2 hours but the rising time should remain the same, as the goal of sleep restriction is to achieve a sleep efficiency of at least 85 percent. Patients will need to keep a sleep diary to keep track of their sleep efficiency. Once they have reached an efficiency level of 85 percent five nights in a row, they can add 15 minutes to bedtime, allowing an additional 15 minutes in bed.

Progressive Relaxation. Visual imagery, self-hypnosis, and progressive muscle relaxation are potentially powerful tools that can enhance the quantity and quality of sleep. It is unlikely that simply providing a relaxation tape will be sufficient; patients should be instructed to learn relaxation techniques during the day prior to implementing them at bedtime.

Cognitive Techniques. Cognitive therapy techniques are based on the premise that thoughts and worries about sleeplessness and its consequences trigger fear and anxiety about not being able to sleep, which further intensify and increase sleeplessness. Cognitive behavioral techniques target the "cognitive distortions" with the goal of reframing them to break the cycle. Cognitive distortions include unrealistic expectations about the number of hours of sleep needed (i.e., "I must get 8 hours of sleep . . . or else"), faulty casual attributions regarding difficulty sleeping (i.e., "I'm genetically predisposed to insomnia"), and exaggeration and "catastrophizing" regarding the consequences of a poor night's sleep (i.e., "Poor sleep will shorten my life"). Therapeutic messages include keeping realistic expectations, not blaming insomnia for all problems with daytime functioning, refraining from "trying to sleep," not giving too much importance to sleep, and developing some tolerance to the effects of insomnia.

SLEEP MOVEMENT DISORDERS

RLS affects approximately 9 percent of the U.S. adult population and is reported twice as often in women than in men (Hening, Walters, Allen, et al., 2004). Patients complain of an uncontrollable and uncomfortable urge to move. Symptoms increase at night and disrupt sleep onset and sleep maintenance. RLS follows a circadian rhythm pattern corresponding with the sleep–wake cycle.

Periodic limb movement disorder (PLMD), also referred to as nocturnal myoclonus, is commonly seen in patients with RLS and is characterized by repetitive, periodic, and stereotypical movements of the legs during non-REM sleep. Myoclonic jerks every 20 to 40 seconds are demonstrated on polysomnography. It is more common in elderly patients with comorbid medical illnesses, and the patients' only complaint may be a sense of restless, disturbed sleep.

Etiology and Diagnosis

Etiology of RLS is thought to be related to impaired CNS iron transport and storage (Connor, Boyer, Menzies, et al., 2003). Iron is a requisite for dopamine synthesis, and a deficit results in a hypodopaminergic state in the motor cortex and extrapyramidal system. Secondary causes of RLS and PLMD include peripheral neuropathy, peripheral vascular disease, and lumbar spine disease.

Women may present in pregnancy with secondary RLS associated with iron deficiency; this also occurs with women who have a chronic disease. RLS is diagnosed by taking a careful history. Diagnosis is supported by abnormal iron studies.

Treatment Options

Supplemental iron 65 mg bid along with vitamin C 250 mg to increase bioavailability and absorption may offer some relief. Administration of a dopamine agonist may reduce the movements of RLS at the risk of side effects and rebound. There are anecdotal reports that off-label use of anticonvulsants, such as gabapentin (Neurontin), may decrease symptoms. Benzodiazepines, particularly temazepam (Restoril), 15 to 30 mg qhs, and clonazepam (Klonopin), 0.5 to 2.0 mg qhs, have demonstrated efficacy and improvement in sleep. However, clinicians must keep in mind attenuated risks of daytime sedation, habituation, tolerance, and withdrawal. Patients with RLS should avoid medications such as SSRIs, antihistamines, and caffeine.

NARCOLEPSY

Narcolepsy is a disorder of excess sleep drive and disturbance in the regulation of sleep wakefulness. Patients with narcolepsy complain of sleepiness or "sleep attacks" occurring at times other than the usual time for sleep (night) despite adequate sleep time and quality of sleep. Episodes of cataplexy with the appearance of REM-like atonia of skeletal muscle occur outside the context of a REM period without loss of consciousness, frequently occurring with a sudden onset, lasting for a few seconds to a few minutes, and sometimes mistaken for a seizure. Other signs and symptoms include excessive daytime sleepiness, disrupted or fragmented nighttime sleep, hypnagogic hallucinations, and sleep paralysis.

Etiology and Diagnosis

The pathophysiology of narcolepsy is related to a deficit of orexin/hypocretin in the hypothalamus, which regulates sleep onset (Saper, Cano, and Scammell, 2005). There is also evidence of an association with the human leukocyte antigen DQB1 0602 gene. Onset of narcolepsy is typically in adolescence, and a definitive diagnosis is made by overnight polysomnography followed by a multiple sleep latency test, which shows sleepiness and sleep-onset REM periods. Narcolepsy will result in a finding of frequent transitioning from wakefulness to REM sleep.

Treatment Options

Treatment strategies include medications that promote wakefulness, such as pemoline (Cylert). Pemoline may be prescribed in dosages of 37.5 to 150.0 mg daily in one or two divided doses. Pemoline is a sympathetic amine and CNS stimulant similar in action to amphetamines. Modafinil (Provigil), starting dose 200 mg qam up to a max of 400 mg/day, has the advantage of low abuse potential but has significant drug–drug interactions. Caution should be used in administering modafinil in the elderly.

Stimluants are also used in the symptomatic treatment of narcolepsy. Methylphenidate and dextroamphetamine, 20 to 60 mg daily in one or two divided doses, available in regular and sustained-release formulations, may offer relief to some patients but carry high risk of abuse. Transdermal patches may offer an alternate form of administration. Severe cataplexy responds to sodium oxybate (Xyrem) 6 to 9 mg bid with a starting dose of 2.25 g po bid. However, this drug has restricted access in the United States. Nonsedating SSRIs that decrease REM sleep such as fluoxetine (Prozac) 20 to 80 mg/day during wakeful periods, TCAs such as clomipramine (Anafranil) 25 to 75 mg/day, or protriptyline (Vivactil) 5 to 20 mg/day may be useful in decreasing the onset of REM sleep and cataplexy but have anticholinergic side effects.

SLEEP APNEA

Sleep apnea is a respiratory disturbance associated with sleep. Apnea is defined as cessation of airflow at the nose and mouth for 10 seconds or longer. The most common apnea is obstructive sleep apnea syndrome, which occurs when impaired airflow in the upper airway causes symptoms. Respiratory effort increases to maintain normal airflow, resulting in recurrent arousal from sleep, the consequence of which is daytime sleepiness. Causes of decreased upper airway caliber include obesity (deposits of adipose tissue around the airway), adenotonsillar hypertrophy (most commonly in children), mandibular deficiency, and macroglossia (often associated with hypothyroidism). Symptoms include snoring, gasping for breath, or choking during sleep. The result is restless sleep and daytime sleepiness.

Diagnosis

When obstructive sleep apnea is suspected, the diagnosis is confirmed by polysomnography if more than five obstructive apneas or hypopneas occur per hour of sleep during at least 6 hours of nocturnal sleep. Laboratory testing that includes arterial blood gas analysis, chest x-ray and electrocardiography (looking for signs of pulmonary hypertension or cor pulmonale), and serum thyroid-stimulating hormone (to rule out hypothyroidism) may be useful. Visualization of the upper airway should be performed to rule out obstructing tumors and anatomical abnormalities.

Treatment Options

Treatment is targeted toward opening the airway and maintaining a patent airway during sleep. This can be accomplished by a mechanical device, a nasal continuous positive airway pressure (nasal CPAP). This device holds the airway open by a pneumatic splint effect. Patients wear a tight-fitting mask attached to a flow generator to maintain positive airway pressure. Nasal CPAP is the optimal and least invasive treatment available but depends on patient compliance. Alternatively, nasal "pillows" can be inserted into the nares and may be preferred over the mask by some patients. There are a number of oral appliances available, including a mandibular advancement orthotic and tongue-retaining devices. Surgical modification of the upper airway can also be performed by uvulopalatopharyngoplasty, which almost always eliminates snoring but corrects the obstructive sleep apnea syndrome in only approximately 50 percent of patients.

More recently, the "pillar procedure," in which splints are inserted into the palate, have also given relief. Surgery on the upper airway has limited success. Patients should be advised to avoid alcohol and muscle relaxants or medications that decrease respiratory drive, and obese patients should be advised to lose weight. Protriptyline (Vivactil) and fluoxetine (Prozac), both nonsedating antidepressants, suppress REM sleep, during which most apneas occur, and may increase upper airway tone.

CONCLUSION

Approximately 40 percent of adults have sleep disorders sporadically, and 15 percent of adults have severe insomnia. Women, elderly patients, and patients with other medical or psychiatric conditions are at higher risk. Women experience a higher prevalence of insomnia across the life span, with increased risk during pregnancy, perimenopause, and menopause. Most patients do not seek treatment or talk to their health care providers about the problems they have sleeping, even though untreated sleep disorders have significant impact on mental health and physical well-being. All too often, patients self-medicate with alcohol and OTC remedies, which leads to an increased risk for substance abuse and dependence. Treatment of sleep disorders and underlying problems can improve patients' physical and mental health, overall sense of well-being, and quality of life. Behavioral therapy and lifestyle modification should always be a part of the treatment for insomnia. The availability of newer benzodiazepine receptor agonists has established a new treatment paradigm for insomnia, and the FDA has approved eszopiclone (Lunesta), zolpidem (Ambien) extended release, and ramelteon (Rozerem) without limiting the duration of treatment, thereby broadening the scope of insomnia management.

Nonbenzodiazepine hypnotics have robust efficacy and a low risk of daytime somnolence and low development of tolerance. Medications in this new class of sedative hypnotics are safer than older compounds such as benzodiazepines and sedating TCAs and antihistamines. Treatment of sleep disorders including insomnia, RLS, narcolepsy, and apnea require ongoing evaluation and follow-up to assess the effectiveness of therapy and response to treatment. PCPs are critical in alleviating the problems of sleep disorders in their patients, and they must consistently maintain their knowledge and expertise in treating these serious health problems in order to maximize the health and well-being of their patients.

Resources for Providers

Sleep Diary: *www.nhlbi.nih.gov/health/public/sleep/starslp/teachers/sleep_diary.htm*

Two Week Sleep Diary: *www.sleepeducation.com/pdf/sleepdiary.pdf*

References

American Psychiatric Association. (2000). Sleep disorders. In *Diagnostic and statistical manual of mental disorders* (Revised 4th ed., pp. 599–604). Washington, DC: Author.

Becker, P. M. (2005). Pharmacologic and nonpharmacologic treatments of insomnia. *Neurologic Clinics, 23,* 1149–1163.

Bjoeklund, C., Bengtssom, C., Lissner, L., et al. (2002). Women's sleep: Longitudinal changes and secular trends in a 24-year perspective. Results of the populations study of women in Gothenburg, Sweden. *Sleep, 25,* 894–896.

Breslau, N., Roth, T., Rosenthal, L., et al. (1996). Sleep disturbance and psychiatric disorders: A longitudinal epidemiological study of young adults. *Biological Psychiatry, 39,* 411–418.

Collier, E., Skitt, G., & Cutts, H. (2003). A study of the experience of insomnia in a psychiatric inpatient population. *Journal of Psychiatric Mental Health Nursing, 10,* 697–704.

Connor, J. R., Boyer, P. J., Menzies, S. L., et al. (2003). Neuropathological examination suggests impaired brain iron acquisition in restless legs syndrome. *Neurology, 61*, 304–309.

Diagnostic Classification Steering Committee. (1990). *International classification of sleep disorders: Diagnostic and coding manual.* Rochester, MN: American Sleep Disorders Association.

Drake, C. I., Roehrs, T. A., Richardson, G. A., et al. (2002). Epidemiology and morbidity of excessive daytime sleepiness. *Sleep, 25*(Suppl), A91.

Du, L., Bakish, D., Ravindran A., et al. (2004). MAO-A gene polymorphisms are associated with major depression and sleep disturbance in males. *Neuroreport, 15*, 2097–2101.

Foley D. J., Monjan A. A., Brown, S. L., et al. (1995). Sleep complaints among elderly persons: An epidemiologic study of three communities. *Sleep, 18*, 425–432.

Hauri, P. J. (1998). Insomnia. *Clinics in Chest Medicine, 19*(1), 157–168.

Hening, W., Walters, A. S., Allen, R. P., et al. (2004). Impact diagnosis and treatment of restless legs syndrome (RLS) in a primary care population: The REST (RLS epidemiology, symptoms and treatment) primary care study. *Sleep, 5*, 237–246.

Ho, A. P., Gillin, J. C., Buchsbaum, M. S., et al. (1996). Brain glucose metabolism during non-rapid eye movement sleep in major depression. A positron emission tomography study. *Archives of General Psychiatry, 53*, 645–652.

Jochelson, P., Scharf, M., & Roth, T. (2004). Efficacy of indiplon in inducing and maintaining sleep in patients with chronic sleep maintenance insomnia. *Sleep*, 27 (Suppl), A262.

Krystal, A. D. (2004). Depression and insomnia in women. *Clinical Cornerstone, 6*(Suppl 1), S19–S28.

Luisi, A. F., & Pawasauskas, J. E. (2003). Treatment of premenstrual dysphoric disorder with selective serotonin reuptake inhibitors. *Pharmacotherapy, 23*, 1131–1140.

Manber, R., & Armitage, R. (1999). Sex, steroids and sleep: A review. *Sleep, 22*, 540–555.

Mauri, M. (1990). Sleep and the reproductive cycle: A review. *Health Care for Women International, 11*, 409–421.

McCall, W. V., Reboussin, B. A., & Cohen, W. (2000). Subjective measurement of insomnia and quality of life in depressed inpatients. *Journal of Sleep Research, 9*, 43–48.

Mindell, J. A., & Jacobson, B. J. (2000). Sleep disturbance during pregnancy. *Journal of Obstetric, Gynecologic, and Neonatal Nursing, 29*, 590–597.

Moline, M. L., Brock, L., & Zack, R. (2004). Sleep in women across the life cycle from adulthood through menopause. *Medical Clinics of North America, 88*, 705–736.

Morgenthaler, T., Kramer, M., Alessi, C., et al. (2007). Practice parameters for the psychological and behavioral treatment of insomnia: An update. An American Academy of Sleep Medicine Report. *Sleep, 29*, 1415–1419.

National Institutes of Health. (2005). National Institutes of Health state-of-the-science conference statement on manifestations and management of chronic insomnia in adults, June 13-15, 2005. *Sleep, 28*, 1049–1057.

National Sleep Foundation. (2006). 2005 Sleep in America poll: Summary of findings. Washington, DC: Author. Retrieved July 1, 2008, from *http://www.sleepfoundation.org/site/c.hulXK;M01xF/b.2419039/k.14E4/2005_sleep_in_America_Poll.htm.*

National Sleep Foundation. (2007). *Melatonin: The basic facts*. Retrieved July 1, 2008, from *http://www.sleepfoundation.org/site/c.hulXK;M01xF/b.2421201/k.5FF7/Melatonin_The_Basic_Facts.htm.*

Nofzinger, E. A., Nichols, T. E., Meltzer, C. C., et al. (1999). Changes in forebrain function from waking to REM sleep in depression: Preliminary analysis of [18]FDG PET studies. *Psychiatry Research, 91*, 59–78.

Nowell, P. D., & Buysse, D. J. (2001). Treatment of insomnia in patients with mood disorders. *Depression and Anxiety, 14*, 7–18.

Owen, J. F., & Matthews, K. A. (1998). Sleep disturbance in healthy middle-aged women. *Maturitas, 30*, 41–50.

Perlis, M, McCall, W. V., Krystal, A. D., et al. (2004). Long-term, non-nightly administration of zolpidem in the treatment of patients with primary insomnia. *Journal of Clinical Psychiatry, 65*, 1128–1137.

Piccinelli, M., & Wilkinson, G. (2000). Gender differences in depression: Critical review. *British Journal of Psychiatry, 177*, 486–492.

Ringdahl, E. N., Pereira, S. L., Delzell, J. E. (2004). Treatment of primary insomnia. *Journal of the American Board of Family Practice, 17(3)*, 212–219.

Roth, T. (2001). The relationship of psychiatric diseases and insomnia. *International Journal of Clinical Practice, 49*(116), 3–8.

Roth, T., & Ancoli-Isreal, S. (1999). Daytime consequences and correlates of insomnia in the United States: Results of the Sleep Foundation Survey. II. *Sleep, 22*(Suppl 2), S354–S358.

Santiago, J. R., Nolledo, M. S., Kinzler, W., et al. (2001). Sleep and sleep disorders in pregnancy. *Annals of Internal Medicine, 134*, 396–408.

Saper, C. B., Cano, G., & Scammell, T. E. (2005). Homeostatic, circadian, and emotional regulation of sleep. *Journal of Comparative Neurology, 493*, 92–98.

Spielman, A. J., Caruso, L. S., & Glovinsky, P. B. (1987). A behavioral perspective on insomnia treatment. *Psychiatric Clinics of North America, 10*(4), 541–553.

Theorell-Haglow, J., Lindberg, E., & Janson, C. (2006). What are the important risk factors for daytime sleepiness and fatigue in women? *Sleep, 29*, 751–757.

Verster, J. C., Volkerts, E. R., Schreuder, A. H., et al. (2002). Residual effects of middle-of-the-night administration of zaleplon and zolpidem on driving ability, memory functions, and psychomotor performance. *Journal of Clinical Psychopharmacology, 22*(6), 576–583.

Voderholzer, U., Al-Shajlawi, A, Weske, G., et al. (2003). Are there gender differences in objective and subjective sleep measures? A study of insomniacs and healthy controls. *Depression and Anxiety, 17*(3), 162–172.

Walsh, J. K. (2006). Insights into the public health burden of insomnia. *Sleep, 29*(2), 142–143.

Walsh, J. K., Vogel, G. W., Scharf, M., et al. (2000). A five week, polysomnographic assessment of zaleplon 10 mg for the treatment of primary insomnia. *Sleep Medicine, 1*(1), 41–49.

Zammit, G., Gillin, J. C., McNabb, L., et al. (2003). Eszopiclone, a novel nonbenzodiazepine. *Sleep Abstract Supplement, 26*, A297.

Janet Baiardi
Peter Wolf

chapter 15

Loss and Bereavement

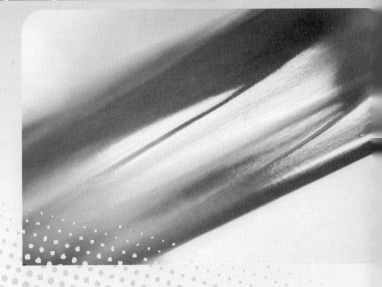

Loss and bereavement due to death is an inevitable human experience that occurs in the life of almost every patient, yet many primary care providers (PCPs) are uncomfortable with and limited in intervening effectively. For the most part, dealing with grief has remained outside of the practice of medicine (Casarett, Kutner, and Abraham, 2001). Death of a loved one presents unique qualities in comparison to other losses such as loss of job, separation in divorce, and loss of physical capabilities. Death's irreversibility changes the meaning and purpose of the survivor's life routines and calls for specialized grief assessment and intervention. The focus of this chapter is on loss and bereavement and, more specifically, how the PCP can effectively intervene with clients who have experienced a loss through death.

BEREAVEMENT, GRIEF, AND MOURNING

There are multiple terms in the literature used to describe the associated sequelae to loss. The terms *bereavement*, *grief*, and *mourning* are often used interchangeably, and although they are associated, there are some conceptual distinctions. Bereavement occurs from loss or deprivation of a significant other (Stroebe, Stroebe, and Hanson, 1993) and causes a physical and emotional reaction that can be termed *grief*. *Grief* is the subjective experience of bereavement. Mourning is the culturally determined set of customs and mores surrounding grief (Bowlby, 1960). For the PCP, bereavement is often a catalyst for seeking treatment, since the symptoms of bereavement manifest in various forms, one of those being somatic complaints.

The burden of cost attached to loss and bereavement is noteworthy. James and Friedman (2003) found that the death of a significant other has the most profound effect on work, with the estimated loss of productivity to employers at $37.5 billion per year. Much of that impact was related to two issues: caregiving, which often affects a significant period of time before the death, and the long-term consequences of the loss, which extend beyond the immediate period surrounding the death. Thus, bereavement, including the physical and emotional consequences, has the potential to impact the workplace both before and long after the loss.

The likelihood of a PCP directly or indirectly encountering medical issues rooted in bereavement occurs perhaps more frequently than thought—or desired. For example, the elderly bereaved are more likely to visit their PCPs after a loss since there is an increase in health consequences, including mortality (Schum, Lyness, and King, 2005; Williams, 2005). Due to various complex reactions to and outcomes of loss, the PCP must be able to accurately assess and diagnose bereavement-related issues. The skills necessary include understanding the influence of gender and culture, identifying the signs and symptoms of bereavement, recognizing complicated grief (CG), and providing treatment options including referral to specialized services when needed.

Even though the specific bereavement responses to death are unpredictable, there are significant distinctions between an unexpected death and an expected death. Sudden death decreases time to prepare, making closure less attainable and particularly difficult (Carr, House, Wortman, et al., 2001). Anticipated death allows time to prepare for the death, yet the long-term stress on caregivers and families can add to the potential of somatic responses. Persons who experience an unexpected death appear to have more difficulty coping (Burton, Haley, and Small, 2006), although there is a great deal of variability in coping and much of the research fails to account for the predeath experience. In their longitudinal study, Burton, Haley, and Small noted survivor resilience across multiple domains of bereavement. Unexpected death was the significant predictor in outcome, particularly for depression. Highly stressed caregivers were prone to social isolation.

INFLUENCE OF GENDER

The connection of gender with grief is rooted in the historical writings of philosophers and lived out in the traditional behaviors and roles of women in the ritual of grief (Secomb, 1999). Women live longer than men and are likely to become widowed and remain widowed (Carr and Ha, 2006). Additionally, women assume multiple social roles, including caregiver, nurturer, and survivor, and historically, women have assumed the role of mourning.

The crisis of loss for women challenges basic learned perspectives that were formed as a part of life with the deceased. Knowing others shapes self-image. Throughout our life, we develop relationships with others, some of which are so intimate that the identity becomes one. Death disrupts relationships and one's meaning, and purpose in life needs to be redefined. Grieving involves reconstructing and rebuilding personal meaning in one's life (Danforth and Glass, 2001).

There is a significant body of literature regarding gender differences in grief that has been inconsistent and challenged (Carr and Ha, 2006). Early research indicated that men suffered greater health consequences from bereavement than women (Stroebe, Stroebe, and Schut, 2001). Skidmore

(1999–2000) examined levels of grief in men and women who experienced the death of a child and found that women experienced more grief than men. In a study of older married and widowed persons, Lee, DeMaris, Bavin, et al. (2001) found that depressive symptomatology was higher in widowed men, but this finding was confounded because married women have higher levels of depression than married men. In contrast, Chen, Bierhals, Prigerson, et al. (1999) found that widows were more likely to experience traumatic grief, depression, and anxiety than widowers.

The inconsistencies related to research findings have been largely due to methodologic issues, which include the lack of longitudinal data, failure to examine the interactional effects of variables, and predisposing gender differences in physical and mental health.

Even though death is unique to each person, men and women approach grief differently. Stroebe, Stroebe, and Schut (2001) conducted an exhaustive review of the literature on gender differences in bereavement. While adjustment to bereavement has often been attributed to levels of social support, they discovered that the difference in adjustment may be more aptly explained by differences in coping styles. Women are more likely to utilize coping strategies that are emotionally expressive and confront their grief. On the other hand, men tend to employ more problem-focused coping strategies. They propose a nonlinear model of bereavement recovery where different coping styles may be more effective at different times.

Women experience the redefining of themselves differently. Gender influences emotional and health outcomes, including reframing purpose in life, processing of emotions, adjusting to being alone, and newly established life routines (Danforth and Glass, 2001). Redefining a woman's purpose in life after the death of a loved one is an all-consuming task. A lack of confidence, increased sense of vulnerability, and detachment can be precipitated by death of a loved one.

A search to regain a sense of equilibrium between self and the world includes gender-specific stressors such as limited financial security and unequal employment, which impact the process of attaining equilibrium. In contrast, women typically experience greater social support networks, including familial support and friendships in addition to a greater sense of spirituality (Carr and Ha, 2006; Falkenstein, 2004; Stroebe et al., 2001).

Secomb (1999) argues that women experience the dying process inherently within life rather than at some future time or event. Therefore, a woman's experience of grief becomes intensely closer and aptly more integrated into her womanhood. The journey a woman shares with the deceased unites her with the other in an experience of her own mortality. Thus, women understand the importance of being with the dying as well as those grieving because of her interconnectedness with others' grief and past experiences of death.

INFLUENCE OF CULTURE

For the PCP to assess and intervene effectively with the bereaved, it is necessary to have a cultural understanding of grief symptoms and mourning practices. The PCP should strive to understand the influence of culture on behaviors (Rosenblatt, 1993). Knowing ethnic and cultural backgrounds does not provide conclusive information about another's cultural perception of death (Gallagher-Thompson, Dillinger, Gray, et al., 2006), so the clinician needs to listen attentively to cultural influences as described by the client.

According to Penderhughes (1989), practitioners develop certain abilities that enhance their work with patients. Culturally sensitive practitioners feel comfortable with various grief responses, appreciate cultural differences, and sort out cultural inaccuracies. Not all behaviors or symptoms are culturally connected; therefore, a PCP with cultural awareness assesses how the behavior fits within the normal grief responses or other psychological conflicts within the person. There has been very little research that has examined cultural variations in response to grief and adjustment (Carr and Ha, 2006). The following section provides some examples of grief perceptions and mourning practices in various cultures. It is important to note that some practices and beliefs may be seen across many cultures; however, you may also see differences in practice within a particular culture.

In the black family, the role of mother is that of sustaining family life by fulfilling the basic needs of survival for children and members of the broader kinship network (Smith, 2002). Prevalent in the black community is the self-perpetuating myth telling individuals that to be strong means refusing to express emotions in an effort to protect those who are dependent (Churn, 2003; Smith). Recognition of this pivotal role and function in the family helps the PCP to understand the difficulty of verbalizing a grief response, as this insinuates weakness (Churn). For black women, extensive social networks and connection to a faith-based community may provide a positive resource to support bereavement.

Expressions of grief in the Hispanic community involve both festive jubilation based in religious belief of the afterlife and intense emotions of sadness due to the void of a significant relationship. The strong Hispanic faith-based belief in the afterlife may create simultaneous feelings of joy and sadness: joy and excitement for the deceased who will join deceased ancestors and sadness about the absence of the loved one (Gallagher-Thompson et al., 2006).

For some cultures, there is no separation between religious beliefs and human affairs. The Native American community perceives grief as a process of achieving balance with nature (Cox, 2005). The ritual of grief is demonstrated by bringing to the grave an object that honors the deceased's life on earth. For example, a woman's grave might have food or clothing, representing her role in the community. Other cultures, such as the Muslim community, exhibit the value of close family bonding especially at the time of death and grieving (Riad, 2005). The community responds immediately with the washing and wrapping of the body as well as with prayers for the forgiveness of the deceased's sins.

Death and grief within the Jewish community is viewed as the body's journey home. Rituals like body washing, shrouding, and using a wooden coffin remind those who grieve of the simplicity of the human body. Those who grieve will be surrounded by the community for 7 days, a tradition called *shiva*, which in Hebrew means "seven" (Cytron, 1993). Not all those who mourn will have completed the grief experience at the end of shiva. In fact, some who continue to feel the loss of a loved one might feel guilt as a result of a continued need to grieve.

Understanding the cultural strengths and assets that influence grief responses of patients is achieved by stepping out of one's own culture and presuppositions (Rosenblatt, 1993). Culturally sensitive knowledge applies to assessing symptoms, strategizing treatment plans, evaluating outcomes, and implementing interventions. Understanding cultural perceptions of death provides the PCP with an informed and insightful response to the patient's needs.

RELATIONAL NATURE OF THE LOSS

The nature of the relationship with the deceased will impact the nature of bereavement. The loss of a child can challenge the core meaning of life itself, as often the child is perceived as an extension of oneself, therefore causing parents to question their purpose and role within the family system. Death of a spouse or partner surfaces identity needs and the task of reframing purpose, recreating life goals, and coping with loneliness. The death of a parent ruptures the attachment and security so essential in achieving developmental milestones, and the death of a sibling shifts birth order and the role within the family system. The following section describes various relational losses in more detail.

Perinatal Loss

Perinatal loss refers to the loss of a child at any time during the pregnancy or the immediate time after birth. It is estimated that approximately 20 percent of all pregnancies result in a loss (Neugebauer and Ritscher, 2005). Perinatal loss is recognized as a significant life event with an associated bereavement (Keefe-Cooperman, 2004–2005).

The experience of perinatal loss has been described as a period of "silence" (Hazen, 2006), an obstetrical event (Neugebauer and Ritscher, 2005), and as medical "objectification" (Jonas-Simpson and McMahon, 2005). Perinatal loss has been considered a taboo subject and, subsequently, not accorded the same rituals of mourning as other types of losses. The reasons for this are varied. From a historically social perspective, miscarriage and stillbirth were described as frequent occurrences throughout history, and the absence of mourning was a socially adaptive mechanism that fell short of providing sufficient bereavement support (Payne, Horn, and Relf, 1999). Another reason for the lack of recognition of a perinatal loss and its associated bereavement is based on Bowlby's (1980) attachment theory. This interpretation of the theory assumes that the attachment between the mother and lost child is not very strong, as the attachment represents a future relationship. To the contrary, research evidence has suggested that there is indeed a relational entity between the mother and child (Neugebauer and Ritscher; Uren and Wastell, 2002). Recognition of perinatal loss and bereavement became evident in the early 1980s with the advent of birthing rooms and more holistic and inclusive birthing practices.

Grief associated with perinatal loss occurs separately and distinctly from depression (Neugebauer and Ritscher, 2005). The nature and intensity of the grief are related to the social context (Hazen, 2003), and there is a concomitant social isolation related to the inability to openly express grief (Uren and Wastell, 2002). Jonas-Simpson and McMahon (2005) describe the language used when discussing the perinatal loss as objectifying the experience and negating the humanhood of the loss, thereby intensifying the suffering. Women need to be provided with opportunities to find meaningful work and connect with their social environments to support the healing process (Hazen).

The death of a child confronts a parent—especially a mother—with the loss of what has been a part of her since conception, not only in the person but in her dreams for the child's future. The child's death leaves an emotional void in the mother's life, ruptures the continuity of generations, and steals the anticipated hopes for the child's future (Payne et al., 1999). The surviving siblings and the potential children in the mother's future cannot replace the deceased child (Worden, 2002).

The devastating loss of a child, regardless of the age of the child, lingers for years. Women are more likely to withdraw and experience depression due to the loss (Lang, Gottlieb, and Amsel, 1996). The grief associated with the loss of a child appears to be more intense and different from normal grief. Kamm and Vandenberg (2001) describe the grief as similar to CG, although it is not a pathologic grief response. The median time of unresolved grief for a parent of a deceased child is 5 years due to the intense and difficult process of grieving (Schatz, 1986). Overwhelming and intense emotional flooding recurs on a routine basis, with little relief beyond the normal 12-month period.

A woman's identity as a mother is personally and socially that of protector, haven of safety, and teacher of basic emotional and physical survival skills. The societal belief that children should not die before their parents increases the possibility of a mother experiencing feelings of guilt and inadequacy.

Worden (2002) points out that when a child dies, the parents gravitate to blame. The person most likely to experience the blame is the mother, who becomes the scapegoat for the death of the child. Marital strain, discord, and social isolation are often consequences of the loss of a child (Kamm and Vandenberg, 2001), although there is no conclusive evidence that divorce rates are influenced by parental grief (Worden).

Women express more value in open discussion of their feelings and struggles with grief than men (Kamm and Vandenberg, 2001; Stroebe et al., 2001). As noted earlier, the ability of women to openly express their grief facilitates resolution (Hazen, 2003).

Loss of a Spouse or Partner

The death of a spouse has been identified as one of the single most stressful life events (Burton et al., 2006; O'Rourke, 2004), and it is estimated that more than 50 percent of women will experience loss of a spouse. Thus, widowhood is primarily a female experience (Charlton, Sheahan, Smith, et al., 2001; Ott, 2003).

Despite the consistent findings that health consequences are greater for men than women (Stroebe et al., 2001), studies have noted that women who lose a spouse are affected by physical and depressive symptomatology. Beem, Maes, Cleiren, et al. (2000) found that widows experienced more psychological dysfunction than nonwidows, including depression, anxiety, somatization, and sleep disorders. Depression is associated with an increase in mortality. Stroebe, Stroebe, and Abakounkin (2005) found suicidal ideation to be higher for widows than widowers and that it was associated with the level of depression and loneliness. Elderly surviving spouses are at greater risk of mortality in the first 12 months after the spouse's death (Williams, 2005).

Women tend to have wider social networks and greater spirituality (Williams, 2005). It is not clear whether increased social support or networks explains the gender difference in bereavement (Stroebe et al., 2001); it may have some relationship to health outcome. Religious beliefs and spirituality have been found to have positive health effects and facilitate positive adjustment to the loss of a spouse (Crowther, Schmid, and Allen, 2003). Gamino and Sewell (2004) found that those with positive feelings of recovery and hope had a better adjustment to the loss, reporting lower levels of negative grief and higher levels of personal growth.

There is very little known about the experience of loss and bereavement among lesbian couples (Carr and Ha, 2006). Much of this may be related to the general lack of knowledge regarding lesbian culture. In a recent qualitative study, Bent and Magilvy (2006) examined the experience of lesbian widows. They found that bereaved lesbians encountered unique challenges related to the lack of recognition by health care providers and family. Also, they were confronted with negative support and legal battles that hindered grief resolution.

Loss of a Parent, Sibling, or Friend

The loss of a parent is often anticipated and expected by women. However, the bereavement associated with that loss may intensify depending on if the death was sudden or anticipated and may be related to the caregiving involved. Carr and Ha (2006) indicate that there is little research examining friend and sibling death. The loss of siblings and friends may be particularly distressing to women due to the close personal relationships and bonds they develop.

CHARACTERISTICS OF GRIEF

The grieving process is variable and difficult to predict, but the symptoms of grief surface most intensely during the first 13 months following the death of a loved one. Symptoms of grief and the bereavement process present intense risks such as increased mortality rates; suicide; diagnosed mental health conditions, especially depressive symptoms (Ott, 2003); impaired or inappropriate coping skills such as substance or alcohol abuse (Carr and Ha, 2006); and social maladjustment behaviors (Falkenstein, 2004). The purpose of grief is to restore a sense of order, control, and meaning to life. PCPs must understand the phases, stages, tasks, or manifestations of grief as part of the disorganizing experience of death.

Grief reflects more than an expression of emotions related to the deceased. Death is the singularly nonnegotiable event in life that forces the survivors to restructure and rebuild perception of self and the world (Matthews and Marwit, 2004). Death severs a relationship that will never be regained or reconstructed. The grief associated with loss involves the suffering of the whole person (Morse, 2000). Therefore, the work of grief continues for a lifetime even for those who would be categorized as experiencing normal grief.

Defining terms of grief reactions provides important distinctions for the sake of clarity and awareness. The effects of grief impair both the physical and psychological well-being of the person (Matthews and Marwit, 2004). Human reaction to the death of someone with a significant personal bond, whether a spouse, parent, child, sibling, partner, or close friend not related through familial connections, tends to follow an anticipated pattern of behaviors. The adjustment period following the death involves an evolution of emotions, perceptions, and adjustments described in various concepts of grief stages (Payne et al., 1999). These stages or phases have been identified to provide a sense of direction and measurement of how far the person has progressed through the grieving process. A complete examination of the models of grief is beyond the scope of this chapter but is briefly summarized.

MODELS OF GRIEF

The earliest model of grief was described by Lindemann (1944) and focused primarily on the bereavement associated with disaster. Bowlby (1980) describes four phases of grief: numbness, yearning, despair, and recovery. During these phases, somatic symptoms are evident. During the recovery phase, somatic symptoms subside and relationships redevelop. Successfully working through the phases is essential for mourning.

Many clinicians are familiar with and have utilized Kubler-Ross's (1969) stages of grief to understand the dying process. These stages, described as denial, anger, bargaining, depression, and acceptance, were developed to help dying patients cope, but they have been used by clinicians in bereavement work as well.

Worden (2002) describes grief as a process and describes the tasks of mourning. The bereaved must integrate the loss and resolve emotional attachment for a successful adjustment. The tasks of mourning include acceptance of the reality of the loss, working through the pain of grief, adjusting to the environment without the deceased, and emotionally relocating the deceased to move on with life.

COMPLICATED GRIEF

Deviation from the normal grief process can occur. This deviation has been described as "abnormal grief" or "pathological grief," but several authors cite the negative connotation of those terms and refer to this as CG (Matthews and Marwitt, 2004; Ott, 2003; Payne et al., 1999; Shear, Frank, Houck, et al., 2005). CG is characterized by intrusive grief symptoms that have been described as distinct from other mental health disorders (Box 15.1).

CG reflects intricate elements of our lives that are left unfinished, and the symptoms of CG are exhibited in longing for the deceased and what those individuals meant to our existence (Ott, 2003). Studies indicate that CG is uniquely different in the sense that the etiology is rooted in the loss of a bonded attachment. The severing of the attachment to a safe, stabilizing, and secure source of a person's identity describes a trauma rooted in the history of that person's meaning of the relationship. An even more intense experience of CG is the trauma of detachment from the other as evidenced in mistrust, anger, shock, and guilt.

Box 15.1 • Symptoms of Complicated Grief

- Sense of disbelief
- Intrusive thoughts of the deceased
- Yearning for the deceased
- Anger
- Bitterness
- Preoccupation with the deceased
- Rumination
- Guilt

Adapted from Payne, S., Horn, S., & Relf, M. (1999); Schum, J., Lyness, J., & King, D. A. (2005); Shear, K., Frank, E., Houck, P. R., et al. (2005).

ASSESSMENT

Assessment occurs at every patient encounter. The provider–patient relationship is based on an understanding of the patient's history and source of symptoms to provide appropriate intervention.

Assessing Normal Grief

For the PCP, assessment is an integral aspect of every patient encounter. For the patient who has experienced a loss, the practitioner must be cognizant of those aspects that are associated with a normal grieving process (Box 15.2).

Box 15.2 • Common Signs and Symptoms Associated with Normal Grief

- Fatigue
- Insomnia
- Headaches
- Back pain
- Anorexia and weight loss
- Constipation or diarrhea
- Preoccupation with physical symptoms
- Numbness
- Searching for the deceased
- Impaired concentration
- Anger
- Anxiety
- Sadness
- Guilt
- Dreams of the deceased
- Mood swings

Adapted from Payne, S., Horn, S., & Relf, M. (1999); Kaplan, H., Sadock, B., & Grebb, J. (1994).

Bereavement is a normal occurrence (Schut and Stroebe, 2005), and according to the *Diagnostic and Statistical Manual of Mental Disorders (DSM-IV)*, the duration varies widely and there is no clear consensus on the length of a normal period of bereavement (American Psychiatric Association, 1994; Payne et al., 1999; Stroebe et al., 1993). Generally, however, it tends to span 12 to 13 months. There is also agreement that normal grief work may never truly end but that the bereaved may continue a timeless emotional attachment to the lost loved one (Stroebe et al.).

There are no universal responses to loss, and the response itself is subject to cultural variation. Bereaved individuals experience both physical and psychological responses. Both men and women will feel distress and depression after the death of a loved one. Women generally have higher levels of depression (Stroebe et al., 2001) than men, but widowed men tend to be at higher risk for health consequences.

There are myriad somatic complaints that accompany normal grief. One of the most common presenting complaints is fatigue related (Payne et al., 1999), followed by sleep-related complaints. Other physical complaints include changes in appetite, muscle aches and pains, abdominal fullness, gastrointestinal changes, headaches, and increased susceptibility to infections. During the bereavement period, patients often present with symptoms of psychological distress including sorrow, despair, and overwhelming sadness. Recent studies have demonstrated that the loss of a loved one, either partner or child, increases the risk of mortality (Schum et al., 2005; Schut and Stroebe, 2005; Williams, 2005).

Assessing Complicated Grief

The PCP must be able to distinguish normal grief from more pervasive issues such as CG, major depressive disorder (MDD), and posttraumatic stress disorder (PTSD). Bereaved individuals who experience any of these disorders require additional interventions and referral to a mental health provider.

There has been much debate as to whether CG is distinct from other depressive or traumatic disorders (Lobb & Monterosso, 2006; Ogrodniczuk, Piper, Joyce, et al., 2003; Ott, 2003; Shear et al., 2005). Discussions continue as to whether CG should be included as a separate *DSM-IV* classification (Horowitz, Siegel, Holen, et al., 1997; Lobb and Monterosso; Matthews and Marwit, 2004; Schut and Stroebe, 2005; Shear et al.), and questions remain regarding whether the symptoms of CG overlap with depressive disorder or anxiety (Horowitz et al.).

CG can occur when the grief is prolonged, usually beyond the first year, or when the initial grief process is absent and appears at later time. It is estimated that approximately 20 percent of bereaved individuals experience CG (Lobb and Monterosso, 2006). There is agreement that the symptoms of CG include yearning for the deceased, rumination, painful intrusive memories, preoccupation, and guilt (Ogrodniczuk et al., 2003; Ott, 2003; Shear et al., 2005).

The CG period tends to resurface intense feelings related to separation anxiety and psychological trauma, which is uniquely different from exposure to a traumatic event (Ott, 2003). The trauma of CG involves the redefinition of a person's identity rather than the intrusive memories of survival characterized by PTSD.

The assessment explores not only the person's presenting life situation in light of the death but the pattern of how the person responds to loss in her whole life. Patients with a history of depression are more likely to demonstrate symptoms of depression and grief (Kaplan, Sadock, and Grebb, 1994); however, a patient might be experiencing grief but not presenting with symptoms of depression. Ogrodniczuk, Piper, Joyce, et al. (2003) note that patients might not present with symptoms of depression but will experience symptoms of intense CG.

There are some distinctions among CG, MDD, and PTSD that can assist the PCP during assessment. MDD can be distinguished from CG by the pervasiveness of the sadness and guilt, intensity of the rumination, suicidal ideation, and psychosis (Schum et al., 2005). PTSD is marked by fear (Shear et al., 2005) and nightmares are common, whereas in CG, nightmares are rare and sadness is the hallmark (Table 15.1).

When symptoms of grief are prolonged, distressing, and begin to interfere with daily functioning, the PCP needs to determine whether the patient is experiencing CG, MDD, or some other mental health issue. Shear, Frank, Houck, et al. (2005) indicate that the Inventory of Complicated Grief (Prigerson, Masiejewski, Reynolds, et al., 1995) is a useful tool for assessing CG, but its use has been primarily limited to the research arena. Casarett, Kutner, and Abraham (2001) describe an interview process that utilizes open-ended questions that focus on the recognition, reaction, relinquishment, readjustment, and reinvestment related to the loss; open-ended questions may provide the PCP with the best option to assess for grief (Table 15.2).

TREATMENT OPTIONS

The complexity of grief reflects the complexity of interventions. Numerous research studies indicate that no one intervention approach is preferred over

Table 15.1 • Distinction Among Complicated Grief, Major Depressive Disorder, and Posttraumatic Stress Disorder

Complicated Grief	Major Depressive Disorder	Posttraumatic Stress Disorder
Death of someone significant	*Causative factors:* Biological, genetic, and psychosocial	Exposure to death due to life-threatening situation
Sadness and intense yearning for the deceased	Pervasive sadness	Restricted range of emotions
Guilt by omission or commission	Rumination about failures	—
Self-isolation	Loss of interest in activities	Diminished interest and feelings of detachment
Eating disturbance and physiologic health changes	Change in eating pattern, either increased or decreased	—
Sleep disturbance due to intrusive thoughts about the deceased and missing the deceased	Hyper- or hyposomnia	Difficult staying asleep or falling asleep due to intrusive thoughts and fears about the event
Dreams of deceased are common	—	Nightmares about the trauma event
Anger and bitterness related to the deceased and events surrounding the death	Fatigue and lack of energy	—
Feelings of worthlessness	Morbid preoccupation with worthlessness	—
Difficulty remembering daily routines and making decisions	Inability to focus and make decisions concerning daily tasks	Difficulty concentrating
Wanting to be with the deceased but not suicidal ideation or intent	Suicidal ideation or thoughts of death that are more than a fear of dying	Sense of hopelessness in future careers, life plans, and normal life span
Conversations with the bereaved	Psychosis	Avoids thoughts, feelings, conversations associated with the trauma

Adapted from American Psychiatric Association (1994). Kaplan, H., Sadock, B., & Grebb, J. (1994).; Shear, K., Frank, E., Houck, P. R., et al. (2005); Schum, J., Lyness, J., & King, D. A. (2005); Worden, J. W. (2002).

Table 15.2 • Open-Ended Questions for a Complicated Grief Interview

Grief Response	Desired Outcome	Suggested Questions
Denial, avoidant, repressing feelings	Verbalizing nonthreatening experience Putting patient at ease with difficult topic Establishing permission to choose what to share about her grief	Tell me about the deceased What do you want me to know about your loved one?
Expressing loss of hope and purpose in life	Helping patient reframe meaning of her life Verbalizing life reflections to allow recognition of what has changed as well as what gives hope	How has your life changed since the death of your loved one? How are you different?
Expressing emotional flooding during holidays, birthdays, anniversaries, etc.	Recollecting and re-experiencing the deceased and the relationship Recalling memories to validate the patient's feelings and life story	What did you enjoy doing with your loved one at that time? What does the *(insert event)* mean to you? How can you remember this date, time, event?
Readjusting, reinvesting in the future An emotional relocation and movement onward with life (Worden, 2002)	Establishing an emotional relationship with the deceased that will not impair daily functioning	What has helped you cope with the loss of your loved one? What are your plans for the future (or, more specific, for this year)? What have you learned about yourself?

Adapted from Casarett, D., Kutner, J. S., & Abraham, J. (2001).

another (Forte, Hill, Pazder, et al., 2004). There is limited evidence that social supports for noncomplicated grief will have a buffer impact on the loss experience or facilitate recovery (Stroebe, Zech, Stroebe, et al., 2005). Some studies conclude that the natural grieving process is sufficient for noncomplicated grief (Schut and Stroebe, 2005), but similar studies indicate that as many as 33 percent of bereaved individuals experience CG—and the more complicated the grief, the better chance social interventions will be effective.

For the majority of patients who experience a normal grief experience, grief intervention will occur in the context of the primary care visit (Payne, Jarrett, Wiles, et al., 2002). Interventions for grief often begin prior to the loss itself (Casarett et al., 2001) due to the anticipation of the loss. Anticipatory grief symptoms are learned by assessing the impact of the life-threatening illness on the primary social system (Casarett et al.), and the intervention begins with an open discussion of the patient's prognosis and quality-of-life decisions. This provides options for the patient and family to decide how to grieve and to explore critical end-of-life decision making while the patient is still able to express desired interventions.

If the PCP is present for the death or has the opportunity to intervene immediately following, it is important that she takes the opportunity to openly share in the experience. Casarett, Kutner, and Abraham (2001) state that sitting quietly with the family or actively listening and acknowledging their grief is important. Follow-up over the next year is critical and provides an opportunity to monitor for adverse health consequences, CG, and other mental health disorders.

Following the death event, the person experiences numbness, disbelief, and flooding of emotions to which the most appropriate response is presence with a minimum exchange of words. Remembering details and medical explanations will probably be meaningless; therefore, outlining a simple plan is important and should include a follow-up appointment. Subsequent interventions over the next several months will include noting concerns about observed symptoms of grief, reassuring individuals about the normal process of grief, and assessing coping strategies and support systems (Box 15.3).

Pharmacotherapy during the grief process has some benefit. The use of an antianxiety agent or short-acting sedative during the initial loss may be appropriate (Casarett et al., 2001). Other agents that may be utilized during the grief process include benzodiazepines, selective serotonin reuptake inhibitors, and norepinephrine dopamine reuptake inhibitors such as bupropion (Zyban, Wellbutrin). Warner, Metcalf, and King (2001) found that a short course of low-dose benzodiazepines had neither a positive or negative effect on bereavement during the first 6 months after the loss. Another study (Zisook, Shuchter, Pedrelli, et al., 2001) found the use of bupropion improved grief intensity and depressive symptoms. Overall, studies indicate that pharmacotherapy has a significant benefit on improving symptoms of depression and sleep (Forte et al., 2004).

The efficacy of grief counseling has been debated (Schut and Stroebe, 2005). However, it appears that it may be more efficacious in the treatment of

Box 15.3 • Grief Interventions for the Primary Care Provider

Anticipatory Grief
- Offer support by providing accurate information.
- Create a culturally sensitive end-of-life plan.
- Identify coping strategies.

Acute and Early Grief
- Provide compassionate presence in listening and validating feelings.
- Allow patient to respond to feelings.
- Set a follow-up appointment.
- Help patient to connect somatic symptoms with grief reaction.
- Support the patient's progress through normal grief.
- Offer grief counseling (support groups, individual).
- Consider short-term pharmacotherapy.
- Assess for mental health disorders and suicidal ideation.

Continued and Chronic Grief
- Explore the meaning of anniversaries and holidays that resurface emotional responses.
- Review the finality of the death.
- Assure the patient regarding the variability of the grief reaction.
- Identify unresolved issues or multiple losses that may be impacting the grief reaction.
- Offer grief counseling (support groups, individual).
- Assess for mental health disorders and suicidal ideation.

Complicated Grief
- Review the grief progress, and discuss observations with the patient.
- Strategize realistic goals and outcomes.
- Assess for other mental health disorders and suicidal ideation.
- Make referrals as necessary.
- Consider pharmacotherapy in conjunction with grief therapy.

Adapted from Casarett, D., Kutner, J. S., & Abraham, J. (2001); Payne, S., Jarrett, N., Wiles, R., et al. (2002); Worden, J. W. (2002).

CG (Jordan & Neimeyer, 2003). The use of grief counseling, whether through the use of support groups or more structured individual therapy, should be a mutual decision made between the patient and provider.

If the PCP determines that the individual is experiencing a CG or other mental health disorder, referral may be appropriate. Approaches that the PCP may utilize in conjunction with outside therapy include active listening and maintaining the supportive relationship (Payne et al., 2002). Treatment of MDD and other mental health disorders requires referral to a mental health specialist for further management. The PCP should work collaboratively to provide for the continuous holistic management of the patient.

CONCLUSION

Health care providers experience loss, bereavement, and grief in their personal and professional lives. The care of grieving patients challenges the provider to utilize culturally sensitive assessment and intervention techniques. The challenge of treating death-related symptoms lies in the reality that no one escapes the limits of human mortality. Therefore, caring for the grieving patient contains an element of caring for the provider's own needs to grieve.

This chapter focused on easing the daunting task of providing healing for those experiencing the pain of death. Each grief story presents an opportunity to explore the rich core of a person's identity and to allow the grieving person to be understood. The key to healing lies in the knowledge of the human need for meaning, purpose, and direction in life, particularly after the death of a loved one. By further exploring the field of thanatology, the PCP can continue to offer the patient the necessary support and treatment.

Resources for Providers

TIME: Toolkit of Instruments to Measure End-of-Life Care:
www.chcr.brown.edu/pcoc/toolkit.htm
Funded by the Robert Wood Johnson Foundation and Nathan Cummings Foundation, this toolkit provides a resource of instruments useful in end-of-life care. The purpose is to provide a bibliography to improve the quality of care and quality of life for dying patients and their families.

Resources for Patients

Center for Loss and Life Transition: *http://www.centerforloss.com*
Dedicated to the further understanding of grief

Compassionate Friends: *http://compassionatefriends.com*
Nonprofit self-help organization dedicated to grief support after the death of a child

Dougy Center for Grieving Children and Families: *www.dougy.org*
Provides support for families to share their experiences as they move through the grieving process

Positive Aging Resource Center: *http://positiveaging.org/provider/overview2.html*
Provides mental health resources related to the aged for caregivers, adults, and health practitioners

References

American Psychiatric Association. (1994). *Diagnostic and statistical manual of mental disorders* (4th ed.). Washington, DC: Author.

Beem, E., Maes, S., Cleiren, M., et al. (2000). Psychological functioning of recently bereaved, middle-aged women: The first 13 months. *Psychological Reports, 87*(1), 243–254.

Bent, K. N., & Magilvy, J. K. (2006). When a partner dies: Lesbian widows. *Issues in Mental Health Nursing, 27*, 447–459.

Bowlby, J. (1960). Grief and mourning in infancy and early childhood. *Psychoanalytic Study of the Child, 15*, 9–52.

Bowlby, J. (1980). *Attachment and loss, Vol. 3: Loss, sadness and depression.* New York: Basic Books.

Burton, A. M., Haley, W. E., & Small, B. J. (2006). Bereavement after caregiving or unexpected death: Effects on elderly spouses. *Aging and Mental Health, 10*(3), 319–326.

Carr, D., & Ha, J-H. (2006). Bereavement. In J. Worell & C. D. Goodheart (Eds.), *Handbook of girls' and women's psychological health* (pp. 397–405). Oxford: University Press.

Carr, D., House, J. S., Wortman, C., et al. (2001). Psychological adjustment to sudden and anticipated spousal death among the older widowed. *Journal of Gerontology: Social Sciences, 56B*(4), S237–S248.

Casarett, D., Kutner, J. S., & Abraham, J. (2001). Life after death: A practical approach to grief and bereavement. *Annals of Internal Medicine, 134*, 208–215.

Charlton, R., Sheahan, K., Smith, G., et al. (2001). Spousal bereavement—Implications for health. *Family Practice, 18*(6), 614–618.

Chen, J. H., Bierhals, A. J., Prigerson, H. G., et al. (1999). Gender differences in the effects of bereavement-related psychological distress in health outcomes. *Psychological Medicine, 29*, 367–380.

Churn, A. (2003). *The end is just the beginning.* New York: Random House.

Cox, G. (2005). Views of death in Native America: The Navajo of the Southwest. *Family Therapy Magazine*, 19–23.

Crowther, M., Schmid, B., & Allen, R. (2003). Widowhood and spirituality: Coping responses to bereavement. *Journal of Women and Aging, 15*(2–3), 145–165.

Cytron, B. (1993). To honor the dead and comfort the mourners: Traditions in Judaism. In D. P. Irish, K. F. Lundquist, & V. J. Nelson (Eds.), *Ethnic variations in dying: Diversity in universality* (pp. 113–123). Washington, DC: Taylor & Francis.

Danforth, M. M., & Glass, J. C. (2001). Listen to my words, give meaning to my sorrow: A study in cognitive constructs in middle-age bereaved widows. *Death Studies, 25*, 513–529.

Falkenstein, C. A. (2004). The relationships between spirituality, coping skills, depression, and social support among acutely bereaved individuals. (Doctoral dissertation, Temple University, 2003). *Dissertation Abstracts International, 64*(7-B), 3520.

Forte, A. L., Hill, M., Pazder, R., et al. (2004). Bereavement care interventions: A systematic review. *BMC Palliative Care, 3*(3). Retrieved June 23, 2008, from *http://www.biomedcentral.com/content/pdf/1472-684X-3-3.pdf.*

Gallagher-Thompson, D., Dillinger, J., Gray, H. L., et al. (2006). Women's issues at the end of life. In J. Worell & C. D. Goodheart (Eds.), *Handbook of girls' and women's psychological health* (pp. 406–415). Oxford: University Press.

Gamino, L. A., & Sewell, K. W. (2004). Meaning constructs as predictors of bereavement adjustment: A report from the Scott & White grief study. *Death Studies, 28*, 397–421.

Hazen, M. (2003). Societal and workplace responses to perinatal loss: Disenfranchised grief or healing connection. *Human Relations*, 56(2), 147–166.

Hazen, M. (2006). Silences, perinatal loss, and polyphony: A post modern perspective. *Journal of Organizational Change Management, 19*(2), 237–249.

Horowitz, M. J., Siegel, B., Holen, A., et al. (1997). Diagnostic criteria for complicated grief disorder. *American Journal of Psychiatry, 154*, 904–910.

James, J. W., & Friedman, R. (2003). *The grief index: The hidden annual costs of grief in America's workplace 2003 survey.* Sherman Oaks, CA: The Grief Recovery Institute Educational Foundation Inc. Retrieved June 23, 2008, from *http://www.grief-recovery.com/The_Grief_Index_2003.pdf.*

Jonas-Simpson, C., & McMahon, E. (2005). The language of loss when a baby dies prior to birth: Cocreating human experience. *Nursing Science Quarterly, 18*(2), 124–130.

Jordan, J. R., & Neimeyer, R. A. (2003). Does grief counseling work? *Death Studies, 27*, 765–786.

Kamm, S., & Vandenberg, B. (2001). Grief communication, grief reactions and marital satisfaction in bereaved parents. *Death Studies, 25*, 569–582.

Kaplan, H., Sadock, B., & Grebb, J. (1994). *Kaplan and Sadock's synopsis of psychiatry* (7th ed.). Baltimore, MD: Williams & Wilkins.

Keefe-Cooperman, K. (2004–2005). A comparison of grief as related to miscarriage and termination for fetal abnormality. *Omega: Journal of Death and Dying, 50*, 281–300.

Kubler-Ross, E. (1969). *On death and dying.* New York: Macmillan.

Lang, A., Gottleib, L. N., & Amsel, R. (1996). Predictors of husbands' and wives' grief reactions following infant death: The role of marital intimacy. *Death Studies, 20*, 33–57.

Lee, G., DeMaris, A., Bavin, S., et al. (2001). Gender differences in the depressive effect of widowhood in later life. *Journal of Gerontology: Social Sciences, 56*, S154–S163.

Lindemann, E. (1944). Symptomatology and management of acute grief. *American Journal of Psychiatry, 101*, 141–148.

Lobb, K. L., & Monterosso, A. S. (2006). *A systematic review of the literature on complicated grief.* Commonwealth of Australia: Department of Aging. Retrieved June 23, 2008, from *http://www.aodgp.gov.au/internet/wcms/publishing.nsf/content/7B67B9ESEBBDA29ECA25716B007662BA/$File/grfall.pdf.*

Matthews, L. T., & Marwit, S. J. (2004). Complicated grief and the trend toward cognitive behavioral therapy. *Death Studies, 28*, 849–863.

Morse, J. (2000). Responding to the cues of suffering. *Health Care for Women International, 21*, 1–9.

Neugebauer, R., & Ritscher, J. (2005). Depression and grief following early pregnancy loss. *International Journal of Childbirth Education, 20*(3), 21–24.

Ogrodniczuk, J., Piper, W., Joyce, A., et al. (2003). Differentiating symptoms of complicated grief and depression among psychiatric outpatients. *Canadian Journal of Psychiatry, 48*(2), 87–93. Retrieved June 23, 2008, from *http://ww1.cpa-apc.org:8080/publications/archives/cjp/2003/march/ogrodniczuk.pdf.*

O'Rourke, N., (2004). Cognitive adaptation and women's adjustment to conjugal bereavement. *Journal of Women and Aging, 16*(1–2), 87–104.

Ott, C. (2003). The impact of complicated grief on mental and physical health at various points in the bereavement process. *Death Studies*, 27, 249–272.

Payne, S., Horn, S., & Relf, M. (1999). *Loss and bereavement.* Buckingham: Open University.

Payne, S., Jarrett, N., Wiles, R., et al. (2002). Counselling strategies for bereaved people offered in primary care. *Counselling Psychology Quarterly, 15*, 161–177.

Penderhughes, E. (1989). *Understanding race, ethnicity, and power. The key to efficacy in clinical practice.* New York: Free Press.

Prigerson, H. G., Maciejewski, P. K., Reynolds, C. F., et al. (1995). Inventory of complicated grief: A scale to measure maladaptive symptoms of loss. *Psychiatry Research, 59*(1–2), 65–79.

Riad, S. (2005). Death and dying: The Islamic view. *Family Therapy Magazine*, 25–27.

Rosenblatt, P. C. (1993). Cross cultural variation in the experience, expression and understanding of grief. In D. P. Irish, K. F. Lundquist, & V. J. Nelson (Eds.), *Ethnic variations in dying: Diversity in universality* (pp. 13–19). Washington, DC: Taylor & Francis.

Schatz, B. (1986). Grief of mothers. In T. A. Rando (Ed.), *Parental loss of a child* (pp. 303–314). Champaign, IL: Research Press Company.

Schum, J., Lyness, J. & King, D. A. (2005). Risk factors for complicated grief. *Geriatrics, 60*(4), 18–20, 24.

Schut, H., & Stroebe, M. (2005). Interventions to enhance adaptation to bereavement. *Journal of Palliative Medicine, 8*(Suppl 1), S140–S147.

Secomb, L. (1999). Philosophical deaths and feminine finitude. *Mortality 4*(2), 111–125.

Shear, K., Frank, E., Houck, P. R., et al. (2005). Treatment of complicated grief: A randomized controlled trial. *Journal of the American Medical Association, 293*(21), 2601–2608.

Skidmore, K. V. (1999–2000). Parental bereavement: Levels of grief as affected by gender issues. *Omega: Journal of Death and Dying, 40*(2), 351–372.

Smith, S. H. (2002). "Fret no more my child . . . For I'm all over heaven all day": Religious beliefs in the bereavement of African American middle-aged daughters coping with the death of an elderly mother. *Death Studies, 26*, 309–323.

Stroebe, M. S., Stroebe, W., & Abakounkin, G. (2005). The broken heart: Suicidal ideation in bereavement. *American Journal of Psychiatry, 162*(11), 2178–2180.

Stroebe, M. S., Stroebe, W., & Hanson, R. O. (Eds.). (1993). *Handbook of bereavement.* Cambridge: Cambridge University Press.

Stroebe, M., Stroebe, W., & Schut, H. (2001). Gender differences in adjustment to bereavement: An empirical and theoretical review. *Review of General Psychology, 5*, 62–83.

Stroebe, W., Zech, E., Stroebe, M., et al. (2005). Does social support help in bereavement? *Journal of Social and Clinical Psychology, 24*, 1030–1050.

Uren, T. H., & Wastell, C. A. (2002). Attachment and meaning-making in perinatal bereavement. *Death Studies, 26*, 279–308.

Warner, J., Metcalf, C., & King, M. (2001). Evaluating the use of benzodiazepines following recent bereavement. *British Journal of Psychiatry, 178*, 36–41.

Williams, J. R. (2005). Depression as a mediator between spousal bereavement and mortality from cardiovascular disease: Appreciating and managing the adverse health consequences of depression in the elderly surviving spouse. *Southern Medical Association, 98*(1), 90–95.

Worden, J. W. (2002). *Grief counseling and grief therapy* (3rd ed.). New York: Springer.

Zisook, S., Shuchter, S., Pedrelli, P., et al. (2001). Bupropion sustained release for bereavement: Results of an open trial. *Journal of Clinical Psychiatry, 62*(4), 227–230.

Carol Mallory
Alice Running
Bernadette Longo

chapter 16

Complementary and Alternative Medicine

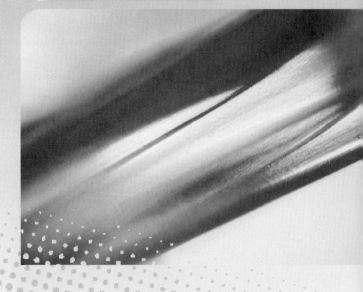

Complementary and alternative medicine (CAM) is a group of practices and products not usually considered part of conventional medicine (National Center for Complementary and Alternative Medicine [NCCAM], 2006). Between 1990 and 1997, users of CAM increased from 33.8 to 42.0 percent of the population, a substantial increase (Eisenberg, Davis, Ettner, et al., 1998), and is likely to continue to increase. Today, at least half of our nation's adult population visits some sort of alternative practitioner each year, exceeding visits made to traditional doctors (Lake, 2007). The many CAM users are college educated and female, who use these modalities in addition to conventional methods (Lake). These women are looking for primary care that includes all methods that are potentially beneficial. Eisenberg, Davis, Etnner, et al. and Unutzer, Klap, Sturm, et al. (2000) reported that most individuals with mental or emotional symptoms use a dual approach to treatment, seeking both conventional and complementary therapies at the same time. Therefore, primary care providers (PCPs) need to be aware of the evidence that exists related to CAM and the potential interactions when combined with conventional approaches to care. PCPs also need to routinely ask patients if they are using CAM modalities, especially botanical and dietary supplements, as 70 percent of women do not tell their clinicians about use of such products (Geller and Studee, 2005). PCPs can work collaboratively with patients to offer the best possible treatments from both CAM and conventional medicine based on individual needs and conditions along with evidence-based practice. If patients and practitioners can work together in this way, patients will be more likely to disclose to the practitioner modalities they previously thought unacceptable.

Although potential interactions between CAM and conventional methods can be dangerous, they can be very effective when used together in a complementary way. In fact, practitioners are moving away from words like *alternative* and instead are using *integrative* and *complementary* to highlight the utility and effectiveness of both modalities. This language brings together the best of conventional and nonconventional (alternative/complementary) methods of care to mental health (Lake, 2007).

As is true with any therapy used in primary care, the limitations and benefits of CAM modalities must be discussed with patients. Women who use herbal products on a day-to-day basis for common symptoms may be under the misconception that the products and other CAM modalities are natural and therefore safe (Geller and Studee, 2005).

Ethnic groups may have different use patterns of CAM modalities. In a study by Lee, Linn, Wrensch, et al. (2000) on women with breast cancer, it was found that whites primarily use nutritional and biologic modalities, Asians primarily use

Table 16.1 • Categories and Modalities for Complementary and Alternative Medicine

Category	Modalities
Alternative systems based	• Homeopathy • Acupuncture • Yoga
Biologic based	• Herbs • Nutritional supplements • Essential oils
Body based	• Massage • Exercise • Light therapy
Mind-Body based	• Biofeedback • Meditation • Relaxation • Music therapy
Energy based	• Therapeutic touch • Healing touch • Reiki

bodywork and herbal preparation, Latinos primarily use nutritional modalities and prayer, and blacks primarily use mind-body modalities (prayer and spirituality).

This chapter will review the five categories of CAM identified by NCCAM (Table 16.1) and includes evidence-based modalities for the treatment of commonly occurring mental health conditions seen in primary care, including depressive and anxiety disorders. For each category, representative modalities will be described, and evidence will be provided for their efficacy.

ALTERNATIVE SYSTEMS–BASED MODALITIES

Three modalities (homeopathy, acupuncture, and yoga) appear to be effective in the treatment of depression and anxiety (Table 16.2).

Homeopathy

Homeopathy, developed by Samuel Hahnemann in the late 1700s, is based on the law of similars—that is, likes cure likes (Steinberg and Beal, 2003). Hahnemann

Table 16.2 • Alternative Systems–Based Modalities

Modality	Interventions	Strength of Evidence*	Recommended Uses	Cautions, Comments
Homeopathy	Depression	Many case reports**	Individual needs determined by trained homeopathic practitioner	Generally too dilute to cause adverse effects. Rare cases of toxicity. Some allergic reactions are noted. Not recommended during pregnancy.
	Anxiety	A few case reports and limited research*	As above	As above
Acupuncture	Depression	Case reports and limited research**	Skilled credible practitioner needed (acupressure can be taught to patients) 30–45 min/wk for 6–8 wk (Freeman et al., 2004)	Caution during pregnancy to avoid uterine stimulation (Motl, 2002). Caution in clotting disorders. Risk of nonsterilized needles.
	Anxiety	**	As above	As above
Yoga	Depression	Large number of medical studies and clinical trials (Massey, 2007)**	Need skilled teacher	Regular practice needed, evolving to a self-directed daily practice (Lake, 2007). Low risk of harm (Massey).
	Anxiety	***	As above	As above

According to Lake (2007):
*Not validated by evidenced-based studies.
**Provisional.
***Substantiated.

believed dilution of a substance increased curative power while decreasing its potential toxicity (Gray, 2000). Immunization is an example that is consistent with the law of similars. Homeopathic remedies, listed in the *Homeopathic Pharmacopoeia of the United States*, are made from plant, animal, and mineral extracts and are available over the counter without a prescription (Steinberg and Beal). It has been difficult to do controlled trials on homeopathic remedies because they are uniquely created for each individual; however, a review of studies done by Linde and Melchart (1998) has shown that homeopathic treatments were on average more effective than placebo.

Homeopathy is compatible with all forms of conventional care. Some conventional medications will reduce the effectiveness of homeopathic remedies, particularly tranquilizers and corticosteroids (Bailey, 2002).

Homeopathic remedies should be treated as medicines, because they can have powerful, energetic effects (Bailey, 2002). Although not backed by controlled studies, low-potency doses are not thought to be harmful even when the remedy is inappropriate. However, this is not the case when the remedies are taken at higher doses (Bailey).

Trained practitioners are needed to determine what is known in homeopathy as the constitution of each client, leading to the correct remedy and potency. Homeopathy is usually safe for children and older adults, but it should not be used during pregnancy (Huebscher and Shuler, 2004).

Depressive disorders can be treated with homeopathic remedies, but this is based on case reports and too few studies (Lake, 2007). In severe and acute major depression, conventional antidepressants should be used first, considering homeopathy when severe symptoms have subsided (Davidson, Morrison, Shore, et al., 1997). Case reports of anxiety disorders successfully treated with homeopathy include social phobia, posttraumatic stress disorder (PTSD), panic attacks, and obsessive-compulsive disorder (Lake).

Acupuncture

It is *believed* that acupuncture stimulates energy channels in the body by way of needles inserted along energetic pathways (Collinge, Wentworth, and Sabo, 2005). Acupuncture is part of traditional Chinese medicine, in which there is a network of energy called *chi* flowing through channels called *meridians* (Mamtani and Cimino, 2002). Needles used in acupuncture may create changes in neurologic mechanisms and a cascade of physiologic events involving the spinal cord, midbrain, and pituitary hypothalamus.

Controlled studies suggest that acupuncture is beneficial for moderate and severe depression (Lake, 2007). More research will soon be available from a 5-year study funded by the National Institutes of Health regarding the efficacy of acupuncture for depression (Huebschner and Shuler, 2004).

Acupressure, where applied pressure can replace needles, can also be effective for depression and is an easy application for patients to learn.

As with depression, there are few studies to substantiate the efficacy of acupuncture for anxiety (Lake, 2007). Motl (2002) suggests that more severe anxiety should be treated with conventional medicine to control symptoms, adding acupuncture and herbs to taper potentially addicting conventional medications. Acupuncture has been used extensively for smoking cessation, but studies suggest that more extensive research is needed (Lake).

Yoga

Yoga has been practiced for more than 5,000 years and includes practice of postures, breathing exercises, and meditation. Several styles of yoga exist. Because patients may be in poor physical condition, PCPs should evaluate each patient's ability to participate.

Yogic breathing and some postures are thought to be beneficial for depression (Lake, 2007). Breathing may decrease depression by vagal nerve stimulation, and breathing and postures create a balance between parasympathetic and sympathetic autonomic tone. Yoga for general anxiety has been substantiated in some studies and anecdotal evidence (Lake). Regular practice results in positive changes in brain activity and reduces serum cortisol, a stress hormone (Lake). There is some evidence that yoga may reduce the need for conventional drugs in patients with general anxiety.

BIOLOGIC-BASED MODALITIES

Herbs are a subset of botanicals and are referred to as *phytomedicines* when they are used to treat disease (Office of Dietary Supplements, 2006). Herbs are identified by the Food and Drug Administration (FDA) as dietary supplements, allowing labels to make "structure and function" claims but no therapeutic or prevention claims (Cass and Cott, 2002). For instance, St. John's wort can claim optimization of mood but cannot claim that it is a natural antidepressant. The World Health Organization (2006) has estimated that 80 percent of the world's population uses herbal medicine.

Herbs are subject to FDA Good Manufacturing Practices, but cases of contamination have been reported. The American Herbal Products Association evaluates manufacturer adherence to high standards.

Herbs can be preferable to pharmaceuticals because they are less likely to cause side effects (Cass and Cott, 2002). When side effects do occur, they are often milder because original plant constituents are more compatible with the chemistry of the human body. Drugs or pharmaceuticals isolate the active ingredient of plants, whereas herbs use the whole plant, relying on the synergistic action of a plant's many constituents. Herbs work to restore balance in the body rather than targeting symptoms, tending to take effect more gradually than pharmaceuticals. Side effects of psychiatric drugs can be serious, including death by overdose. Although overdose or withdrawal is typically not a problem with herbs, patients still need to report side effects so that the herbal preparation can be stopped or the dosage reduced.

Nearly one in five prescription drug users also uses supplements but fails to tell her PCP (Eisenberg et al., 1998). It is essential that providers get a complete drug and herbal history, because some drug–herb combinations work well while others are contraindicated (Cass and Cott, 2002). Box 16.1 contains a questionnaire that can be used to discover the patient's use of CAM. This type of questionnaire lets patients know that their PCP is interested and concerned about the supplements and herbs they may be taking.

Herbs come as teas, tinctures, and, more commonly, tablets and capsules (Cass and Cott, 2002). Each individual has different needs in regard to dosage, but most will fall in the middle range. Starting at the low end and watching for wanted and unwanted responses is advised in adjusting dosage of herbs. Most herbs can safely be used with children, with a good resource being *Smart Medicine for a Healthier Child* (Zand, Walton, and Rountree, 1998).

Treatment Options for Depressive Disorders

Herbs

The most compelling evidence for the use of herbs in the treatment of depression can be found for the herb *Hypericum perforatum* or St. John's wort (Freeman, Helgason, and Hill, 2004). *H. perforatum* is an herb that works as an antidepressant by possibly blocking reuptake of serotonin, norepinephrine, and dopamine (Huebscher and Shuler, 2004). Freeman, Helgason, and Hill and Lake (2007) did extensive literature reviews and found that St. John's wort was as effective as standard antidepressants in current research for mild to moderate depression. St. John's wort may also improve sleep quality in depressed patients.

Box 16.1 • Questionnaire for Current and Past Use of Complementary Modalities

To help us provide comprehensive health care, please provide the following information regarding your use of complementary modalities.

1. Have you used or have you considered using any dietary supplements (vitamins, minerals, amino acids, fatty acids, etc.), herbal preparations, or essential oils in the past?
2. Have you had or have you considered using any body-based therapies, such as massage or light therapy? Do you exercise?
3. Have you had any mind-body type therapy, such as biofeedback? Do you meditate or pray? Do you do any type of relaxation, such as progressive muscle relaxation, guided imagery? What do you do for relaxation?
4. Have you had therapeutic touch, healing touch, Reiki, or any other form of energy therapy?
5. Have you experienced any other type of complementary or alternative therapy?

Lake (2007) recommends a dose of 300 mg tid, which is comparable to conventional antidepressants for moderate depression. Severe depression may need higher doses (1,800 mg/day), and improvement may take several weeks. Side effects include photosensitivity, premature cataract formation, infertility, and neuropathy (Diamond, 2001). Uncommon side effects include upset stomach, restlessness, and mild sedation (Lake). Newborns whose mothers used St. John's wort during pregnancy were found to have increased colic, drowsiness, and lethargy; however, Lee, Minhas, Matsuda, et al. (2003) did not find these conditions in breast-fed infants. Because St. John's wort is similar in action to selective serotonin reuptake inhibitor (SSRI) antidepressants (Diamond) and monoamine oxidase inhibitors (MAOIs) (Lake), it should not be used in conjunction with these drugs. St. John's wort needs to be used with caution in women who are taking oral contraceptives because it can increase the risk of unintended pregnancy by decreasing plasma levels of oral contraceptives. St John's wort may also decrease the effectiveness of hormone replacement therapy (Freeman et al., 2004) and can reduce digoxin levels in healthy people (Diamond).

Nutritional Supplements for Depressive Disorders

The FDA regulates dietary supplements in a manner different from drug products (NCCAM, 2004). The FDA requires drug products to be safe and efficacious prior to marketing, whereas dietary supplements are not subject to premarket approval (NCCAM). Nutritional supplements can be purchased over the counter and online without being prescribed in a formal manner. The FDA is in the process of developing Good Manufacturing Practices for dietary supplements, but until these are in place, companies must follow existing manufacturing requirements for food (NCCAM). Nutritional supplements found to be beneficial for depression include S-adenosyl methionine (SAMe), folic acid and B_{12} (vitamins), 5-hydroxytryptophan (5-http), and omega-3 fatty acids.

S-Adenosyl Methionine. SAMe is a natural substance in the body, and its effectiveness may be due to alleviation of deficiencies (Freeman et al., 2004). Freeman, Helgason, and Hill and Lake (2007) extensively reviewed the literature and found evidence that SAMe is effective for depression, with decreases in postmenopausal depression. The safety of SAMe in breast-feeding and pregnant women has not been established (Freeman et al.).

Dosages of 400 to 1,600 mg/day are comparable to conventional antidepressants, and it is synergistic with folic acid 1 mg, vitamin B_{12}, and conventional antidepressants, accentuating their effects (Lake, 2007). Lower doses of conventional antidepressants can be tried when SAMe is also prescribed (Lake). SAMe has relatively rapid onset, usually 1 week, giving it an advantage over more conventional medicines, which tend to take longer. SAMe needs to be used with caution in patients with certain preexisting conditions or in patients on MAOIs. Patients with cardiac arrhythmias may experience an increase in palpitations, and those with panic attacks may be affected by the stimulating side effects of SAMe. Lastly, because there is insufficient research, patients with type 1 diabetes should be cautioned against using this supplement (Settle, 2002a).

Side effects for SAMe are typically mild and transient and include headache, loose stools or constipation, nausea, vomiting, anxiety, agitation, insomnia, jitteriness, dry mouth, reduced appetite, heart palpitations, sweating, and dizziness. Starting at lower doses and titrating up gradually can help to decrease gastrointestinal (GI) symptoms (Huebscher and Shuler, 2004).

Folic acid and vitamin B_{12} should be taken with SAMe, as they are cofactors in the synthesis of SAMe (Lake, 2007). Bottiglieri, Carnery, Laundy, et al. (2000) found that the severely depressed have low folate levels. Patients with low folate levels do not respond well to antidepressants and therefore should be encouraged to take folic acid (Lake). Folic acid dosages of 0.5 to 1.0 mg/day and vitamin B_{12} 1 mg/day augment conventional antidepressants (Lake), are well tolerated, and are particularly favorable in women (Freeman et al., 2004). Low vitamin B_{12} and E levels are often found in depressed patients, so supplementation may be needed (Lake). In addition, low serum triglycerides and total cholesterol are sometimes found in depressed patients. Diets may need to be modified when patients have total cholesterol lower than 160 mg/dL (Lake).

5-Hydroxytryptophan. 5-HTP is an amino acid precursor of serotonin (Lake, 2007). Amino acids are the building blocks of the neurotransmitter serotonin, which is necessary for improving brain function (Settle, 2002a). Although 5-HTP is not found in foods, it occurs naturally in the body. 5-HTP is easily absorbed and readily available to the brain via the bloodstream. Limited studies have proven the efficacy of 5-HTP for depression (Settle), and data are lacking for use in depression for pregnant, breast-feeding, or perimenopausal women (Freeman et al., 2004).

5-HTP can be as effective as conventional antidepressants at doses of 300 mg/day for moderate depression (Lake, 2007). Although not well studied, starting doses of 50 mg tid are typical, decreasing the dose if nausea develops (Settle, 2002a). Results can be seen in as few as 3 days and typically are seen within 2 weeks. If patients are also taking prescribed antidepressants, the two drugs in combination can potentate each other, so careful assessment is needed. Taking 5-HTP 20 minutes before meals—on an empty stomach—can reduce nausea. The most common side effects of 5-HTP are nausea, heartburn, and GI upset, with the less common side effects being headache, drowsiness, insomnia, palpitations, dry mouth, dizziness, and constipation (Settle).

Adequate B vitamins (especially B_6) are needed for maximum absorption of amino acids (Huebscher and Shuler, 2004). If 5-HTP is combined with other SSRIs, be aware of serotonin syndrome (confusion, shivering, fever, muscle spasms, diarrhea, agitation, increased heart rate), which can be fatal. Safety has not been determined for pregnant or lactating women (Freeman et al., 2004), and 5-HTP is not recommended for bipolar disorders (Huebscher and Shuler).

Omega-3 Fatty Acids. Omega-3 fatty acids are long-chain polyunsaturated fatty acids that are found in fish and some plants (Freeman et al., 2004). Their antidepressant effects are similar to conventional antidepressants (Lake, 2007). Some research has shown a relationship between depression and low-fat diets, suspected to be an omega-3 deficiency (Huebscher and Shuler, 2004).

Overall, omega-3 fatty acids are effective as an adjunctive treatment at 1 to 3 g/day up to 3 g/day as reported in studies reviewed in Freeman, Helgason, and Hill (2004) and are found to be safe for women who are pregnant or breast-feeding. Combined with conventional antidepressants, omega-3 fatty acids may accelerate response time (Lake, 2007). According to Benisek, Shabert, and

Skornik (2000), lactating and pregnant women in the United States have an inadequate intake of omega-3 fatty acids. Omega-3 is essential for normal fetal brain development, and with a deficiency in diets, pregnant women sacrifice their own omega-3 stores, possibly contributing to depression in postpartum periods (Settle, 2002b). Adverse effects (occurring with doses over 3 g/day) include fishy breath, belching, mild nausea, GI upset, possible increased low-density lipoprotein (LDL) and improvement of other lipoproteins, increased bleeding time, exacerbation of asthma in aspirin-sensitive patients, and additive effects with anticoagulants such as aspirin and warfarin (Stoll, 2001). Omega-3 may alter glucose metabolism in diabetics (Lake) by increasing insulin sensitivity and improving glucose tolerance (Pharmacist's Letter/Prescriber's Letter, 2000). Foods with omega-3 include cold-water fish (salmon, tuna, trout, mackerel, sardines, herring, and anchovy), flaxseed oil, and pecans (Huebscher and Shuler, 2004). Omega-3s should be taken with vitamins C 1 g/day and E 800 U/day to reduce oxidative fatty acids damage (Settle).

Treatment Options for Anxiety Disorders

Anxiety is another disorder in which biologic modalities are effective. Psychiatry identifies five categories where anxiety plays a central role:

1. Generalized anxiety disorder
2. Panic disorder
3. Social phobia and other phobias,
4. Obsessive-compulsive disorder
5. Post-traumatic stress disorder (Lake, 2007)

Generalized anxiety is seen most often in primary care and can be any one of the above categories of anxiety. Conventional treatments of anxiety are effective if used in the short term, but those who have longer-term anxiety can become dependent on benzodiazepines, which commonly are used to control anxiety.

Dietary changes are important in the treatment of anxiety and include the avoidance of refined sugar and caffeine and increasing protein and foods containing tryptophan (dairy, eggs, poultry, red meat, soybeans, tofu, and nuts) (Lake, 2007). Along with diet changes, and depending on lab values, supplementation of niacin, vitamins B_6 and E, magnesium, selenium, and phosphorus may also be useful in the reduction of anxiety (Table 16.3).

In addition, there are several biologic modalities effective in the treatment of anxiety, including the use of herbs, nutritional supplements, and some essential oils.

Table 16.3 • Biologic-Based Modalities

Modality	Interventions	Strength of Evidence*	Recommended Uses	Cautions, Comments
Herbs				
St. John's wort	Depression	Compelling evidence from high-quality studies (Lakem 2007)***	For moderate depressed mood, 300 mg tid; for severe depression, up to 1,800 mg/day. Improvement may take several weeks.	Photosynsensitivity, infertility, neuropathy. Do not take with MAOIs or SSRI antidepressants. Caution with HRT and oral contraceptive use. Contraindicated in patients taking immunosuppressive agents (for HIV) and theophylline. Possible serotonin syndrome when used in conjunction with conventional antidepressants (Lake).
Kava Kava	Anxiety	***	70–240 mg/day for stress and moderate anxiety. In menopausal women, 100–200 mg/day to reduce anxiety	Do not use with benzodiazepines. With large doses and long term, may cause dermatitis. May cause liver toxicity (contraindicated for those taking hepatotoxic medications or consuming

(*Continued*)

Table 16.3 • (Continued)

Modality	Interventions	Strength of Evidence*	Recommended Uses	Cautions, Comments
				excess alcohol). Do not use longer than 6–8 wk.
Valerian	Alcohol and substance abuse (anxiety by improving sleep according to Huebscher & Shuler, 2004)	**	400–900 mg up to 2 hr before bed for as long as 28 days or drink as a tea (Huebscher & Shuler).	Impaired alertness (do not drive or operate machinery). Can interact with other sedatives (Huebscher & Shuler).
Nutritional Supplements				
SAMe	Depression	***	400–1,600 mg/day, comparable to conventional antidepressants. Benefits in postpartum and postmenopausal depression. Can use SAMe when beginning a conventional antidepressant to minimize latency period (Schneider & Lovett, 2007)	GI upset (start at lower doses). Caution with cardiac arrhythmias, panic attack, bipolar (stimulating effects), type 1 diabetics (insufficient research). Do not use with MAOIs.
Folic acid B_{12}	Depression	***	0.5–1.0 mg/day folic acid and 1 mg/day vitamin B_{12} in conjunction with SAMe	No adverse effects at recommended doses.

(*Continued*)

Table 16.3 • (Continued)

Modality	Interventions	Strength of Evidence*	Recommended Uses	Cautions, Comments
5-htp	Depression	**	Starting dose 50 mg tid (less if nauseated). Potentiates effects of conventional antidepressants.	Most common side effects are nausea, heartburn, GI upset (take 20 min before meals on an empty stomach). Take doses larger than 100 mg at bedtime due to moderate sedation. Be aware of serotonin syndrome if combined with other SSRIs.
	Anxiety	**	25–100 mg up to tid	As above
Omega-3 fatty acids	Depression	As adjunct***	1–3 g/day. Take with vitamins C 1 g/day and E 800 U/day to reduce oxidative fatty acid damage.	Over 3 g/day: Fishy breath, belching, mild nausea, GI upset, possibly increases LDL, increased bleeding time, exacerbation of asthma in the aspirin sensitive, additive effects with anticoagulants. Alters glucose metabolism in diabetics. Alcohol depletes omega-3.

(Continued)

Table 16.3 • (Continued)

Modality	Interventions	Strength of Evidence*	Recommended Uses	Cautions, Comments
L-theanine	Anxiety	***	50–200 mg/day for moderate anxiety, up to 800 mg/day in divided doses for more severe anxiety (Lake, 2007).	None reported; can be used with conventional or nonconventional biologic treatments (Lake).
Melatonin	Anxiety	No long-term studies done*	2-mg controlled-release may help with benzodiazepine withdrawal.	Side effects include sedation, drowsiness, headache, & depression. Do not drive or operate machinery within 5 hr.
Magnesium	Anxiety	*	200 mg/day	Calming effects enhanced when taken with calcium 400 mg/day.
Essential Oils				
Rosemary	Anxiety	*	A few drops on a tissue inhaled, in bathwater, in massage oil, or in a diffuser	Do not use on patients with hypertension.
Lavender	Anxiety	*	Same as rosemary	Do not use on patients with epilepsy.

According to Lake (2007):
*Not validated by evidence-based studies.
**Provisional.
***Substantiated.

Herbs

Kava Kava. Kava Kava has serotonin blockade abilities and may reduce vagal heart tone in anxious patients (Lake, 2007). Kava Kava has been shown to be more effective than placebo for anxiety in a review of studies done as cited in Lake (2007) and has been compared favorably to benzodiazepines (Cass and Cott, 2002). However, Kava Kava should not be used for severe anxiety or agitation, as it has not been found to be effective. With doses of 60 to 300 mg/day, most patients will not experience reduced cognitive functioning or mental slowing (Lake). Menopausal women can use 100 to 200 mg/day to reduce anxiety. Stress reduction techniques should be considered along with a 3-month trial of Kava Kava (Cass and Cott).

Kava Kava may create psychological dependence but is not physically addicting (Huebscher and Shuler, 2004). However, because Kava Kava is mood altering, there is potential for abuse. A dose of 70 to 240 mg/day has been shown to be as effective as conventional drugs used for generalized anxiety (Lake, 2007). At large doses with long-term use, dermatitis can develop. Kava Kava should not be mixed with alcohol, benzodiazepines, barbiturates, or central nervous system depressants because of its sedating effects. Safety in pregnant and lactating women has not been established. Due to recent cases showing liver toxicity, patients taking other substances that affect the liver should not take Kava Kava. Kava Kava should not be taken longer than 6 to 8 weeks due to the rare but potentially serious risk of liver injury (Geller and Studee, 2005).

Valerian. Valerian has been shown to reduce the severity of benzodiazepine withdrawal by assisting the body to return to a normal sleep pattern (Lake, 2007). Also useful in menopause, doses of 400 to 900 mg can be given up to 2 hours before bed for as long as 28 days (Huebscher and Shuler, 2004).

Nutritional Supplements

L-Theanine. L-theanine is an amino acid found in green tea (Lake, 2007) that has been found effective in the treatment of anxiety. Recent studies have shown that L-theanine enhances alpha brain wave activity, increases gamma-aminobutyric acid (GABA), reduces serotonin, and increases brain levels of dopamine resulting in decreased anxiety. Doses of 50 to 200 mg can last 8 to 10 hours. Moderate anxiety improves with 200 mg 1 to 2 times a day, although severe anxiety can require 600 to 800 mg/day in divided doses. L-theanine does not cause drowsiness, slowed reflexes, impaired concentration, tolerance, or dependence. L-theanine can be combined with conventional synthetic drugs, and there have been no reports of serious side effects.

5-Hydroxytryptophan. The amino acid 5-HTP has been shown to be effective for generalized anxiety. 5-HTP is an essential precursor for serotonin synthesis (Lake, 2007). Serotonin is a neurotransmitter responsible for regulation of mood and anxiety. According to Lake, 5-HTP may be safely combined with conventional antidepressants. If the patient becomes agitated or nervous or has insomnia, this may be due to serotonin syndrome. Starting at the lower doses of 25 mg/day with a gradual increase over several weeks to 100 mg tid can minimize adverse effects. Bedtime doses of up to 400 mg can reduce daytime anxiety, thus improving sleep.

Magnesium. Magnesium has been used commonly to treat anxiety, but there are few studies to substantiate its use (Lake, 2007). Settle (2002a) reported that magnesium deficiencies could prevent tryptophan from increasing brain serotonin. If patients are deficient in magnesium, 200 mg/day may improve anxiety. Effects may be enhanced with the addition of calcium 400 mg/day.

Melatonin. A hormone that comes from the pineal gland and is useful as a sleep aid (Huebscher and Shuler, 2004), melatonin levels are synthesized from tryptophan and serotonin and rise in the evening. Studies have shown that melatonin is effective in decreasing the time it takes to fall asleep as well as increasing total sleep time (Lake, 2007). Limited studies have been done looking at effectiveness in facilitating benzodiazepine discontinuation; however, one study noted that controlled-release melatonin, 2 mg at bedtime, is useful in helping patients discontinue benzodiazepines (Garfinkel, Zisapel, Wainstein, et al., 1999). Dose ranges are from 0.3 mg (to replace normal melatonin levels) up to 3 mg. Melatonin should not be used during the day because of reduced response time with problem solving.

Omega-3 Fatty Acids. In addition to omega-6, omega-3 fatty acids may be helpful in reducing alcohol withdrawal, since chronic alcohol use can deplete omega-3s, thus predisposing to depressed mood (Lake, 2007).

Essential Oils

The essential oils of rosemary and lavender have been found to reduce general anxiety (Lake, 2007) and produce a relaxed alert state. Lavender and rosemary oils can be placed on a tissue and inhaled for effect. Other methods of delivery include placing drops in bathwater, using as massage oil, or placing the oil in a diffuser (Huebscher and Shuler, 2004). Lavender should not be used on patients with epilepsy, while rosemary should not be used in patients with hypertension or asthma (D'Angelo, 2002). If used appropriately, essential oils are considered safe; however, some individuals may exhibit allergies. Appropriate use includes inhalation with a few drops of pure oil in a diffuser, in bath water, or in massage oil. Oils need to be pure without additions or deletions from natural content, and they should be stored in amber bottles away from light to help decrease decomposition (Huebscher and Shuler).

BODY-BASED MODALITIES

Massage Therapy

Massage therapy manipulates muscle and connective tissue, enhancing their function and promoting relaxation. Limited research has shown it to benefit depression as well as reduce stress and anxiety (Lake, 2007). Anxiety is probably reduced by decreasing cortisol and increasing parasympathetic tone. Massage is also beneficial for premenstrual and postpartum depression (Table 16.4).

Massage therapy needs to be regular to gain maximum effectiveness; clients should be encouraged to schedule weekly appointments for an extended period of time. When recommending massage, it is important to remember that some patients may be allergic to the lotions or oils used, and some may not be comfortable with the idea of being touched (Huebscher and Shuler, 2004).

Exercise

Exercise has been shown to reduce depression in numerous studies (Freeman et al., 2004). Sustained exercise increases brain levels of the mood elevators endorphins, dopamine, norepinephrine, and serotonin (Lake, 2007). Length of time varies with age and conditioning, but 30 minutes 3 times a week is considered a standard recommendation. According to Lake, studies have found that exercise can be as beneficial as conventional treatments. One study of older adults found that exercise was equal to or more beneficial than sertraline (Zoloft) (Blumenthal, Babyak, Craighead, et al., 1999). Aerobic exercise and strength training may be equally effective at improving mood (Huebscher and Shuler, 2004) (Table 16.4).

For menopausal women, exercise improves mood and vasomotor symptoms, and it has the added benefit of increasing bone mass (Slaven and Lee, 1997). Regular exercise is beneficial for anxiety and for recovering alcoholics, with as little as 20 to 30 minutes daily significantly reducing symptoms (Lake, 2007). Exercise plans need to start with a physical and cardiovascular workups, especially for those older than 50 years of age.

Table 16.4 • Body-Based Modalities

Modalities	Interventions	Strength of Evidence	Recommended Uses	Cautions, Comments
Massage	Depression (stress reduction)	*	Premenstrual and postpartum depression. Weekly for an extended time, generally weekly for 6–8 wk.	Patients with chronic pain, elderly, or disabilities may need gentle massages.
	Anxiety	Chronic moderate anxiety**	As above	As above
Exercise	Depression	***	30 min 3 times weekly is as effective as conventional antidepressants.	Heart disease, chronic pain, etc., or physically impaired
	Anxiety	**	Regular aerobic exercise or strengthening 20–30 min/day	As above
Light therapy	Depression	***	For SAD, in the morning sitting in front of full-spectrum light (10,000 lux) for 30 min/day	Evening exposure can cause insomnia. Nausea, irritability, headache (sit farther away from the light).

According to Lake (2007):
*Not validated by evidence-based studies.
**Provisional.
***Substantiated.

Light Therapy

Light therapy is known to be effective for depression. The mechanism of action for light is believed to reside in the serotonin neurotransmitter system. Like nonseasonal depression, seasonal affective disorder (SAD), may stem from a dysregulation of the pineal gland due to lack of sunlight (Huebscher and Shuler, 2004). The lack of full-spectrum light received from sunlight results in the dysregulation of hormones, mainly melatonin. Studies have shown that bright light can be as effective as conventional antidepressants for nonseasonal depression (Golden, Gaynes, Ekstrom, et al., 2005). For women who are pregnant or breast-feeding and do not want to take medications, light therapy is a good option (Freeman et al., 2004). Bright light therapy has also been found to be beneficial for premenstrual symptoms, and there is limited evidence that dim light exposure (250 lux daily) may reduce relapse in recovering alcoholics with SAD (Lake, 2007). Evidence shows that sitting in front of 10,000 lux full-spectrum lights in the morning for at least 30 minutes every day can be effective (exposure to light in the evening can result in insomnia; Lake). Possible side effects include nausea, irritability, headache, and eyestrain. To address eyestrain, the patient should sit away from the lights and not look directly at them (Table 16.4).

MIND-BODY MODALITIES

Biofeedback

Biofeedback is a training technique in which patients are taught to use information from their own bodies to improve their health and performance (Association for Applied Psychophysiology and Biofeedback [AAPB], 2006). Biofeedback uses sensors for detecting various physiologic functions, which are converted into a visual or audio signal (Huebscher and Shuler, 2004). Biofeedback modalities include electromyography (EMG), galvanic skin response (GSR), and electroencephalography (EEG). These modalities measure muscle tension (EMG), skin temperature, autonomic nervous tension reflected by stimulation of sweat glands (GSR), and electrical activity in the brain (EEG) (Moss, 2002). Credible practitioners are certified by the AAPB.

In general, biofeedback is beneficial for stress reduction, which is a known precursor to many diseases, including mental health disorders (Moss, 2002). Biofeedback is a safe alternative to medications; however, because biofeedback modifies body functions, PCPs must work closely with therapists for people with chronic illness. Potential barriers to the use of biofeedback may include dementia, mental retardation, certain medical disorders, or personality disorders.

Biofeedback is effective for depression, in particular EEG biofeedback (Lake, 2007), but the mechanism of action is unknown. EMG, GSR, and EEG biofeedback are beneficial for reducing anxiety, and the treatment effects can be similar to anxiety medication. Multiple studies document the effectiveness of biofeedback for anxiety, but the treatment is typically longer than usual (Table 16.5).

Table 16.5 • Mind-Body Modalities

Modalities	Interventions	Strength of Evidence	Recommended Uses	Cautions, Comments
Biofeedback	Depression	EEG **	Number of sessions determined by biofeedback practitioner and patient	Treatments highly individualized. Long-term effects may not be maintained.
	Anxiety	EEG, EMG, GSR, and thermal***	As above	As above
Meditation	Anxiety	***	Mindfulness training, ideally 2 times daily for 15 min. Focus on breath 5–30 min/day.	Reduces the symptoms of chronic anxiety, including irritable bowel syndrome
Relaxation	Depression	*	Guided imagery combined with antidepressants	Greater improvements than with conventional medications alone (Lake, 2007)
	Anxiety	***	Progressive muscle relaxation	Reduces muscle tension
	Benzodiazepine withdrawal	*	Practicing on a regular basis deep breathing and guided imagery	As above
Music therapy	Depression	**	Daily routines best	Positive and negative depending on culture and preferences (Lake)
	Anxiety	Most studies combined with relaxation techniques (Lake)**	Regular listening	Better without distractions. Encourage anxious patients to become absorbed in music.

According to Lake (2007):
*Not validated by evidence-based studies.
**Provisional.
***Substantiated.

Meditation

Meditation, a self-regulatory technique, is a state of inward attention on an object, breath, mantra, or thought process (Fortney and Bonus, 2007). Relaxation and concentration are the foundations of meditation (Lowenstein, 2002). Many studies have been done using meditation as a treatment for anxiety (Lake, 2007). Beneficial effects include decreased oxygen consumption, decreased respiratory rate and blood pressure, and decreased autonomic arousal. Studies in self-regulatory techniques have shown meditation to be effective in psychosomatic illness, pain disorders, PTSD, attention deficit disorder, substance abuse, anxiety disorder, and obsessive-compulsive disorder. Once learned, meditation can be used throughout the life span (Lowenstein).

Mindfulness meditation, developed by Kabat-Zinn (1990), has been shown to decrease chronic stress. Mindfulness meditation involves observing thoughts from a detached state of mind, which increases self-awareness (Lake, 2007). Relapse prevention programs for alcohol and drug abuse offer mindfulness and meditation training.

Meditation is safe and compatible with conventional medicine (Lowenstein, 2002). Patients can be taught to meditate by focusing on breathing 5 to 30 minutes/day (Huebscher and Shuler, 2004). Ideally, meditation should be practiced twice a day for 15 minutes (Lowenstein). Anyone with a sincere intent can meditate (Table 16.5).

Relaxation Techniques

Relaxation techniques include such modalities as progressive muscle relaxation, imagery, and sustained deep breathing (Lake, 2007) (Table 16.5). Relaxation techniques have been substantiated in the treatment of anxiety, and guided imagery is often used for depressed mood. One study on postpartum women diagnosed with depression and anxiety showed significant reductions in both anxiety and depressed mood when relaxation and guided imagery were combined (Rees, 1995).

Imagery uses words that can create a picture in the subject's mind using the five senses (sight, touch, smell, hearing, and taste) (Rossman, 2007). Guided imagery refers to being guided by another voice to create a sense of relaxation. Some imagery scripts involve visualizing physiologic changes that occur with anxiety and relaxation, and other scripts create an inner sense of calm and safety (Huebscher and Shuler, 2004).

Diaphragmatic breathing is an example of a deep-breathing technique, and it is known to reduce anxiety symptoms such as rapid pulse, hyperventilation, and elevated blood pressure. Progressive muscle relaxation involves tensing and releasing each muscle group, holding the tension long enough to feel the tension and then releasing slowly, and noticing the difference between tension and relaxation. Relaxation techniques are effective for mild to moderate anxiety, but they may not be beneficial for patients who hyperventilate or who have panic attacks. Relaxation done regularly has been found to reduce withdrawal symptoms in patients who stop taking conventional sedative-hypnotic medications (Lake, 2007).

Music Therapy

Music therapy has been used for thousands of years in Eastern and Western traditions (Diamond, 2002). Music specifically intended for healing is more effective than music that was not created with that intention (Huebscher and Shuler, 2004). Headphones enhance the experience of soothing music, where the brain can experience binaural sounds (Lake, 2007). Diamond suggests that music therapy needs to be guided by a practitioner, but patients may intuitively listen to music to help them feel better (Lake). Kerr, Walsh, and Marshall (2001) found that patients who had conventional therapy and music therapy had a greater reduction in their anxiety (Table 16.5).

ENERGY MODALITIES

According to NCCAM (2006), energy therapies involve the use of energy fields around the body. Therapeutic touch, healing touch, and Reiki are referred to as biofield energy therapies that affect energy fields thought to surround and penetrate the human body. These therapies affect the biofield by using the hands on the body or the field surrounding the body.

Therapeutic Touch and Healing Touch

Therapeutic touch and healing touch are similar in efficacy and effectiveness (Lake, 2007) (Table 16.6). Multiple studies have been done using both therapeutic and healing touch, but many have design flaws. In a small study evaluating the effectiveness of healing touch and mood (Bradway, 2003), the healing touch patients improved significantly compared with a control group. In both modalities, trained practitioners are required (Bonadonna, 2002).

Table 16.6 • Energy Modalities

Modalities	Interventions	Strength of Evidence	Recommended Uses	Cautions, Comments
Therapeutic touch and healing touch	Depression	**	Regular treatments	Study design flaws. Experienced practitioners are needed.
	Anxiety	*	As above	As above
Reiki	Depression	*	Weekly treatments Weekly treatments	Hands on and distance Reiki For chronically stressed
	Anxiety	**	As above	As above

According to Lake (2007):
*Not validated by evidence-based studies.
**Provisional,
***Substantiated.

Reiki

Reiki has been found to be beneficial for depression and anxiety (Lake, 2007). A limited number of studies have shown a decrease in anxiety in chronically stressed individuals. For patients with anxiety and depression, significant reductions in anxiety were found (Shore, 2004) (Table 16.6).

CONCLUSION

As PCPs more commonly prescribe CAM therapies with an evidence base, their benefits will be further exemplified and proven. This chapter described those modalities found to be useful for the conditions of depression and anxiety. Therapies that have trained and credentialed practitioners should be chosen to assure quality and to know what can be expected in the treatment (Collinge et al., 2005).

Resources for Providers

Association for Applied Psychophysiology and Biofeedback (AAPB): *www.aapb.org*
Facilitates access to a provider directory

Cochrane Collaboration, Complementary Medicine:
www.compmed.umm.edu/cochrane.asp
Complementary and alternative medicine reviews

Healing Touch: *www.healingtouch.net*
Offers a list of qualified practitioners

Holistic Remedies: *www.holisticonline.com/Remedies/depression/dep_acupressure.htm*
Descriptions of specific acupressure points for use in patients with depression

Homeopathic Pharmacopoeia of the United States: www.hpus.com
Official website for standard preparations of homeopathic remedies

Mind Body Institute: *www.mbmi.org/home/*
Information for health professionals—what they treat and mind-body basics

National Center for Complementary and Alternative Medicine (NCCAM): *www.nccam.nih.gov*
National Institutes of Health website with links for research; clinical trials; training; and health information, including acupuncture, depression, homeopathy, dietary supplements, Kava Kava, St. John's wort, and more, with information also available in Spanish

National Center for Homeopathy: *www.homeopathic.org*
Information about homeopathy with links to research, resources, and how to find a homeopath

Natural Medicines, Comprehensive Database: *www.naturaldatabase.com*

Nurse Healers–Professional Associates International (Therapeutic Touch): *www.therapeutic-touch.org*
Offers a list of qualified practitioners

Research Council for Complementary Medicine: *www.rccm.org.uk/cameol/Default.aspx*
Access to summaries on research done on complementary and alternative medicine

Resources for Patients

American Herbal Products Association: *www.ahpa.org*
Herbal information

Complementary and Alternative Medicine, MayoClinic.com: *www.mayoclinic.com/health/alternative-medicine/CM99999*
Information on alternative therapies with links to diseases and conditions, drugs and supplements, and treatment decisions; provides link to answers to patients' questions

Holisticonline.com: *www.holisticonline.com/herb_home.htm*
Offers links to several complementary therapies including self-care

Office of Dietary Supplements: *www.ods.od.nih.gov/index.aspx*
National Institutes of Health website; provides links to health information on dietary supplement use, safety, and research

References

Association for Applied Psychophysiology and Biofeedback (AAPB), an International Society for Mind-Body Interactions. Retrieved November 12, 2006, from *ww.aapb.org*.

Bailey, P. (2002). Homeopathy. In S. Shannon (Ed.), *Handbook of complementary and alternative therapies in mental health* (pp. 402–429). San Francisco, CA: Academic Press.

Benisek, D., Shabert, J., & Skornik, R. (2000). Dietary intake of polyunsaturated fatty acids by pregnant or lactating women in the United States. *Obstetrics and Gynecology, 95*, 77–78.

Blumenthal, J., Babyak, M., Craighead, W., et al. (1999). Effects of exercise training on older patients with major depression. *Archives of Internal Medicine, 159*(19), 2349–2356.

Bonadonna, J. (2002). Therapeutic touch. In S. Shannon (Ed.), *Handbook of complementary and alternative therapies in mental health* (pp. 231–248). San Francisco, CA: Academic Press.

Bottiglieri, T., Carnery, M., Laundy, M., et al. (2000). Homocysteine, folate, methylation, and monoamine metabolism in depression. *Journal of Neurology, Neurosurgery and Psychiatry, 69*(2), 228–232.

Bradway, C. (2003). The effects of healing touch on depression. In *Healing Touch Research Summary*. Healing Touch International/Depression, Retrieved July 5, 2008, from *http://www.healingtouchinternational.org/index.php?option-com_content&task-view&id-88&Itemid-192*

Cass, H., & Cott, J. (2002). Herbal medicine. In S. Shannon (Ed.), *Handbook of complementary and alternative therapies in mental health* (pp. 377–400). San Francisco, CA: Academic Press.

Collinge, W., Wentworth, R., & Sabo, S. (2005). Integrating complementary therapies into community mental health practice: An exploration. *Journal of Alternative and Complementary Medicine, 11*(3), 569–574.

D'Angelo, R. (2002). Aromatherapy. In S. Shannon (Ed.), *Handbook of complementary and alternative therapies in mental health* (pp. 72–92). San Francisco, CA: Academic Press.

Davidson, J., Morrison, R., Shore, J., et al. (1997). Homeopathic treatment of depression and anxiety. *Alternative Therapies in Health Medicine, 3*(1), 46–49.

Diamond, J. (2001). *The clinical practice of complementary, alternative, and Western medicine*. Boca Raton, FL: CRC Press.

Diamond, J. (2002). The therapeutic power of music. In S. Shannon (Ed.), *Handbook of complementary and alternative therapies in mental health* (pp. 517–537). San Francisco, CA: Academic Press.

Eisenberg, D., Davis, R., Ettner, S., et al. (1998). Trends in alternative medicine use in the United States, 1990-1997: Results of a follow-up national survey. *Journal of American Medical Association, 280*(18), 1569–1575.

Fortney, L., & Bonus, K. (2007). Recommending meditation. In D. Rakel (Ed.), *Integrative medicine* (pp. 1051–1064). Philadelphia: WB Saunders.

Freeman, M., Helgason, C., & Hill, R. (2004). Selected integrative medicine treatments for depression: Considerations for women. *Journal of the American Medical Women's Association, 59*, 216–224.

Garfinkel, D., Zisapel, N., Wainstein, J., et al. (1999). Facilitation of benzodiazepine discontinuation by melatonin. *Archives of Internal Medicine, 159*, 2456.

Geller, S., & Studee, L. (2005). Botanical and dietary supplements for menopausal symptoms: What works, what does not. *Journal of Women's Health, 14*(7), 634–639.

Golden, R., Gaynes, B., Ekstrom, R., et al. (2005). The efficacy of light therapy in the treatment of mood disorders: A review and meta-analysis of the evidence. *American Journal of Psychiatry, 162*(4), 656–662.

Gray, B. (2000). *Homeopathy: Science or myth?* Berkeley, CA: North Atlantic Books.

Huebscher, R., & Shuler, P. (2004) *Natural, alternative, and complementary health care practices.* St. Louis: Mosby.

Kabat-Zinn, J. (1990). *Full catastrophe living: Using the wisdom of your body and mind to face stress, pain and illness.* New York: Delacorte.

Kerr, T., Walsh, J., & Marshall, A. (2001). Emotional change processes in music-assisted reframing. *Journal of Music Therapy, 38*(3), 193–211.

Lake, J. (2007). *Textbook of integrative mental health care.* New York: Thieme Medical Publishers.

Lee, A., Minhas, R., Matsuda, N., et al. (2003). The safety of St. John's wort (*Hypericum perforatum*) during breastfeeding, *Journal of Clinical Psychiatry, 64,* 966–968.

Lee, M., Lin, S., Wrensch, M., et al. (2000). Alternative therapies used by women with breast cancer in four ethnic populations. *Journal of National Cancer Institute, 92,* 42–47.

Linde, K., & Melchart, D. (1998). Randomized controlled trials of individualized homeopathy: A state-of-the-art review. *Journal of Alternative and Complementary Medicine, 4*(4), 371–388.

Lowenstein, K. (2002). Meditation and self-regulatory techniques. In S. Shannon (Ed.), *Handbook of complementary and alternative therapies in mental health* (pp. 159–181). San Francisco, CA: Academic Press.

Mamtani, R., & Cimino, A. (2002). A primer of complementary and alternative medicine and its relevance in the treatment of mental health problems. *Psychiatric Quarterly, 73*(4), 367–381.

Massey, P. (2007). Prescribing movement therapies. In D. Rakel (Ed.), *Integrative medicine* (pp. 999–1007). Philadelphia: WB Saunders.

Moss, D. (2002). Biofeedback. In S. Shannon (Ed.), *Handbook of complementary and alternative therapies in mental health* (pp. 136–158). San Francisco, CA: Academic Press.

Motl, J. (2002). Acupuncture. In S. Shannon (Ed.), *Handbook of complementary and alternative therapies in mental health.* San Francisco, CA: Academic Press.

National Center for Complementary and Alternative Medicine (NCCAM), National Institutes of Health. (2004). *Backgrounder: Biologically based practices: An overview.* Retrieved January 27, 2007, from *www.nccam.nih.gov/health/backgrounds/biobasedprac.htm.*

National Center for Complementary and Alternative Medicine (NCCAM), National Institutes of Health. (2006). *Get the facts: What is CAM?* Retrieved January 30, 2007, from *www.nccam.nih.gov/health/whatiscam.*

Office of Dietary Supplements, National Institutes of Health. (2006). *Botanical dietary supplements: Background information.* Retrieved December 17, 2006, from *http://ods.od.nih.gov/factsheets/botanicalbackground.asp.*

Pharmacist's Letter/Prescriber's Letter. (2000). Continuing education booklet: Natural medicines in clinical management of diabetes. *Natural Medicine Clinical Management, 2*(6).

Rees, B. (1995). Effect of relaxation with guided imagery on anxiety, depression, and self-esteem in primiparas. *Journal of Holistic Nursing, 13,* 255–267.

Rossman, M. (2007). Guided imagery and interactive guided imagery. In D. Rakel (Ed.), *Integrative medicine* (pp. 1031–1037). Philadelphia: WB Saunders.

Schneider, C., & Lovett, E. (2007). Depression. In D. Rakel (Ed.), *Integrative medicine.* Philadelphia: WB Saunders.

Settle, J. (2002a). Nutritional supplements. In S. Shannon (Ed.), *Handbook of complementary and alternative therapies in mental health* (pp. 115–131). San Francisco, CA: Academic Press.

Settle, J. (2002b). Diet and essential fatty acids. In S. Shannon (Ed.), *Handbook of complementary and alternative therapies in mental health* (pp. 93–113). San Francisco, CA: Academic Press.

Shore, A. (2004). Long-term effects of energetic healing on symptoms of psychological depression and self-perceived stress. *Alternative Therapies in Health Medicine, 10*(3), 42–48.

Slaven, L., & Lee, C. (1997). Mood and symptom reporting among middle-aged women: The relationship between menopausal status, hormone replacement therapy, and exercise participation. *Health Psychology, 16,* 203–208.

Steinberg, D., & Beal, M. (2003). Homeopathy and women's health care. *Journal of Obstetric, Gynecologic, and Neonatal Nursing, 32*(2), 207–214.

Stoll, A. (2001). *The omega-3 connection: The groundbreaking Omega-3 Antidepression-Diet and Brain Program.* New York: Simon & Schuster.

Unutzer, J., Klap, R., Sturm, R., et al. (2000). Mental disorders and the use of alternative medicine: Results from a national survey. *American Journal of Psychiatry, 157,* 1851–1857.

World Health Organization. (2006). *Data and statistics.* Retrieved December 17, 2006, from *www.who.int/research/en.*

Zand, J., Walton, R., & Rountree, R. (1998). *Smart medicine for a healthier child.* New York: Avery.

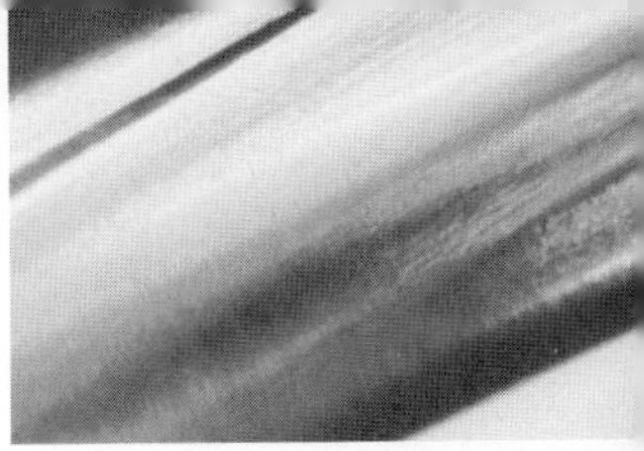

Index

C

D

E

F

G

H

N

O

P

R

S

T

U